The New Leadership Challenge

Creating the Future of Nursing

FOURTH EDITION

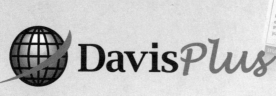

 **Davis***Plus*

Online Resource Center

Davis*Plus* is your online source for a wealth of learning resources and teaching tools, as well as electronic and mobile versions of our products.

Visit **davisplus.fadavis.com**

STUDENTS

Unlimited FREE access.
Sign up today to see what's available for your title.

INSTRUCTORS

Upon Adoption.
Password-protected library of title-specific, online course content.

T **Taber's** online resources are now available across many of the **Davis***Plus* resource pages.

Look for this icon **T** to find Taber's resources!

Explore more online resources from F.A.Davis

DAVIS'S DRUG GUIDE ONLINE

www.DrugGuide.com

The complete Davis's Drug Guide for Nurses® database with over 1,100 monographs on the web.

Taber's Online

www.Tabers.com

The power of Taber's® Cyclo-pedic Medical Dictionary on the web. Find more than 60,000 terms, 1,000 images, and more.

DAVIS'S Laboratory and Diagnostic Tests with Nursing Implications

www.LabDxTest.com

The complete database for Davis's Comprehensive Handbook of Laboratory and Diagnostic Tests with Nursing Implications online. Access hundreds of detailed monographs.

powered by
unbound
MEDICINE

www.FADavis.com

F.A. DAVIS COMPANY

The New Leadership Challenge

Creating the Future of Nursing

FOURTH EDITION

Sheila C. Grossman, PhD, APRN-BC, FNP
Professor & Director of Family Nurse Practitioner Track
School of Nursing
Fairfield University
Fairfield, Connecticut

Theresa M. "Terry" Valiga, EdD, RN, ANEF, FAAN
Professor & Director, Institute for Educational Excellence
Duke University School of Nursing
Durham, North Carolina

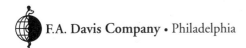
F.A. Davis Company • Philadelphia

F. A. Davis Company
1915 Arch Street
Philadelphia, PA 19103
www.fadavis.com

Printed in the United States of America

Last digit indicates print number: 10 9 8 7 6 5 4 3 2 1

Publisher, Nursing: Joanne P. DaCunha
Director of Content Development: Darlene D. Pedersen
Project Editor: Elizabeth Hart
Electronic Project Editor: Alexis Zanetti
Design and Illustration Manager: Carolyn O'Brien

As new scientific information becomes available through basic and clinical research, recommended treatments and drug therapies undergo changes. The author(s) and publisher have done everything possible to make this book accurate, up to date, and in accord with accepted standards at the time of publication. The author(s), editors, and publisher are not responsible for errors or omissions or for consequences from application of the book, and make no warranty, expressed or implied, in regard to the contents of the book. Any practice described in this book should be applied by the reader in accordance with professional standards of care used in regard to the unique circumstances that may apply in each situation. The reader is advised always to check product information (package inserts) for changes and new information regarding dose and contraindications before administering any drug. Caution is especially urged when using new or infrequently ordered drugs.

Library of Congress Cataloging-in-Publication Data

Grossman, Sheila.
  The new leadership challenge : creating the future of nursing / Sheila C. Grossman, Theresa M. Valiga. — 4th ed.
      p. ; cm.
  Includes bibliographical references and index.
  ISBN 978-0-8036-2606-5
  I. Valiga, Theresa M. II. Title.
  [DNLM: 1. Nursing, Supervisory. 2. Leadership. 3. Nurse Administrators. WY 105]

  610.73068—dc23

                                   2012016048

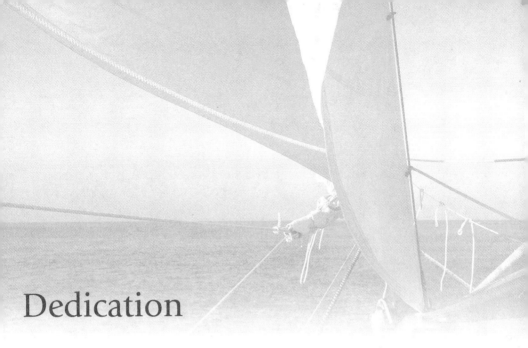

Dedication

This book is dedicated to each and every nurse who is leading the profession to a preferred future and to my students, patients, mentors, and colleagues who have taught me so much about staying committed to a vision of enhancing leadership and followership. Also, I want to thank my husband, Bob, and our daughters, Lisa and Beth, who have always inspired me to keep on task and do my best.

SCG

This book is dedicated to the many faculty and other professional colleagues, as well as the hundreds of students I have known, who have helped me crystallize my thinking about leadership and who, themselves, have taken on the challenge of providing leadership. Through dialogues in the classroom and in the online environment, papers that have been written, conversations in each other's offices, sharing of resources and ideas, and observations of these individuals functioning as leaders, I have come to understand more fully the true meaning of what it means to be a leader. I also dedicate this book to my husband, Bob, who continues to support me in all my professional pursuits and whose patience and understanding have meant the world to me. This book also is dedicated to my sister, Diane Czerepuszko, a nurse, a leader, a friend. Finally, I dedicate this book to my mother and father. Although neither of them is here to see its publication, they were a tremendous influence in my development as a professional and, hopefully, a leader; for that and for all they have given me, I will be forever grateful.

TMV

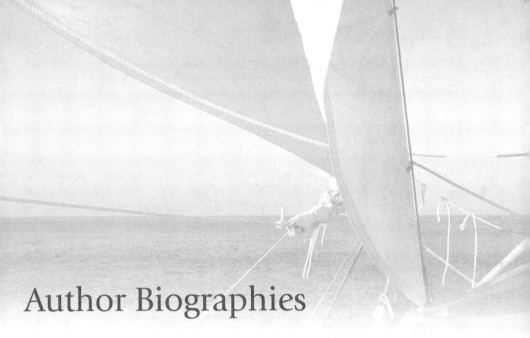

Author Biographies

Sheila C. Grossman, PhD, APRN-BC, received her baccalaureate degree in nursing and her doctoral degree in higher education professional administration from the University of Connecticut, her master's degree from the University of Massachusetts in biophysiological nursing with a clinical nurse specialty in respiratory nursing, and her post master's certificate as a Family Nurse Practitioner from Fairfield University. She has been a staff, charge, and supervisor nurse on a variety of medical-surgical units and intensive care units. She has been a critical care nursing instructor at Hartford Hospital and St. Francis Hospital and Medical Center, both in Hartford, CT. She has taught nursing at the University of Connecticut and currently is Professor and Director, Family Nurse Practitioner Track in the School of Nursing at Fairfield University (CT). She works as a nurse practitioner one day per week at an urban primary care clinic in Hartford, CT.

Dr. Grossman has produced multiple international, national, and regional presentations and publications in the areas of pathophysiology, palliative care, primary care and critical care nursing outcome studies, mentoring, leadership, and evidence-based practice. She is a past member of the Connecticut State Board of Nursing; a member of Sigma Theta Tau International; a Commissioner on the American Nurses Credentialing Center Commission on Certification; and a member of the National Organization of Nurse Practitioner Faculties, American Association of Critical Care Nurses, American College of Nurse Practitioners, and American Academy of Nurse Practitioners. She serves on multiple Manuscript Review Boards, is a Mentoring Expert Resource for the American Nurses Association, and is a frequent keynote speaker on leadership and mentoring.

Dr. Grossman has received several awards, including the NONPF Outstanding NP Educator Award, 2011; Josephine Dolan Award for Outstanding Contributions to Nursing Education sponsored by the CT Nurses Association, 10/09; and two AJN Book of the Year Awards.

Theresa M. "Terry" Valiga, EdD, RN, ANEF, FAAN, received her bachelor's degree in nursing from Trenton State College (now The College of New Jersey) and her master's and doctoral degrees, both in nursing education, from Teachers College, Columbia University. She has been a faculty member at Trenton State College, Georgetown University, Seton Hall University, Villanova University, and Fairfield University, where she served as Dean of the School of Nursing. At present, she is the Director of the Institute for Educational Excellence in the School of Nursing at Duke University (North Carolina). Before holding this position, Dr. Valiga served for 9 years as the Chief Program Officer at the National League for Nursing. Dr. Valiga's primary research interests relate to students' cognitive/intellectual development, critical thinking, and leadership development. Her publications, presentations, and consultations center around these topics, as well as curriculum development, creative teaching strategies, and various issues related to nursing education. She is the author of numerous articles and has coauthored several other books: *The Nurse Educator in Academe: Strategies for Success, Using the Arts and Humanities to Teach Nursing: A Creative Approach, Achieving Excellence in Nursing Education,* and *Clinical Nursing Education: Current Reflections.* She has served as Vice President of Sigma Theta Tau International and National Vice President of the Interdisciplinary Honor Society of Phi Kappa Phi, and she has held numerous leadership positions in nursing throughout her career. Dr. Valiga also is the recipient of several awards, including the Sigma Theta Tau International Founders Award for Excellence in Education and the National League for Nursing Isabel Stewart Award for Excellence in Nursing Education, and she is a Fellow in the Academy of Nurse Educators and the American Academy of Nursing.

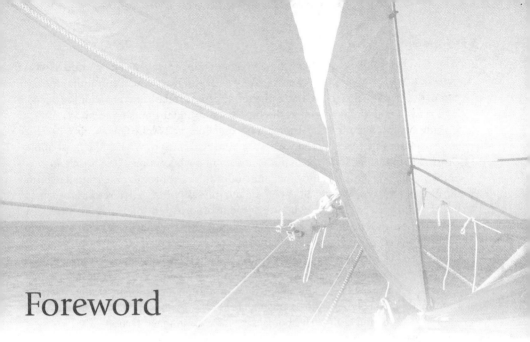

Foreword

This fourth edition of Grossman and Valiga's book on *The New Leadership Challenge* comes at a time when the call for nurse leadership is louder than ever before in history. The Institute of Medicine (IOM), created by Congress to be our nation's think tank for health policy, has published two reports focusing on how essential nurse leadership is to the health of our nation in the 21st century. The 2004 IOM report entitled *Keeping Patients Safe* urges nurses to exert transformational leadership, take responsibility for the design of work and workspace to prevent and mitigate error, and serve as prime movers in the development of organizational cultures of safety. The 2011 report on *The Future of Nursing* encourages nurses to act as full partners with physicians and other health care professionals in redesigning and leading health change, including the policy-setting work of serving on boards. Gone are the days when nurses could reasonably bemoan the fact that their services weren't appreciated. We are now living in a time when the onus is on us to step up to the challenge of meeting rising expectations for our profession, expectations that summon us to exert intraprofessional and interprofessional leadership.

And this book certainly helps us rise to the challenge by providing the resources necessary to succeed in this endeavor. Grossman and Valiga do not confuse leadership with having an administrative title, but expect all nurses throughout their careers to internalize the equation, nurse = leader, no matter what segment of nursing practice they intend to make their own. This edition once again tackles important basics—similarities and differences between leadership and management; the inter-relationship between followership and leadership; the importance of emotional intelligence, creativity, and networking in personal effectiveness—but there are some new emphases too—the importance of reflective practice in the leadership journey and the link between quality improvement and the leader's striving for excellence. The easy-to-read tables make the complicated easy to grasp, and the exercises at the end of each chapter enable the reader to apply the subject matter personally to her or his situation. The pithy quotes sprinkled liberally throughout the book—from Winston Churchill to Martin Luther

King, Jr.—do a good job of linking thoughts about nursing with the larger world of ideas over time. What is more, the extensive annotated bibliography that constitutes the last part of this book points those with a whetted appetite for the subject to additional readings, classics in both the overall leadership literature and the nursing literature.

Traditionally, becoming a leader might be something you aspired to over time because you wanted a title or higher pay or respect and recognition. What I like most about Grossman and Valiga's book is that it focuses on how becoming a leader isn't an endpoint; it is the means to creating the future of health care, by fashioning and designing the future of nursing. We will all have to do our innovative best wherever we are planted if we are collectively going to address the graying of society, the pressures occasioned by globalization and the increasing diversity of our patients, and the changes that need to be made to deliver quality accessible care in a period of severely constrained resources (human and financial). Opinion leaders throughout the United States overwhelmingly said that they would like nurses to have even more influence than they now do in preventing medical errors, providing quality care, promoting wellness, increasing efficiency, coordinating patients, and addressing the needs of an aging population (Robert Wood Johnson Foundation, 2010). This book helps move us in that direction.

Angela Barron McBride, PhD, RN, FAAN
Distinguished Professor–University Dean Emerita
Indiana University School of Nursing

References

Institute of Medicine. (2004). In A. Page (Ed.), *Keeping patients safe. Transforming the work environment of nurses.* Washington, DC: National Academies Press.

Institute of Medicine. (2011). *The future of nursing: Leading change, advancing health.* Washington, DC: National Academies Press.

Robert Wood Johnson Foundation. (2010, January 20). *Nursing leadership from bedside to boardroom. Opinion leaders' perceptions.* Retrieved from http://www.rwjf.org/humancapital/product.jsp?id=54491.

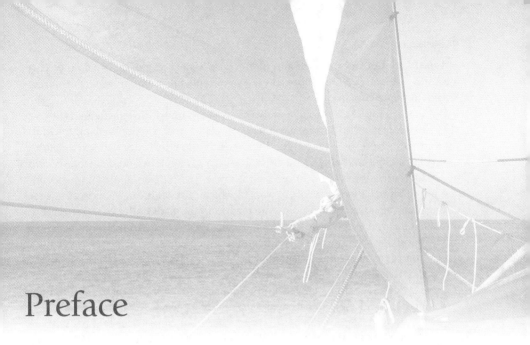

Preface

The New Leadership Challenge: Creating the Future of Nursing has been written as a reference book and textbook for students in nursing, as well as for nurses in any practice role. The book should be particularly helpful for nurses pursuing graduate study, including those preparing as clinical nurse leaders and those pursuing a doctorate of nursing practice. It provides an overview of major ideas related to the multidimensional concept of "leadership" and explores those ideas at various levels of one's career development: beginning, intermediate, and advanced.

Each chapter includes learning objectives, a synthesis of extensive readings (classics and contemporary, from nursing and, more often, non-nursing literature) on the specific topic, a case study, and a variety of critical thinking exercises that are designed to help the reader better understand the topic and its relation to leadership and the development of individuals as leaders. Resources from the arts and humanities that relate to the specific topic and that enhance learning about it are provided, and examples from clinical practice, education, and administration are included.

Unlike many other textbooks and resource books that claim to address leadership, this book takes that charge seriously. In many other books, particularly those written by and for nurses and nursing students, the authors confuse leadership with management and end up focusing more on management than on leadership. Perhaps that is because the phenomenon of leadership is more elusive than that of management and because one cannot outline "steps" of leadership as one can do to some extent with management (e.g., planning, delegating, budgeting).

This book takes on the challenge of exploring the elements of true leadership, particularly in the "new world" context we face continually. It explores various definitions and conceptualizations of leadership, examines extant theories of leadership, analyzes the notion of vision and visionary leadership, and tackles the intricacies of leader–follower relationships. The importance of followership, the facilitation of change, the management of conflict, the use and abuse of power, gender perspectives related to leadership, and the development of oneself and of others as leaders all are discussed. In essence, then, this book takes a broad look at the complex phenomenon of leadership and examines multiple dimensions of it.

The major points made throughout this book and its unifying elements are as follows: (1) although leadership and management are related, they are not one and the same; (2) leadership is not an innate ability, but rather one that can be learned and developed through conscious and purposeful effort; (3) each of us can be and, perhaps, needs to be a leader if nursing is to advance as a profession and have a significant impact now and in the future; and (4) there are ways in which each of us can develop as a leader throughout our careers. These points are made and the goals of the book are achieved through a balance of theoretical exploration; the extensive use of real-world examples from clinical practice, education, and administration; self-assessment exercises; and the integration of creative learning activities.

The New Leadership Challenge: Creating the Future of Nursing focuses on nurses and nursing. It does not confuse leadership and management. It also explores the multifaceted concept of leadership in depth. As such, it is of value to several audiences.

Most undergraduate programs include a course in nursing leadership. A study conducted by one of the authors and another colleague revealed, however, that although many courses carried the title "Nursing Leadership," most actually dealt with management and delegation. In a world where experts recognize clearly that true leadership is needed for the future, *The New Leadership Challenge: Creating the Future of Nursing* meets a need, particularly for those undergraduate programs that already have or will soon have a course that addresses true leadership.

Most graduate programs (both master's and doctoral) focus on the preparation of graduates for leadership roles in the profession, so a book that addresses just that is most appropriate. Students preparing as advanced practice nurses, clinical nurse leaders, nurse administrators, or educators do not want to use a text that "advertises" leadership but "delivers" management; if they wanted management, they would have pursued an MBA or a graduate degree in health-care administration. Instead, they want a text that helps them understand what leadership is and how it relates to the nursing roles for which they are preparing. This book meets that need.

Finally, this book serves as a valuable resource for nurses in clinical practice, nurse researchers, nurse educators, and nurse administrators who see the need to learn more about the phenomenon of leadership and how to develop those abilities in themselves and in others (e.g., fellow clinicians, students, staff). One's ongoing education in an ever-changing world cannot be limited to clinical, teaching, or administrative knowledge and skills alone. It also must address broader knowledge and skills—such as those related to leadership—that are integral to one's practice.

One of the most important features of this book is the exposure to and integration of the extensive writings about leadership done by experts in that field; thus, the literature base for this book is not limited to nursing. This is designed to broaden readers' perspectives and expose them to a much wider range of resources that can be tapped for ongoing personal development. The reader will note that there are a number of references that some will consider "old." They have been retained deliberately because they are classics in the field, are primary sources, have been written by leadership scholars, and are elegant, saying the most with the least amount of effort. The annotated summaries of "must-read" books on leadership included in this fourth edition are intended to help readers expand their horizons about leadership resources.

The New Leadership Challenge: Creating the Future of Nursing, as the title implies, also presents a clear orientation to the future. Using the writings of Wheatley as a basis, the entire book is "framed" in the context of the future—what organizations are expected to look like in the future, the skills that people associated with those organizations will need in order to survive and thrive, the need to plan for a blending of professional and personal commitments, and so on. The old-model, hierarchical organization that characterizes so many health-care agencies is expected to "die" very quickly, and people in those organizations will need to be able to function and provide leadership in a totally new kind of environment. This book is designed to help professional nurses make this transition.

In addition to these important features, *The New Leadership Challenge: Creating the Future of Nursing* offers several other unique features. First, it is accompanied by an electronic instructor's guide that offers numerous teaching approaches that might be used with undergraduate or graduate students and with nurses in practice. Overall, this book—conceptualized in its broadest sense—is designed to be interactive, stimulating, creative, challenging, and thought-provoking.

The intent of this book is to help nurses and nursing students explore the many facets of leadership and examine strategies that will aid them in (1) seeing themselves as potential leaders, (2) developing skills needed to function as leaders, and (3) taking on the challenges of a leadership role in the current and future health-care setting. It challenges the reader's thinking, presents new ways to conceptualize leadership, and prepares nurses for their role as leaders in creating a preferred future for nursing. Readers are invited to open their minds to new perspectives; entertain the notion that the chaotic, uncertain world of today and tomorrow presents tremendous opportunities for nurse leaders to influence the future of our profession; and think of themselves as leaders who can develop in that role throughout their careers. We welcome you to the world of *The New Leadership Challenge: Creating the Future of Nursing*.

Sheila C. Grossman
Theresa M. "Terry" Valiga

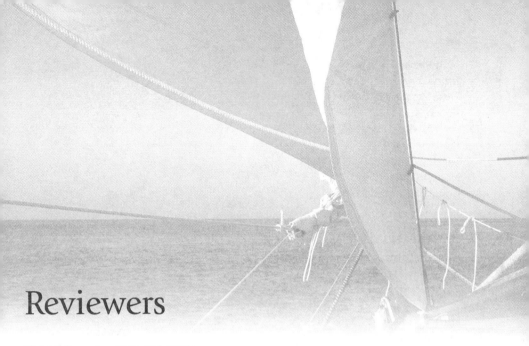

Reviewers

Vicki J. Coombs, PhD, RN, FAHA
University Department Chair
Keiser University
Ft. Lauderdale, Florida

Suzanne Farrell, RN, BSN, MSN
Lecturer
Thompson Rivers University
Kamloops, British Columbia
CANADA

Diane Porretta Fox, RN, MSN, CNE, EdD candidate
Associate Professor
Eastern Michigan University
Ypsilanti, Michigan

Andrew Frados, DNP, MSN, ARNP, BSN, RN
Associate Professor
Miami-Dade College
Miami, Florida

Diane Haleem, PhD, RN
Professor of Nursing
Marywood University
Scranton, Pennsylvania

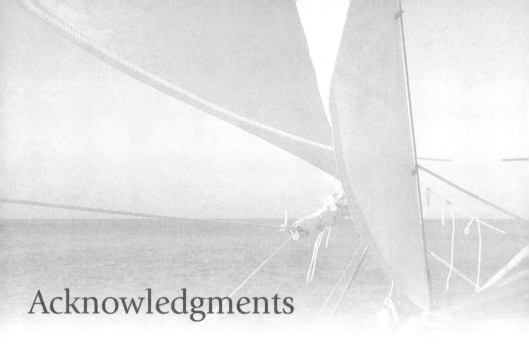

Acknowledgments

The authors wish to thank Joanne DaCunha for inviting us to explore the concept of leadership through a textbook and for her innovative ideas about what this book could be. We will always be grateful for her inspiration, her faith in us, and her ongoing support with the project and the revised editions. Also we thank Elizabeth Hart, Jennifer Schmidt, and Lisa Thompson for all of their assistance in the editing and publishing process of this book. We would like to add our gratitude also to Dr. Angela McBride for her thoughtful reflections in the Foreword to this book. Finally, we thank our families and friends for their love and support throughout the process of developing and writing this book.

SCG
TMV

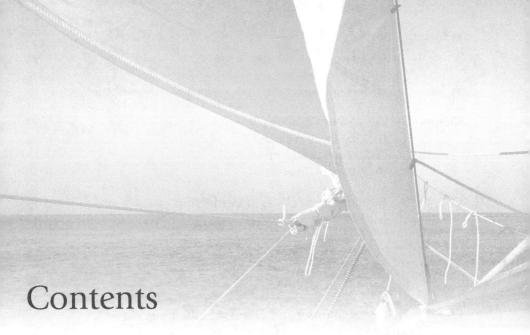

Contents

CHAPTER 1

The Nature of Leadership
Distinguishing Leadership From Management

LEARNING OBJECTIVES
- Compare and contrast major theoretical ideas about leadership.
- Discuss the essential elements of leadership.
- Describe the nine tasks of leadership.
- Distinguish leadership from management.
- Create a personal definition of leadership that reflects its essential elements.

INTRODUCTION

Chaos. Uncertainty. Unpredictability. Constant change. These are all characteristics of the world in which we now live, and all indications are that the world of the future will be even more chaotic, more uncertain, more unpredictable, and in even greater states of constant and unprecedented change and flux. Such circumstances desperately call for new leaders, even though "being an effective leader in today's tumultuous world is almost impossible" (Tetenbaum & Laurence, 2011, p. 48). Indeed, "if there was ever a moment in history when a comprehensive strategic view of leadership was needed, . . . this is certainly it" (Bennis & Nanus, 1985, p. 2).

Defining just what leadership is, who leaders are, what leaders do, and how leadership is different from management—a phenomenon with which it often is confused—is no easy task. This chapter is intended to address these questions and help the reader understand the complex, multidimensional concept we refer to as leadership. It is also intended to challenge readers to consider the leadership needed in nursing today, to think about themselves as leaders, and to reflect on how leadership responsibilities can be integrated into their roles as professional nurses.

1

For almost a century, writers have attempted to describe leadership, and researchers have attempted to identify the defining characteristics of leaders. The outcome has been one very clear conclusion: "Leadership is one of the most observed and least understood phenomena on earth" (Burns, 1978, p. 2). It is multidimensional and multifaceted—a universal human phenomenon that many know when they see it but that few can define clearly.

In fact, there are almost as many different definitions of leadership as there are people who write about it. According to Bennis and Nanus (1985, p. 4): "Decades of academic analysis have given us more than 350 definitions of leadership. Literally thousands of empirical investigations of leaders have been conducted in the last seventy-five years alone, but no clear and unequivocal understanding exists as to what distinguishes leaders from non-leaders, and perhaps more important, what distinguishes *effective* leaders from *ineffective* leaders" (p. 11).

The lack of a "clear and unequivocal understanding" of leadership has led these experts on the subject to assert that "never have so many labored so long to say so little" (p. 4). Despite this situation, however, there is increasing clarity about what true leadership is and how it is different from the related concept of management.

BRIEF OVERVIEW OF SELECTED THEORIES OF LEADERSHIP
Great Man Theory

Theories of leadership have evolved tremendously over the years (Bass, 2008). Among the earliest was the "Great Man Theory," which asserted that one was a leader if one was born into the "right" family—usually a family of nobility—and possessed unique characteristics, most of which were inherited. Although some individuals who were born into the "right" family did accomplish extraordinary things and did, in fact, change the course of history, the notion that "leaders are born, not made" did not capture the imagination of the masses, and it failed to recognize that there was more to leadership than having royal blood. Thus began the search for the traits or cluster of traits that would determine whether a person would be a leader.

Trait Theories

Personal trait theories of leadership attempted to distinguish leaders from other people and identify the universal characteristics of leadership. Not surprisingly, no qualities were found that were universal to all leaders, although a number of traits did seem to correlate with leadership (Bass, 2008): above average height and weight, an abundant reserve of energy, an ability to maintain a high level of activity, a better education, superior judgment, decisiveness, a breadth of knowledge, a high degree of verbal facility, good interpersonal skills, self-confidence, and creativity. In addition to the fact that these theories revealed no universal traits among leaders, they also failed to acknowledge the importance of the situation in which leadership occurred.

Situational Theories

Situational theories, in comparison, gave clear recognition to the significance of the environment and the particular situation as factors in the effectiveness of a leader. They asserted that the leader was the individual who was in a position to institute change when a situation was ready for change. In other words, the leader did not plan for a change, nor was the leader chosen by a group of followers; he or she just "happened to be in the right place at the right time" and took the action that was needed to resolve a crisis or manage a problem. Although this view of leadership was broader than merely looking at one's heritage or specific traits, it still did not capture the complexity of the phenomenon and failed to acknowledge one very important element in a leadership "event"—the followers.

Contemporary Theories

More contemporary theories of leadership clearly recognize that effective leadership depends partly on the person of the leader, partly on the situation at hand, and partly on the qualities and maturity of the followers. In fact, most recent writings (Bennis, 2004, 2006; Burns, 2003; Chaleff, 2009; Collins, 2001; Corona, 1986; DePree, 1992; DiRienzo, 1994; Kellerman, 2008; Kelley, 1992, 1993; Keohane, 2010; Lee, 1993; Parse, 2009; Pickens, 2000) assert that without followers, there is no leadership; followers therefore are a most significant element in the leadership "equation." Their needs, goals, abilities, sense of responsibility, degree of involvement, potential, and so forth are all important in determining the effectiveness of a leader.

In addition to acknowledging the significance of followers, more modern theories recognize that leadership is not a random occurrence. Instead, it very much involves having a vision, communicating that vision to others, planning with followers on how to make the vision a reality, effecting change, managing conflict, empowering followers, serving as a symbol for the group, serving as a source of energy and renewal for the group, and taking responsibility for facilitating the ongoing development of followers.

A recent content analysis of leadership studies published in peer-reviewed journals between 1999 and 2008 was undertaken to identify salient characteristics often associated with leadership traits. As a result of this rigorous analysis, the researchers (Brocato, Jelen, Schmidt, & Gold, 2011) developed a matrix and concluded that focusing on complex behavioral decision making and the group performance that results from it is more important than focusing on the leader's behavioral traits.

Tetenbaum and Laurence (2011) acknowledged that there has been little change in leadership styles and practices despite the current paradigm of chaos, disequilibrium, and change in organizational structures. They endorsed the model of leadership proposed by Heifetz (Heifetz, Grashow, & Linsky, 2009), which outlines the role of the leader as disturbing equilibrium and engaging followers in solving an organization's problems—a theory, they assert, that is useful in the face of chaos, ambiguity, and rapid change. None of the common theories of leadership, including trait, skills, style, situational, leader–member exchange, contingency, and even transformational, "is sufficiently rigorous to address today's volatile environment" (p. 48), they note, and more modern theories must be relevant for today's world.

The notion of leaders disturbing equilibrium also is advanced by Gryskiewicz (2005). He notes that "probably the most important challenge a leader faces today is building an organization that continually renews itself—an organization of which creativity . . . and innovation . . . are ongoing" (p. 8). Thus, engendering "positive turbulence" is a critical factor in contemporary theories of leadership.

The theory of appreciative inquiry also has relevance to new ways of thinking about leadership. According to Havens, Wood, and Leeman (2006), appreciative inquiry "is a philosophy and methodology for promoting positive organizational change through creating meaningful dialogue, inspiring hope, and inviting action" (p. 464). It is a perspective that focuses on successes and involves a cycle of discovery (appreciating what is), dreaming (imagining what might be), designing (determining what should be), and delivering (creating what will be). This view, therefore, requires the formulation of a vision and engagement with followers to articulate and realize that vision, both of which are key ingredients of leadership.

Much attention is being paid recently to complexity theory (Crowell, 2010), which asserts that we must think about people and organizations as nonlinear, complex adaptive systems and respond appropriately. Complexity can be thought of as lying between static order at one end and chaos at the other, where in seemingly unpredictable situations, predictions can be made and some degree of order and focus can be attained. Such perspectives have relevance for guiding leaders who must live at the edge of chaos and collaborate with others to create new futures.

Finally, in our own field, Parse (2009) has proposed the humanbecoming leading-following model that challenges traditional notions of leadership. She asserts that "power resides with the constituents of a situation and . . . there are at least three essentials inherent in leading: commitment to a vision, willingness to risk, and reverence for others" (p. 369). This model, therefore, places high value on all those who interact (i.e., what we typically think of as "leaders" and "followers") to create change, innovate, and "cocreate infinite possibilities" (p. 375).

Leadership is, indeed, a complex, multifaceted phenomenon that does not "just happen" and is not limited to an elite few. It can be learned. It is deliberative. And it is not necessarily tied to a position of authority. A leadership role is something each one of us has the potential to fulfill.

LEADERSHIP AND MANAGEMENT

The vast array of textbooks on leadership—particularly in nursing—often is titled "leadership and management." A careful analysis of the content of those textbooks often reveals, however, that a great deal of attention is given to management and very little to leadership. In fact, although the authors of many such textbooks make a point at the outset that leadership and management are not the same thing, they often go on to use the terms interchangeably and imply that the only person who is providing leadership to a group is the person who is in the management position. Nothing can be farther from the truth.

It is true that leadership and management are related and that many managers are also leaders. In fact, Jennings, Scalzi, Rodgers, and Keane (2007) report that their review of 140 articles about leadership and management led them to conclude that there are more commonalities than differences between the two concepts. However, these phenomena are not the same and should not be confused. Most important, one must remember that **leadership is not necessarily tied to a position of authority** and that each of us has the potential, and perhaps the responsibility, to provide leadership in our specific area of practice, our institution, our professional organizations, our community, and our profession as a whole. Leadership, therefore, should be thought of as a skill, rather than as a role.

TASKS OF LEADERSHIP

Several years ago, one of the most noted experts in the field of leadership, John Gardner, outlined nine tasks of leadership that help distinguish it from management. Those tasks of leadership (Gardner, 1989), which still have relevance today, are as follows:

1. *Envisioning goals:* Pointing others in the right direction and helping the group members balance and deal with any tension between long- and short-term goals
2. *Affirming values:* Regenerating and revitalizing the beliefs, values, purposes, and vision shared by members of the group, and challenging the values held by some
3. *Motivating:* Unlocking or channeling motives that exist within members of the group, having and promoting positive attitudes, being creative, and encouraging others to be excited about the future and about how they can be a part of it
4. *Managing:* Planning, setting priorities, making decisions, facilitating change, and keeping the system functioning, all in an effort to move the group toward achieving the goals and realizing the vision
5. *Achieving a workable unity:* Establishing trust, striving toward cohesion and mutual tolerance, managing conflict, and "creating loyalty to the larger venture" (p. 29)
6. *Explaining:* Helping others understand what the vision is, why they are being asked to do certain things, and how they relate to the larger picture
7. *Serving as a symbol:* Serving as a risk taker and acting as the group's source of unity, voice of anger, collective identity, and continuity, as well as its source of hope
8. *Representing the group:* Speaking and acting for or on behalf of the group and being an advocate for the group
9. *Renewing:* Blending continuity and change and breaking routines, habits, fixed attitudes, perceptions, assumptions, and unwritten rules . . . and keeping hope alive

One can see how the task of motivating is congruent with concepts espoused by appreciative inquiry (Havens et al, 2006). Additionally, the notion of trust inherent in the task of achieving a workable unity is highly congruent with the concepts of trustworthy leadership, integrity, and authenticity espoused by the Center for Courage and Renewal (Jackson, 2011), an educational nonprofit organization whose mission is to nurture personal and professional integrity and the courage to act on it.

Gardner (1989) asserted that the "*sine qua non* of leadership" (p. 29) is the ability to achieve a workable unity in the group and build community, a perspective supported by Schweitzer (2006), who talked about the leader moving from being a soloist to being an orchestrator. And as Gardner noted (1989, p. 33), in the process of renewing, the leader must "keep a measure of diversity and dissent in the system [as a way to avoid] the trance of nonrenewal."

In essence, "leadership is not tidy" (Gardner, 1989, p. 33); it is more of an art than a science. Management, in comparison, often is thought of as a science in which a series of steps can be followed to implement the role. Elements of the tasks of leadership will be explored in greater depth, but a careful look at how leadership differs from management can facilitate a more thorough understanding of leadership.

SPECIFIC DISTINCTIONS BETWEEN LEADERSHIP AND MANAGEMENT

Abraham Zaleznik (1981) has written extensively about the differences between leadership and management. In his classic work, Zaleznik asserted that leaders and managers are very different kinds of people: they differ in their motivation, their personal history, and how they think and act; they differ in their orientation toward goals, work, human relationships, and themselves; and they differ in their worldviews.

Goals

Leaders are proactive in formulating goals, primarily because they typically arise out of some personal passion for a better world. The goals are developed through dialogue with others, engagement with the literature, and self-reflection. Leaders shape ideas instead of merely responding to the ideas of others. They act to change the way people think about what is desirable, possible, and necessary. Managers, by comparison, adopt impersonal attitudes toward goals because someone higher in the organizational hierarchy often formulates those goals, which are deeply embedded in the history and culture of the organization and arise out of necessity rather than passion and desire.

Conceptions of Work

Regarding their conceptions of work, leaders act to develop fresh approaches to long-standing problems and to open issues for new options. They are not satisfied with the status quo and tend to create excitement in their work. Their instinct is to take risks, challenge "sacred cows," challenge existing assumptions, and ask "Why not?" Managers see work as a task to be accomplished with the least amount of turmoil and the greatest amount of coordination, balance, and efficiency. They act to limit choices and "rock the boat" as little as possible. Their instinct, in contrast to that of leaders, is for survival.

> *The cautious seldom err.* —Confucius

Relationships With Others

In their relationships with others, leaders are concerned with what events and decisions mean to those who are affected by them. They care about the people with whom they work, and they want to promote the development and individual creativity of their followers. They facilitate, focus on personal issues, and encourage the growth of others. Relationships with leaders may appear turbulent, intense, and at times even disorganized because of the involvement of all concerned. Despite this ability to work effectively with others, leaders are comfortable with solitary activity because it provides time for reflection, creative thinking, and incubation of ideas. Although managers are often thought of as "human engineers" (Holle & Blatchley, 1987) and like working with people, they tend to maintain a lower level of emotional involvement in their relationships with employees. They assign, focus on personnel issues, and promote the growth of the organization. They prefer to reconcile differences, seek compromises, and not become involved with what events mean to others. Instead, managers are concerned with how events occur, how things get done, and whether tasks are accomplished, preferably in the most efficient, cost-effective manner.

Sense of Self

Managers and leaders also have a different sense of self, according to Zaleznik (1981). Using the terms coined by William James many years ago, Zaleznik says leaders are "twice born" individuals—those who are separate from their environment, never "belong" to organizations, and have had many challenges in life. They are not threatened by the ideas of others because their sense of self comes from within, not from their roles or the expectations of others. Managers, on the other hand, often define themselves in terms of the organization and prefer not to have their ideas challenged. According to Zaleznik, they are "once born" individuals, whose lives are rather harmonious and who are very much influenced by others' opinions.

Table 1–1 summarizes these and other differences between leaders and managers. It is important to note that this table compares the extreme "ideal" leader with the extremely "organization-focused" manager for purposes of illustration. Although it may be difficult to do, many managers also serve as leaders in their organizations, and people in positions of authority are often leaders; therefore, the distinctions are not as clearcut as Table 1–1 may suggest. In fact, a recent analysis (Jennings et al, 2007) suggested that today's health-care environment requires managers/administrators to be leaders; therefore, the distinctions between these two roles are becoming increasingly blurred.

An important point to emphasize, however, is that **one can be a leader without being in a position of authority**. It is this aspect that professional nurses need to keep in mind when they face challenges in the practice arena: each one of us has the potential to provide leadership that will create new futures, and one need not be in a hierarchical position of authority to do that. In fact, if one considers how leaders "rock the boat," challenge existing ways of doing things, constantly ask "Why not?" questions, and are comfortable with—and indeed, thrive on—turmoil, one can see that it is sometimes easier to be a leader if one is *not* in a hierarchical position of authority.

Managers are people who do things right. Leaders are people who do the right thing. —Warren Bennis & Burt Nanus

ELEMENTS OF LEADERSHIP

As noted, leadership is a complex, multifaceted phenomenon that has been defined in hundreds of ways. Ken Robinson (2009), one of the world's leading thinkers on

TABLE 1-1 Differences Between Leadership and Management

	LEADERSHIP	MANAGEMENT
Position	Selected or allowed by a group of followers	Appointed by someone higher in the organizational hierarchy
Power base	Comes from knowledge, credibility, and ability to motivate followers	Arises from one's position of authority
Goals/visions	Arise from personal interests and passion that may not be synonymous with the goals of the organization	Espoused or prescribed by the organization
Innovative ideas	Developed, tested, and encouraged among all members of the group	Allowed, provided they do not interfere with task accomplishment, but not necessarily encouraged
Risk level	High risk, creativity, innovation	Low risk, balance, maintaining the status quo
Degree of order	Relative disorder seems to be generated	Rationality and control prevail
Nature of activities	Related to vision and judgment	Related to efficiency and cost-effectiveness
Focus	People	Systems and structure
Perspective	Long-range, with an eye on the horizon	Short-range, with an eye on the bottom line
Degree of "freedom"	Freestanding and not limited to an organizational position of authority	Tied to a designated position in an organization
Actions	Does the right thing (Bennis & Nanus, 1985, p. 21).	Does things right (Bennis & Nanus, 1985, p. 21)

creativity and innovation, is convinced that finding one's passion is all that is needed to change the world. Although he does not frame this discussion in the context of leadership, Robinson makes a strong case for the power of passion.

"Coach K," longstanding coach of the Duke University men's basketball team and the "winningest" coach in college basketball history, asserted that the key elements of successful leadership are knowing, understanding, and trusting people; "constantly improving to reach maximum potential" (Krzyzewski, 2000, p. 28); having passion, quiet courage and heart; communicating directly; being honest and of the highest integrity; creating a sense of "collective responsibility" (p. 76); caring . . . about the individual, about the team, about the team's performance, and about excellence; working effectively as a team; having realistic, attainable, and shared goals; and "thinking as one" (p. 71).

Despite these myriad definitions, however, several fundamental elements of leadership recur in writings about the concept. Those elements—vision, communication skills, change, stewardship, and developing and renewing followers (Box 1–1)—are discussed in depth to help the reader gain a better understanding of leadership.

BOX 1-1 **Elements of Leadership**

Vision
Communication skills
Change
Stewardship
Developing and renewing followers

Vision

Few would argue that having, creating, and expressing a vision is an important element of leadership. Manfredi (1995) asserted that one of the primary roles of leaders is that of creating visions—"engag[ing] in the process of traveling into the future" (p. 62). Leadership involves dreaming of possibilities, believing that there can be a better world, exploring uncharted waters, and asking questions such as " Why not?" Indeed, "great leaders create dreams that galvanize people into action" (Yeh, 2005, p. 13).

> *Leaders can conceive and articulate goals that lift people out of their petty preoccupations, carry them above the conflicts that tear a society apart, and unite them in a pursuit of objectives worthy of their best efforts. —John Gardner*

The significance of vision to leadership has been identified by numerous experts in the field (Bennis, 1989, 2004; DePree, 1989; Gardner, 1990; Hesselbein, Goldsmith, & Somerville, 1999; Jackman, 2005; Kouses & Posner, 2008; Nanus, 1992; Phillips, 1997; Thornberry, 2006). In fact, the ability to see a new world, or a different world, and mobilize others to help make it a reality is one of the hallmarks of leadership. Consider the following examples of individuals and their dreams, many of which became realities as a result of the individual's determination, persistence, and passion:

- **Henry Ford:** Affordable cars for "common" people
- **Mahatma Gandhi:** Freedom of the people of India
- **Steve Jobs:** Desktop computers for personal use
- **Martin Luther King, Jr.:** Racial equality
- **Candy Lightner:** Reduced drunk-driving fatalities
- **Mother Teresa:** Compassionate care for the poorest of the poor
- **Florence Nightingale:** Reduced battlefield fatalities resulting from poor care
- **Robert Pittman:** A "marriage" between rock music and television

- **Fred Smith:** Overnight mail and package delivery, 365 days of the year
- **Sam Walton:** Affordable shopping in a family-oriented store

Although we think of these individuals today as major figures in our nation's or world's history, they were little-known men and women when their visions began to take shape, when they began talking to others about their vision, and when they initiated actions to turn those dreams into reality. As a result, we now see most people owning cars; the worldwide impact of the Sisters of Charity; greater racial equality; the effectiveness of Mothers Against Drunk Driving (MADD); the positive outcomes of nonviolence; freedom of people in various parts of the world; the success of Wal-Mart and Federal Express; a computer in many homes and offices; the impact of Music Television (MTV) on our nation's youth; and more scientific and nursing-oriented approaches to health care. It has been said that "in creating a vision, we are creating a power, not a place, an influence, not a destination" (Wheatley, 1999, p. 55). Surely, individuals like these have created a power and an influence that have touched millions.

As professional nurses in practice, each envisions a better world. One might think of ways to promote greater involvement of patients' families in care decisions or a more powerful role for the professional nurse on the health-care team. Another might see a more effective way to prepare patients for the transition from the critical care unit to a step-down unit or from the hospital to home care. And yet another may look at ways to increase hospital stays for certain patients, such as those undergoing mastectomy, or encourage greater autonomy for the nurse in making referrals to needed services.

> *Cautious, careful people always casting about to preserve their reputation and social standing, never can bring about a reform. Those who are really in earnest must be willing to be anything or nothing in the world's estimation.* —Susan B. Anthony

Whatever the vision, if it is something about which one cares, as a leader, one cannot sit idle waiting for others to "make it happen." Instead, one must "think outside the box and . . . imagine all the places [we] can go" (Sturman, 2002, p. 36). As leaders, nurses must talk about their vision to other nurses, nurse managers and administrators, patients, patients' families, other health professionals, members of the media, legislators—in fact, anyone who will or should listen. Nurses must be passionate about the "little corner of the world" that needs change and take every opportunity to do something to make that change happen. They must move beyond "the walls of current policy, practice, procedure, and assumptions [as well as] the walls of the past—safe, familiar, and secure" (Hesselbein et al, 1999, p. 2). Nurses do not have to be in positions of authority to raise the issues, to argue the necessity for the change, to elicit support for the idea, to speak eloquently and enthusiastically about possible solutions, or to convince others that it is a vision worth working toward. But they must have the vision.

The secret of leadership is . . . enthusiasm: winning others to your ideas by the joy you yourself feel in them. —J. Donald Walters

Communication Skills

As can be seen from the preceding discussion and from a review of Gardner's (1989) tasks of leadership, leadership involves communicating one's ideas and visions, explaining to others (e.g., followers, group members) how that vision has relevance for them and how they can be a part of making it a reality, and inspiring others to invest their energies on behalf of the group and the goal. In essence, excellent communication skills are essential for effective leadership.

Individuals who have great ideas but refuse to share them with others or who communicate them in a way that does not generate excitement in others are not likely to see their visions become reality. Individuals who cannot help others clearly see the vision probably will not be very effective in convincing those potential followers to "join in the struggle." Likewise, individuals who are unable to listen to the ideas of others, respond to their suggestions, and convey enthusiasm for input from all group members are not likely to be able to facilitate change, sustain an effort over time, or effectively manage the conflict that is almost certain to arise as new goals are being realized.

Nurses excel in communication. They know how to listen and how to encourage people to keep trying when there seems to be no hope of success or when the effort is extraordinarily difficult. They know how to encourage others to respond openly and how to overcome barriers to communication. Nurses are, therefore, particularly advantaged in this element of leadership, and they should use this skill to its fullest.

The public puts a great deal of trust in nurses, and the credibility of nurses is strong in the eyes of patients, families, legislators, and the general public. Nurses who provide leadership can benefit from this favorable perception by communicating their vision at every opportunity. Such opportunities are, in fact, more readily available than many nurses realize: serving on a committee at one's institution or professional association, speaking at a conference, writing for a professional journal or a local newspaper or organizational newsletter, meeting with a legislator, talking with patients and their families, being interviewed on a local radio station, holding office in one's professional association, campaigning for a candidate or a particular issue, confronting a health-care team member, networking at professional meetings, forming alliances with other health-care professionals, seeking and using a mentor, and so on. We are limited only by our imaginations and willingness to take risks.

Change

If leadership involves articulating and realizing visions, the process by which that happens is change. Indeed, "learning to lead is, on one level, learning to manage change" (Bennis, 1989, p. 145). Leaders, therefore, need to be effective change agents, knowing when change is needed, "stretch[ing] the imagination of followers" (Manfredi, 1995, p. 63) to appreciate the need for change, planning effectively for change to occur, involving those who will be affected by change in the process, helping others realize their role in making change and creating new worlds, maintaining a positive attitude throughout the challenges of change, and knowing when to maintain the status quo.

As Gardner (1990) noted, "[L]eaders must understand the interweaving of continuity and change" (p. 124). They must realize that not all change is good or necessary and that changing only for the sake of changing is not always healthy. Therefore, continuity often is what a group needs, at least for a certain period. But leadership also involves a willingness to create change and manage the chaos that often is associated with change. It involves a willingness to embrace uncertainty (Clampitt & Dekoch, 2001) and risk failure rather than waiting for "guaranteed" success, and it involves keeping focused on the goal or vision.

Professional nurses have a responsibility to create change in their work or professional arenas. Nurses who are dissatisfied with the intake form used for new patients, for example, thinking it is not complete enough to provide an adequate database to plan long-term home care, can complain about the form to their colleagues and "blame" someone else for its inadequacies. But the professional nurse who is a leader will do more than just complain. He or she will outline what is needed to make the form complete, perhaps test it out in practice (by informally adapting the existing form), develop a plan for pilot testing on a wider scale, and propose how the new form could be integrated into the admission standards for nurses in that agency. Such an approach creates change that is intended to improve the overall quality of patient care, and although it takes more effort than merely complaining about the inadequacies of the existing intake form, the outcomes are worth the effort. As previously mentioned, leaders do not need to be in positions of authority, and they do not need to wait for "guaranteed" success before trying new approaches and creating change.

> *Leadership is action, not position.* —Donald H. McGannon

Stewardship

"Stewardship is to hold something in trust for another" (Block, 1993, p. xx) and being responsible for something more than just oneself. It has to do with serving others, rather than serving our own self-interests or attempting to control others, and it involves a balance of power. In essence, stewardship incorporates "engendering partnerships" (Block, 1993, p. 6) and empowerment, and it occurs when one leads "with soul" (Bolman & Deal, 2011).

Block (1993) titled his first chapter "Replacing Leadership with Stewardship" and described leadership as "inevitably associated with behaviors of control, direction, and knowing what is best for others" (p. 13), noting that it "does not leave much room for the concept of partnership" (p. 17). Based on the previous discussion, Block's definition may be an appropriate one for management, but it is not at all consistent with leadership as it has been described here. Leadership and stewardship, therefore, are not necessarily opposites or incompatible phenomena. In fact, Block's discussion of stewardship as "creating something we care about so we can endure the sacrifice, risk, and adventure that commitment entails" (p. 10) is congruent with the elements of leadership described previously: deep commitment, risk taking, high energy, working with others, and an enormous investment of self.

If leaders are to move forward with creating new worlds and helping visions become realities, they must have a sense of stewardship. They must feel responsible for the "larger picture," oversee the implementation of change, ensure that it is the overarching vision that drives decisions and actions, establish partnerships with followers or group members, and give their personal self-interests a "back seat." They must, in the words of Robert Greenleaf (1977), be servant-leaders, those who "first serve others [and] whose primary motivation is a desire to help others" (Spears, 1995, p. 3).

Professional nurses at all levels need to have a sense of stewardship about their practice arenas—whether in the clinical area, education, administration, or research—and be concerned with overall excellence in those arenas. Educators, for example, who have a vision of creating positive learning experiences for students—where they are fully engaged in the learning process, work collaboratively with each other, are excited about what they are learning, use their creative and other potentials to the fullest, and use the teacher as a guide and a resource to facilitate their own learning—cannot be concerned with doing this only in their own courses. If they are to be leaders and demonstrate the essential element of stewardship, there must be an effort to see that such positive learning experiences are provided for students throughout the curriculum and a willingness to oversee that what is being done in the name of "positive learning experiences" is based on theory and research.

Developing and Renewing Followers

Finally, leadership involves the continual development of followers and ongoing renewal of their commitment, understanding, and involvement. In fact, Tichy (1997) asserted that one of the truly defining characteristics of leaders is their investment in creating leaders all around them.

More than accomplishing tasks or meeting deadlines, "leadership is about taking people to places where they have never dared to go . . . and building into the future by developing the abilities of others" (Tichy, 1997, p. xiv). Leaders who have a vision for the future need to ensure that there are people to carry that vision forward and continue to work to make it become a reality. Building toward a vision requires collaboration between leaders and followers, as well as a cadre of effective followers who provide leadership.

It is the leader's responsibility to build such a cadre and develop the next generation of leaders. Because "all people have untapped leadership potential" (Tichy, 1997, p. 6), part of the leader's role is to recognize that potential and capitalize on it so that an effort or change can be sustained. Developing and renewing others can occur through personal attention, role modeling, precepting, and mentoring, each of which is described briefly to show their similarities and differences.

Personal Attention

Personal attention involves the personal guidance one gives to another. It requires that the strengths, limitations, and goals of the "recipients" are known and are used as a basis for the challenges presented to those individuals, the opportunities made available to them, and the expectations that are set regarding their contributions to the group.

Role Modeling

Role modeling occurs when a more experienced individual performs a role in such a way that novice leaders follow the individual's actions, style, values, behaviors, and so on. Because one can be a role model for another without even knowing it, this method of developing and renewing others is considered a more passive approach.

Precepting

Precepting is a strategy often used in nursing in which an experienced individual may be "assigned" to teach, guide, and assist another who is learning a role. The preceptor relationship often has a specific time limitation, and specific responsibilities of the preceptor and preceptee are clearly outlined.

Mentoring

Mentoring, in comparison, is a purposeful relationship in which an experienced, accomplished individual chooses to enter into a relationship with a less experienced individual who shares certain values or goals, is seen as having potential, shares a certain "chemistry" with the mentor, and is willing to work with the mentor. Mentors "open doors" for protégés, give critical feedback and personal guidance about career goals and other significant matters, and are willing to enter into a relationship that may last for many years. When true mentoring occurs, protégés may accomplish professional goals that far exceed those of the mentor.

It is clear that there are many approaches to developing and renewing followers. Some are conscious and purposeful (e.g., mentoring, personal attention), some are "assigned" (e.g., precepting), and some may occur without the leader even being aware of their occurrence (e.g., role modeling). Regardless of the strategy used, the leader is committed to the development of the followers and to their continued renewal and involvement.

CONCLUSION

Leadership is a complex, multifaceted phenomenon that is quite different from management. It is a potential that each of us has and a set of skills that can be learned, developed, and nurtured. Most important, it is not necessarily tied to a position of authority in an organization.

Opportunities exist in all aspects of our lives to exercise leadership and to make a difference in the lives of others and in the directions of groups and organizations. Leaders do not need to be appointed or even "invited" to exercise leadership; they do it because they "care more than others think is wise; risk more than others think is safe; dream more than others think is practical; and expect more than others think is possible" (anonymous quote about attaining excellence).

Never, never, never quit. —Winston Churchill

Leadership is needed for growth and progress—of individuals, groups, organizations, and institutions. As Harry Truman once said, "In periods where there is no leadership, society stands still. Progress occurs when courageous, skillful leaders seize the opportunity to change things for the better." In this world of increasing chaos, uncertainty, unpredictability, interdependence, and constant change, leadership is desperately needed. Nowhere is this more evident than in today's health-care arena.

Professional nurses are in an excellent position to provide leadership within their work settings, professional associations, communities, and society at large. Their communication skills, ability to work collaboratively with others, sense of service to others, well-established credibility, and commitment to high-quality patient care make them excellent candidates to provide this much-needed leadership. But they need to think about leadership in different ways.

Tanner and Weinman (2011) noted that the Carnegie Foundation's report on the preparation of nurses (Benner, Sutphen, Leonard, & Day, 2009) stresses the importance of helping nurses integrate an identity that defines themselves as nurses who are scholarly in their practices and who provide leadership in their arenas of practice. She also referenced *The Future of Nursing* report (Institute of Medicine, 2010) that clearly calls for nursing to shape its own future, which requires nurses to be prepared as leaders who can lead change to improve the nation's health, particularly through the powerful influence of nurses.

Broome (2011) emphasized the need for new visions of what leadership is and how they must be developed. She acknowledged the power of followers and the importance of the leader–follower relationship in creating change, and she stressed the importance of deliberately and systematically helping nurses develop as leaders. Such a generation of "bold, dynamic leaders, who know when to lead and when to follow" (p. 254) will shape effective organizations in which all nurses can make a difference. This book presents such a challenge to readers.

CRITICAL THINKING EXERCISES

Given the opportunity to publish "the definitive definition of leadership," what would you write? How does your definition reflect the nine tasks of leadership and the essential elements of leadership?

_____

_____

_____

Ask several nursing colleagues and several people outside the health professions (including children) to define leadership. What are the similarities in the definitions offered by these individuals? Are there any significant differences in their definitions? If so, what are they? How do you explain those differences?

_____

_____

_____

If an alien came to earth, approached you, and said, "I see you are a nurse. Take me to your leader," to whom would you take the alien? Who, in your opinion, is providing true leadership within the profession or even within your own institution? Why would you take the alien to this person?

_____

_____

_____

Read *The Velveteen Rabbit* (Williams, 1975). What leadership concepts can you identify in this children's story? What can we learn about leadership from this story?

_____

_____

_____

CRITICAL THINKING
EXERCISES —cont'd

Read the poem "If" by Rudyard Kipling. How do you think this relates to leadership and to the art of becoming a leader?

If

If you can keep your head when all about you
Are losing theirs and blaming it on you;
If you can trust yourself when all men doubt you
Yet make allowance for their doubting, too;
If you can wait and not be tired of waiting,
Or being lied about, don't deal in lies.
Or being hated, don't give way to hating,
And yet not look too good nor talk too wise;
If you can dream and not make dreams your master;
If you can think and not make thoughts your aim;
If you can meet with triumphs and disaster
And treat those two impostors just the same;
If you can bear to hear the truths you've spoken
Twisted by knaves to make a trap for fools,
Or see the things you gave your life to, broken
And stoop to build them up with worn-out tools;
If you can make one heap of all your winnings
And risk it on one turn of pitch and toss,
And lose and start again at your beginnings
And never breathe a word about your loss;
If you can force your heart and nerve and sinew
To serve your turn long after they are gone,
And so hold on when there's nothing in you
Except the will that says to them "hold on;"
If you can talk with crowds and keep your virtue,
Or walk with kings nor lose the common touch;
If neither foes nor loving friends can hurt you;
If all men count with you but none too much,
If you can fill the unforgiving minute
With sixty seconds worth of distance run—
Yours is the world and everything that's in it,
And—which is more—you'll be a man, my son!

—Rudyard Kipling

_____

_____

Continued

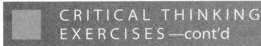

CRITICAL THINKING
EXERCISES —cont'd

Complete the self-assessment tool included below—the *Grossman & Valiga Leadership Characteristics and Skills Assessment* tool—to get a sense of how you "measure up" as a leader. How did you score? Were your scores consistent with how you think of yourself as a leader? Where were your greatest areas of strength?

_____

_____

APPENDIX

GROSSMAN & VALIGA LEADERSHIP CHARACTERISTICS AND SKILLS ASSESSMENT

Directions: Part 1 lists statements that are useful in determining a person's perception of what makes a good leader. **Part 2** lists skills that are useful in determining a person's ability to lead. Answer "SA" to those statements with which you Strongly Agree and "A" to those statements with which you Agree. Answer "D" to those statements with which you Disagree and "SD" to those statements with which you Strongly Disagree.

	PART 1				
	STATEMENT	SA	A	D	SD
1.	Leaders are very creative.				
2.	The most important goal of a leader is to be sure the job gets done.				
3.	Leaders should focus on people, not on the system.				
4.	One does not need to be in a position of authority to be a leader.				
5.	Credibility is an important characteristic of a leader.				
6.	Leaders tend to be people with high energy who are passionate about their work.				
7.	Leaders focus more on being creative than on accomplishing their vision or goal(s).				
8.	Persistence is a trademark of an effective leader.				
9.	Leaders are committed to their vision and tend not to adapt to change well.				
10.	Leaders are good at empowering others to grow.				

	PART 1—cont'd				
	STATEMENT	SA	A	D	SD
11.	It is important for leaders to have a dream and to be future-oriented.				
12.	A person's ability to lead in a professional setting depends on his or her self-esteem.				
13.	A leader's style of leading is determined by the situation and/or task at hand.				
14.	A good leader must have integrity.				
15.	Leaders mentor others to assist them in pursuing their dreams.				
16.	Leadership is a quality one is born with, and it cannot be acquired.				
17.	Good leaders help others to resolve conflict.				
18.	One does not need to be an excellent critical thinker in order to be a great leader.				
19.	A good leader should have excellent communication skills.				
20.	Leaders always follow the rules.				

	PART 2				
	STATEMENT	SA	A	D	SD
1.	I value integrity higher than power.				
2.	People tend to think I have the ability to influence others.				
3.	I feel confident about my knowledge base and skills, given my years of experience.				
4.	I have a definite dream for where I want to be in my profession.				
5.	I have mentored another person and found the experience rewarding.				
6.	Change usually makes me feel nervous, and I tend to lose my self-confidence.				
7.	I feel energized taking risks unless they are life-threatening.				

Continued

	PART 2—cont'd				
	STATEMENT	SA	A	D	SD
8.	I do not feel confident calling a physician about my patient's status.				
9.	When I experience conflict, I usually give in and accommodate the other person.				
10.	I feel I do make a difference as a nurse and plan to continue to do so.				
11.	Since I am only a nurse, I am not responsible for patient care errors.				
12.	I often follow others when I am not sure what to do about something.				
13.	I notice I agree with others easily unless the issue is very dear to my heart.				
14.	I attempt to empower ancillary workers because I find the team spirit is enhanced.				
15.	Personally, I do not really have a vision as to where I plan to be in a few years.				
16.	I enjoy conflict and rarely compromise my needs.				
17.	I am an autonomous person.				
18.	I have been told I am extremely reliable and dependable.				
19.	I have great passion for my nursing career.				
20.	It is important to me to think about and plan for the future.				

Scoring. Assign the number shown in the box below to the response you gave to each question in **Part 1** and each question in **Part 2**.

	PART 1				
	STATEMENT	SA	A	D	SD
1.	Leaders are very creative.	4	3	0	0
2.	The most important goal of a leader is to be sure the job gets done.	4	3	2	1
3.	Leaders should focus on people, not on the system.	4	3	2	1

	STATEMENT	SA	A	D	SD
	PART 1—cont'd				
4.	One does not need to be in a position of authority to be a leader.	4	3	0	0
5.	Credibility is an important characteristic of a leader.	4	3	0	0
6.	Leaders tend to be people with high energy who are passionate about their work.	4	3	0	0
7.	Leaders focus more on being creative than on accomplishing their vision or goal(s).	4	3	3	4
8.	Persistence is a trademark of an effective leader.	1	2	3	4
9.	Leaders are committed to their vision and tend not to adapt to change well.	0	0	3	4
10.	Leaders are good at empowering others to grow.	4	3	0	0
11.	It is important for leaders to have a dream and to be future-oriented.	4	3	0	0
12.	A person's ability to lead in a professional setting depends on his or her self-esteem.	4	3	0	0
13.	A leader's style of leading is determined by the situation and/or task at hand.	4	3	0	4
14.	A good leader must have integrity.	4	3	2	1
15.	Leaders mentor others to assist them in pursuing their dreams.	4	3	0	0
16.	Leadership is a quality one is born with, and it cannot be acquired.	0	0	3	4
17.	Good leaders help others to resolve conflict.	4	3	2	1
18.	One does not need to be an excellent critical thinker in order to be a great leader.	0	0	3	4
19.	A good leader should have excellent communication skills.	4	3	0	0
20.	Leaders always follow the rules.	0	0	3	4

Interpretation of Scores
Part 1: Perception of what makes a good leader
Add up your score for Part 1. Here's what the scores indicate:

70 to 80 = Excellent perception of a good leader.
60 to 69 = Good perception of a good leader.
50 to 59 = Probably mixing up the difference between management and leadership.
40 to 49 = Definitely mixing up the difference between management and leadership.
39 or less = Need to do some reading on what good leadership is.

	PART 2				
	STATEMENT	SA	A	D	SD
1.	I value integrity higher than power.	4	3	0	0
2.	People tend to think I have the ability to influence others.	4	3	0	0
3.	I feel confident about my knowledge base and skills, given my years of experience.	4	3	0	0
4.	I have a definite dream for where I want to be in my profession.	4	3	3	4
5.	I have mentored another person and found the experience rewarding.	4	3	0	0
6.	Change usually makes me feel nervous, and I tend to lose my self-confidence.	4	3	0	0
7.	I feel energized taking risks unless they are life-threatening.	4	3	0	0
8.	I do not feel confident calling a physician about my patient's status.	0	0	3	4
9.	When I experience conflict, I usually give in and accommodate the other person.	0	0	3	4
10.	I feel I do make a difference as a nurse and plan to continue to do so.	4	3	0	0
11.	Since I am only a nurse, I am not responsible for patient care errors.	0	0	3	4
12.	I often follow others when I am not sure what to do about something.	0	0	3	4
13.	I notice I agree with others easily unless the issue is very dear to my heart.	4	3	3	4
14.	I attempt to empower ancillary workers because I find the team spirit is enhanced.	4	3	0	0
15.	Personally, I do not really have a vision as to where I plan to be in a few years.	4	3	2	2
16.	I enjoy conflict and rarely compromise my needs.	4	3	0	0
17.	I am an autonomous person.	4	3	0	0
18.	I have been told I am extremely reliable and dependable.	4	3	0	0
19.	I have great passion for my nursing career.	4	3	0	0
20.	It is important to me to think about and plan for the future.	4	3	0	0

Part 2: Perception of your own ability to lead

Add up your score for Part 2. Here's what the scores indicate:

70 to 80 = Extremely high perceived leadership ability.
60 to 69 = High perceived leadership ability.
50 to 59 = Moderate perceived leadership ability.
40 to 49 = Low perceived leadership ability.
39 or less = Extremely low perceived leadership ability.

References

Bass, B. M. (2008). *The Bass handbook of leadership: Theory, research, and managerial applications* (4th ed.). New York, NY: Free Press.

Benner, P., Sutphen, M., Leonard, V., & Day, L. (2009). *Educating nurses: A call for radical transformation*. San Francisco, CA: Jossey-Bass.

Bennis, W. (1989). *On becoming a leader*. Reading, MA: Addison-Wesley.

Bennis, W. (2004). A leadership discussion with Warren Bennis. Webcast sponsored by the American Society of Association Executives Foundation, April 20, 2004.

Bennis, W. (2006). The end of leadership: Exemplary leadership is impossible without full inclusion, initiatives, and cooperation of followers. In W. E. Rosenbach & R. L. Taylor (Eds.), *Contemporary issues in leadership* (6th ed., pp. 129–142). Boulder, CO: Westview Press.

Bennis, W., & Nanus, B. (1985). *Leaders: The strategies for taking charge*. New York, NY: Harper & Row.

Block, P. (1993). *Stewardship: Choosing service over self interest*. San Francisco, CA: Berrett-Koehler.

Bolman, L. G., & Deal, T. E. (2011). *Leading with soul: An uncommon journey of spirit* (3rd ed.). San Francisco CA: Jossey-Bass.

Brocato, B., Jelen, J., Schmidt, T., & Gold, S. S. (2011). Leadership conceptual ambiguities: A post-positivistic critique. *Journal of Leadership Studies, 5*(1), 35-47.

Broome, M.E. (2011). Leadership: Old concept, new visions (Editorial). *Nursing Outlook, 59*(5), 253-255.

Burns, J. M. (1978). *Leadership*. New York, NY: Harper Torchbooks.

Burns, J. M. (2003). *Transforming leadership: A new pursuit of happiness*. New York, NY: Atlantic Monthly Press.

Chaleff, I. (2009). *The courageous follower: Standing up to and for our leaders* (3rd ed.). San Francisco, CA: Berrett-Koehler.

Clampitt, P. G., & Dekoch, R. J. (2001). *Embracing uncertainty: The essence of leadership*. Armonk, NY: M. E. Sharp.

Collins, J. (2001). Good to great. Retrieved from http://www.fastcompany.com.

Corona, D. F. (1986). Followership: The indispensable corollary to leadership. In E. C. Hein & M. J. Nicholson (Eds.), *Contemporary leadership behavior: Selected readings* (3rd ed., pp. 87–91). Boston, MA: Little, Brown.

Crowell, D. (2010). *Complexity leadership: Nursing's role in health care delivery*. Philadelphia, PA: F. A. Davis.

DePree, M. (1989). *Leadership is an art*. New York, NY: Dell.

DePree, M. (1992). *Leadership jazz*. New York, NY: Doubleday Currency.

DiRienzo, S. M. (1994). A challenge to nursing: Promoting followers as well as leaders. *Holistic Nursing Practice, 9*(1), 26–30.

Gardner, J. W. (1989). The tasks of leadership. In W. E. Rosenbach & R. L. Taylor (Eds.), *Contemporary issues in leadership* (2nd ed., pp. 24–33). Boulder, CO: Westview Press.

Gardner, J. W. (1990). *On leadership*. New York, NY: Free Press.

Greenleaf, R. K. (1977). *Servant leadership: A journey into the nature of legitimate power and greatness*. New York, NY: Paulist Press.

Gryskiewicz, S. S. (2005). Leading renewal: The value of positive turbulence. *Leadership in Action, 25*(1), 8-12.

Havens, D. S., Wood, S. O., & Leeman, J. (2006). Improving nursing practice and patient care: Building capacity with appreciative inquiry. *Journal of Nursing Administration, 36*(10), 463-470.

Heifetz, R. A., Grashow, A., & Linsky, M. (2009). *The practice of adaptive leadership: Tools and tactics for changing your organization and the world*. Boston, MA: Harvard Business Review Press.

Hesselbein, F., Goldsmith, M., & Somerville, I. (Eds.). (1999). *Leading beyond the walls*. San Francisco, CA: Jossey-Bass.

Holle, M. L., & Blatchley, M. E. (1987). *Introduction to leadership and management in nursing* (2nd ed.). Boston, MA: Jones & Bartlett.

Institute of Medicine. (2010). *The future of nursing: Leading change, advancing health*. Washington, DC: National Academies Press.

Jackman, I. (Ed.). (2005). *The leader's mentor: Inspiration from the world's most effective leaders*. New York, NY: Random House.

Jackson, R. (2011). Leadership: Integrity, authenticity, and courage. Retrieved from http://www.couragerenewal.org/newsletter/spring2011/314-leadership-integrity-authenticity-and-courage

Jennings, B. M., Scalzi, C. C., Rodgers, J. D., & Keane, A. (2007). Differentiating nursing leadership and management competencies. *Nursing Outlook, 55*(4), 169–175.

Kellerman, B. (2008). *Followership: How followers are creating change and changing leaders*. Boston, MA: Harvard Business Press.

Kelley, R. (1992). *The power of followership: How to create leaders people want to follow and followers who lead themselves*. New York, NY: Doubleday Currency.

Kelley, R. (1993). How followers weave a web of relationships. In W. E. Rosenbach & R. L. Taylor (Eds.), *Contemporary issues in leadership* (3rd ed., pp. 122–133). Boulder, CO: Westview Press.

Keohane, N.O. (2010). *Thinking about leadership*. Princeton, NJ: Princeton University Press.

Kouses, J. M., & Posner, B. Z. (2008). *The leadership challenge: How to keep getting extraordinary things done in organizations* (4th ed.). San Francisco, CA: Jossey-Bass.

Krzyzewski, M. (2000). *Leading with the heart*. New York, NY: Warner Business Books.

Lee, C. (1993). Followership: The essence of leadership. In W. E. Rosenbach & R. L. Taylor (Eds.), *Contemporary issues in leadership* (3rd ed., pp. 113–121). Boulder, CO: Westview Press.

Manfredi, C. (1995). The art of legendary leadership. *Nursing Leadership Forum, 1*(2), 62–64.

Nanus, B. (1992). *Visionary leadership*. San Francisco, CA: Jossey-Bass.

Parse, R. R. (2009). The humanbecoming leading-following model. *Nursing Science Quarterly, 21*(4), 369–375.

Phillips, D. T. (1997). *The founding fathers on leadership*. New York, NY: Warner Books.

Pickens, T. (2000). What makes a good leader? *Creative Living, 29*(4), 13–16.

Robinson, K. (2009). *The element: How finding your passion changes everything*. New York, NY: The Penguin Group (Viking).

Schweitzer, C. (2006). From soloist to orchestrator. *Associations Now*, March, 33–36.

Spears, L. C. (Ed.). (1995). *Reflections on leadership: How Robert K. Greenleaf's theory of servant-leadership influenced today's top management thinkers*. New York, NY: John Wiley & Sons.

Sturman, C. (2002). Dare to dream. *Leader to Leader, 23*(Winter), 35–39.

Tanner, C., & Weinman, J. (2011). It's all about leadership (2011). *Journal of Nursing Education, 50*(5), 239–241.

Tetenbaum, T., & Laurence, H. (2011). Leading in the chaos of the 21st century. *Journal of Leadership Studies, 4*(4), 41–49.

Thornberry, N. (2006). A view about "vision." In W. E. Rosenbach & R. L. Taylor (Eds.). *Contemporary issues in leadership* (6th ed., pp. 31–43). Boulder, CO: Westview Press.

Tichy, N. M. (1997). *The leadership engine: How winning companies build leaders at every level*. New York, NY: HarperBusiness.

Wheatley, M. J. (1999). *Leadership and the new science: Discovering order in a chaotic world* (2nd ed.). San Francisco, CA: Berrett-Koehler.

Williams, M. (1975). *The velveteen rabbit*. New York, NY: Avon Books.

Yeh, R. T. (2005, November/December). 7 essential qualities of leadership. *Association Executive*, 13.

Zaleznik, A. (1981). Managers and leaders: Are they different? *Journal of Nursing Administration, 11*(7), 25–31.

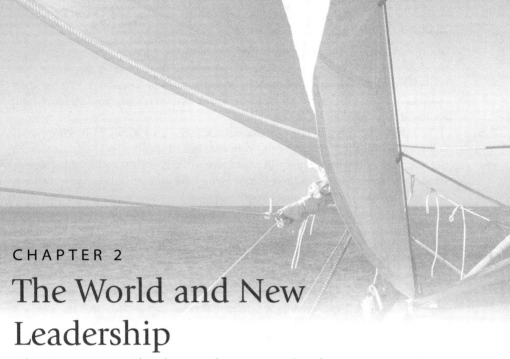

CHAPTER 2

The World and New Leadership

Changing Our Thinking About Leadership

INTRODUCTION

Evidence-based practice, patient outcomes, quality and safety, accountability, information management, interdisciplinary collaboration, partnerships, acquisitions, and affiliations—these are terms we hear, read about, and discuss. All organizations, particularly those in health care, are experiencing change. To continue to participate successfully in health care, nursing will need to continue to evolve in finding ways to use resources wisely, validating the effects of nursing interventions on patient outcomes, developing strong partnerships, and providing high-quality and cost-effective care. These goals can be accomplished if nurses focus on health promotion in all types of care settings, encourage multidisciplinary collaboration, integrate outcome assessment into our daily work as nurses, and "retool" so that we can practice even more autonomously and accountably.

To achieve such goals, all registered nurses (RNs) and advanced practice nurses (APNs) must think in a new way. Being confident as well as competent is consistent with the new view of leadership that will help nurses solidify their roles in the health-care arena. Indeed, it is time to embrace the problems of organizational change and look at each one of these as a challenging opportunity.

To bring change, we must develop a new way of achieving health-care reform. We are now in a new age of health care. A plethora of articles and books discuss nurses and medical assistants in terms of staff mix, patient outcome–driven health care, self-care, cultural awareness, quality improvement, the move to health promotion and disease prevention, patient safety, and multidisciplinary team building, to name some of the issues. Studies evaluating the effects of changes in these areas on care quality or specific ways in which health care providers, especially nurses, need to retool and think in new ways in order to remain significant players in this new age of health care are being emphasized (Porter-O'Grady & Malloch, 2011). Nurses, in all settings, must deliver quality care to diverse populations (The Joint Commission, 2008) and need to be educated to provide safe care to all (Institute of Medicine [IOM], 2002; Quality and Safety Education for Nurses, 2010). These mandates recommend that nurses change their thinking so that they are able to accomplish the following:

- Engage in more independent decision making
- Think in a multidimensional, rather than linear, fashion
- Collaborate more effectively with nurse and non-nurse partners
- Provide leadership (Buerhaus, Donelan, DesRoches, & Hess, 2009; Needleman, Kurtzman, & Kizer; 2007)

A recent IOM report, *The Future of Nursing: Leading Change, Advancing Health* (2010), recommends that nurses work to foster professional collaboration within the health-care team, increasing the percentage of nurses with baccalaureate degrees, doubling the number of nurses with doctorates by 2020, and advocating nursing leadership at every level of the profession (Hassmiller, 2010). It is clear that nurses are essential to changing health care.

> *Do not follow where the path may lead. Go instead where there is no path and leave a trail.* —Anonymous

PREPARING NURSE LEADERS

Many nurses are not prepared for the role they will need to assume in acute care institutions, home care, or other settings, and they may become overwhelmed all too quickly. This chapter is designed to help nurses rethink the notion of leadership and their roles as leaders so that they can participate more effectively in the new and evolving health-care field. Manfredi and Valiga (1990) reviewed a sample of baccalaureate programs to evaluate whether the curricula focused more on the art of leadership or on the science of management. These authors found that most of the programs were teaching management skills, such as how to delegate to a team member, organize one's day, or staff an exceptionally ill patient awaiting transfer to the intensive care unit, and that faculty generally viewed "leadership" and "management" as synonymous. No more recent comparative studies have been published regarding what leadership versus management content is being taught in baccalaureate programs. This book specifically focuses on the art of leadership and not the science of management. Nurse educators need to provide students with the knowledge and experiences that will prepare them to work in multidisciplinary teams. Several studies recommend that nurses need to increase their communication and leadership skills so that they can become effective members of multidisciplinary health-care teams and serve as fully participating partners in negotiations at all levels (Sorensen, Iedema, & Severinsson, 2008; Grossman, 2007). Thus, there is work to be done if we are to prepare each and every nurse as a leader.

Developing Leadership

We are moving from the Scientific Age, with its emphasis on short- and long-term planning, predicting patient acuity, using formulas to provide staff coverage, and following bureaucratic procedures and policies to get tasks done, to a New Science Age that stresses empowerment of all, creating while doing, evaluating processes and outcomes, and collaborating as a team. Such change requires us to exercise leadership in an entirely new way.

Covey (2004) described three characteristics a leader must possess for a successful experience in growing and learning: vision, courage, and humility. Having a dream or vision is imperative, but one must have courage to continue to define that vision to a group and, at the same time, be humble enough to know when to redefine it to meet the needs of the changing times and prepare for the future. Covey also developed the term "co-missioning," which suggests that a staff member must have not only a vision or mission but also a way of measuring the outcomes of the vision. This, in turn, will assist in improving the future outcomes. Bennis and Nanus (1997) described leadership as encompassing vision, the ability to communicate effectively, the ability to be steadfast, and the ability to demonstrate positive self-regard. Having the ability to consistently propel a vision in a group or organization takes self-confidence and assertiveness. McBride (2010) echoed the thoughts of Bennis and Nanus when she described leadership as a process to move a profession or some type of health-care organization "down a new path with different expectations, structures, and ways of conceptualizing how to achieve the mission in light of changing conditions" (p. 165).

For example, to change the nursing task orientation to a patient outcome focus, nurses can use leadership skills. If the desired vision was one of nurses working collaboratively with other health-care members to provide care that best facilitates positive patient outcomes, the monitoring of clients for beneficial or untoward sequelae of nursing, medical, and pharmacological interventions would be done in collaboration with physicians and pharmacists, rather than in isolation. Practices that challenge the traditional "sacred cows" of the medical model have to be adopted so that the vision of nursing care takes center-stage and the profession of nursing is recognized as a primary means to obtaining positive patient outcomes.

Nursing leaders have been developing nursing diagnoses and a taxonomy of nursing interventions since the 1980s, yet they are still carrying out medical orders. Nurses need to define what nursing is and wants to be, then work as a unified body to achieve those goals. The current chaotic state of health care provides a window of opportunity for realization of this vision. (See Chapter 7 for strategies leaders can use to take advantage of these opportunities and to read more in depth about chaos theory.) Nurses need to work to ensure a focus on excellence as well as on cost-effectiveness. Nursing leaders must clearly identify responsibilities of RNs, APNs, and nonlicensed assistive personnel, and they must guide us in creating and strengthening new roles for nurses. With leaders who employ a new way of thinking about leadership, all nurses can be successful in advancing the profession.

CHAOS THEORY

Most nurses acknowledge that the entire health-care system is in chaos, but chaos theory implies that hidden within this seemingly total disorganization are patterns of order. So, if nurses, representing the largest group of professional health-care workers, can create a culture willing to accept change and use innovative and creative ideas, then nurses can be the leaders in health care in these times of uncertainty. "Chaos" is a scientific term meaning to be in a state of complete confusion. Chaos theory is a part of complexity science, which involves the "modelling of living systems" (Capra, 2002). Wheatley (2006) said computers have awakened us to the true definition of chaos because of their ability to store mega data. Millions of pieces of data can be displayed at any one time on any screen. The system allows the millions of bytes of data to be displayed in what appears to be a chaotic jumble, but as one tracks the computer screen, rapidly moving lines seem to appear and connect the data. Thus, what appeared to be chaos actually takes on an orderly shape.

Certainly, each and every nurse has experienced the process of change, either a planned initiative or a spontaneous one in the work setting. What is important for nurses to gain from these change movements is that the innovative and creative thinking that fostered the change must continue to grow and cannot be thought of in an organized, step-by-step linear process. The patterns that emerge during the evaluation process of the change will need to be viewed in the same creative and innovative fashion that triggered the change. By participating in change, allowing time for change to occur, and being aware of the need for more change to evolve, the nurse leaders on the unit or department can create a culture that welcomes continuous change, innovation, and creativity. By creating this culture of uncertainty, the entire staff will bond and work more cohesively. Chaos theory is saying that nurses must continue to adjust to small fluctuations in a dynamic system (their specific nursing unit), such as with late delivery of medications, shortage of supplies, and staff shortages. Using chaos theory, nurses can visualize in a creative manner, and perhaps in an autonomous and calm fashion, that the medications will not cause life-threatening problems if they are administered *slightly* later than the prescribed time, that they can creatively use resources to stretch them, and that they can deliver care in a different manner depending on the number of staff and skill set available.

Think about the last time you had an emergency patient situation—didn't everyone pitch in? There were no formalities, and if the patient's situation deteriorated, the team probably became more collegial and informal as everyone tried harder. This is easily correlated to what happens in a bureaucratic organization when uncertainty increases. People tend to use more personal and group approaches (Kouzes & Posner, 2007) as they come together for the *common good*, and this often occurs unconsciously. Leaders can be instrumental at times like this by using the chaos and the changes it ultimately produces as a positive opportunity. In other words, it seems that "growth appears from disequilibrium, not balance" (Wheatley, 2006, p. 21).

Challenging problems provide people with opportunities for great success. Sweating a bit or being a little anxious about something usually leaves us exhilarated after the problem has been resolved. The health-care chaos that currently surrounds us is one such problem. This can result in an even stronger role for nurses and the identification of more creative ways to provide high-quality and cost-effective care. An example may help illustrate this point.

Many in nursing bemoan the loss of the 80% professional staff and 20% nonprofessional staff mix we enjoyed in the past and the reality of the current 60% professional staff and 40% nonprofessional staff mix in most hospitals today. However, studies conducted by Needleman, Buerhaus, Stewart, Zelevinsky, and Matki (2006) and Aiken, Clarke, Sloane, Sochalski, and Silver (2002) document that care is better with RN staff, but until it is more evident that costs can be maintained with more RN staff, it is unlikely that the proportion of professional staff will increase. It would be contrary to the new science of leadership philosophy, however, to propose a quantitative study measuring cost-effectiveness. Instead, the new science perspective would encourage the emergence of creative leaders who are willing to stray from set formulas and achieve the "right" mix of staff for their individual units by experimenting until that ideal mix is found. For example, a proposal of gradually decreasing professional staff and increasing unlicensed personnel would be more tolerable than just eliminating RN positions. In addition, having an available RN "pool" would allow nurses to be called in when the acuteness of the patient's condition justified professional care. The old bureaucratic way of thinking about having a consistent number of staff members for every unit with a certain number of full-time equivalents (FTEs) of professional and nonprofessional staff just does not work in a world characterized by chaos.

The new science philosophy recommends less prediction, prejudgment, and compartmentalization. Wheatley (2006, 2005) suggested that nurses stop dwelling on tasks and instead focus on facilitating the processes needed to obtain desired goals. For example, nurse managers need to try new staffing patterns that acknowledge that a 60% professional and 40% nonprofessional staff mix (or an 80/20, 30/70, or any other mix) is not ideal for every unit, but that any number of patterns could work if staff worked with each other in new ways. Also, the idea of using teams of RNs, LPNs, and nurse assistants may need to be reassessed, along with teams of multidisciplinary workers. Leaders need to concentrate first on the people who are working to achieve the goals and establishing positive relationships between and among them. Any number of tasks can then be accomplished. When people have positive working relationships with one another, they are more likely to respect one another and to achieve great things. As Wheatley said, "What gives power its charge, positive or negative, is the nature of the relationship" (2006, p. 40).

Some organizations are calling on nurses to navigate their institutions through this chaotic time, and nursing leaders are using a number of creative strategies to influence change, survive, and even grow. Skills such as creativity, patient-centeredness, coordination, multiple priority management, problem solving, critical thinking, and system navigation are identified as being necessary for nurses to use throughout their careers. Quantum theory and the new science, developmental theory, cognitive theory, complexity theory, and perspective transformation support a new holistic view of leadership and find growth in chaos. We must come to the realization that chaos is actually good and can assist a unit or department to use innovative ideas in leading change.

QUANTUM THEORY AND THE NEW SCIENCE

Wheatley (2006) was among the first to relate the changes we have witnessed in science to the need for a new view of leadership. She noted that "if we are to continue to draw from science to create and manage organizations, to design research, and to formulate hypotheses about organizational design, planning, economics, human nature, and change processes, then we need to at least ground our work in the science of our times" (p. 8). By "the science of our times," Wheatley is referring to new research in the disciplines of physics, biology, and chemistry, as well as to the theories of chaos and evolution, which span several disciplines. This new science focuses on relationships and a nonlinear approach, in which the real and the potentially real are visualized simultaneously. It is a method of thinking that replaces our standard, orderly, goal-oriented perspective with a free-flowing, open-space, always-moving, anything-can-happen philosophy. For example, instead of thinking APNs provide holistic care and can perform all of the care of their primary care patients, including phlebotomy, obtaining specimens, faxing prescriptions, following up on laboratory results, and so forth, why not trial the use of an RN and/or nonlicensed medical assistant teamed with each MD/APN? By creating a new delivery system method with more than one person involved, it may be possible to deliver better outcomes, foster greater self-care interest and patient compliance, be more cost-effective, and increase (or at least not decrease) provider and staff morale. These teams could allow for more one-on-one phone or e-mail interaction between visits, an evening support group, quick checks at the clinic practice, and maybe even home visits if necessary. All of these "extra" meetings with patients/families could be instrumental in preventing recidivism with hospital admissions and even primary care visits.

Leadership and Quantum Theory

Wheatley (2006) recommended that we approach leadership through the lens provided by the new science and naturally occurring events. For example, after a storm, meteorologists can review storm patterns on a computer and visualize a pattern in what initially appeared to be chaos. We can also reflect on the fact that a stream, which initially seems to be little more than a random collection of water, sand, rocks, and silt, actually is not random at all but is a carefully designed system in which all parts work together to allow flexibility and the capacity for change as the natural elements of storms, animals, and humans affect its path.

The new science says that living systems organize themselves by seeking order, but this order is not linear or predictive. Organizations, said Wheatley (2006), operate in the same way. They seek order, but not in a linear, hierarchical way. Thus, leadership in an organization may best be provided by a social system comprising many leaders, not only one. Those who relate through coercion or with a disregard for others create negative energy, whereas those who are open to others and see others in their fullness create positive energy. Perhaps by focusing on one nonprofessional staff member at a time and allowing a "connectedness" to occur between that individual and the other staff, a we-versus-they situation can be avoided. If each staff member can be empowered to visualize his or her own potential as well as that of others, a more positive outlook regarding workload and quality of patient care is likely to prevail. Buerhaus and colleagues (2009) offer several recommendations for nurses to continue to make changes in improving the hospital workplace setting. These changes appear to affect patient outcomes and also to heighten the more valued role of the nurse collaborating in a multidisciplinary team effort in health-care delivery in the 21st century.

Quantum Theory and Growth

Quantum theory suggests that an interface among all members of a group is critical. Each person needs to be acknowledged for his or her talents and potential, and each needs to be helped to grow. Perhaps nurses need to visualize the workforce as germinating seeds in space rather than on earth, where gravity pulls the roots toward it and the stem grows away from gravity. In space, seeds grow every which way because there is no gravity to direct them in only a ground-up direction. Likewise, people are not fixed entities gravitating toward one spot and able to be predicted by a set of rules and expectations.

People need to be given the opportunity to grow in all kinds of ways—ways that are unknown to anyone until they happen. It is the task of the leader to encourage and facilitate such growth. Perhaps, visualizing an organization as composed of Gumby-like figures that stretch and overlap with each other in a three-dimensional, rather than linear, structure would allow for greater diversity and uniqueness and open more avenues for communication and effective outcomes. Work productivity cannot be predicted based on a given number of FTEs, certain types of patient hours, and acuity levels. Such task-oriented thinking is not what patient care is all about. Instead, mindsets need to be more multidimensional and open to new possibilities and things that no one has thought of yet. Leaders are the key to success because they facilitate relationships, encourage growth, enjoy uncertainty, and are willing to take risks. Leaders also know how to deal with "toxic" people or those with whom it is difficult to communicate, develop outstanding leaders, and transform organizations (Porter-O'Grady & Malloch, 2011).

The new way of thinking about leadership in a global and almost limitless fashion, and realizing that each individual has a contribution to make, is necessary if nursing is to succeed in delivering the highest-quality care. Valuing hard work and respecting one another are qualities that need to be revived and that must be pervasive. In other words, the whole culture of the practice settings needs reawakening. A job should be viewed as a piece of an ever-changing plan that affects the overall functioning of the organization. Each person must be respected as crucial to the greater goal. Biases, prejudices, insecurities, and preconceived judgments need to be worked out or left behind. When such an atmosphere exists, communication, mentoring, and collaboration are more likely to occur, and self-empowerment and group empowerment dominate. The change from a task-focused setting to more of a process-focused one allows followers and leaders to propel organizations and the individuals within them forward.

From Task-Focused to Holistic Care

The world is moving out of the Industrial or Newtonian Age in which things were described in a linear way and where we became accustomed to separating every system into parts, rather than dealing with the whole. As the world moves toward this greater concern for wholeness, complexity, and interaction, leaders are needed. An example of a health-care organization being more process-focused and implementing a holistic approach to leadership is provided in the accompanying case study.

We must use our imaginations and embrace the idea that there is more to our work than assessing, planning, implementing, and evaluating. Nurses can no longer

Case Study

The senior nurse leaders at an acute care institution were working on integration of the six issues delineated by the Institute of Medicine (IOM) *Crossing the Quality Chasm—A New Health System for the 21st Century* (2001): patient safety, patient-centeredness, efficiency, effectiveness, timeliness, and equity. The nurse leaders also wanted to enforce the newest mandate from IOM (2010), which is to increase nursing leadership at every level. One of the nurse leaders suggested the development of a Patient/Family Advisory Board, which would allow volunteers who served to be integrated into the infrastructure of the hospital. This would entail representatives from this Board sitting in on the hospital's executive leadership sessions, the Hospital Governing Board meetings, and other similar group discussions with an aim toward setting a new standard of care in order to obtain a meaningful voice for patients and families. The nurse leader, the Vice President of Patient Outcomes, marketed the idea, sought volunteers from the community, established the Board, assisted in developing bylaws for the board, integrated the board members into the hospital's organization, and now meets monthly with the board and other groups to receive feedback. Members of the Patient/Family Advisory Board include previous hospital patients and family members of patients who had been hospitalized or died. Outcomes include assisting in promoting a patient safety culture to advance optimal care by establishing priorities, developing specific action plans, and allocating appropriate resources. The Joint Commission and the Institute for Healthcare Improvement recognize that effective leadership is essential in creating a safe, patient outcome–focused delivery system (Aspden, Corrigan, Wolcott, & Erickson, 2004; Institute for Healthcare Improvement, 2007). This is a most innovative way to provide a meaningful voice to health-care consumers.

Eadie (2009) shares actual examples of how to maximize one's contributions toward making a change in an institution/agency as a member of a Board. Just by volunteering to serve on a Board, a nurse will be able to network with other Board members who could assist in enhancing the nurse's career or in accomplishing goals for a specific health-care initiative. Nurses could increase their leadership skills and contribute to the mission of an agency/institution by serving on a governing board such as a Community Health Center, Hospital Issues Board, or some topic-focused Board such as the Northeast Multiple Sclerosis Society Board.

have tunnel vision and be task-oriented. Instead, we need a more in-depth analysis of the data collected before we can decide on what to include in the plan of care. Our whole philosophy of caring for patients must be broadened, and for most of us, our way of simply moving from one task to another will have to change. Most RNs, the average of whom is 42.3 years old and has worked most of her or his 20-plus-year career in a very rigid organizational structure carrying out another profession's orders, will have to reorient themselves to nursing and to leading with a new science of leadership perspective. The quantum mechanics framework of attending to naturally occurring events appreciates individuals for their knowledge and recognizes that they need tools and support, not direction and control (Malloch & Porter-O'Grady, 2009).

SUPPORTING PERSPECTIVES AND PERSPECTIVE TRANSFORMATION THEORY

The idea that people and organizations grow and evolve in response to challenges, disequilibrium, and change is not new, nor is it restricted to quantum mechanics or new science thinking. In fact, it is an idea that has been addressed by psychologists, educators, and nurse theorists. Examples of these follow.

Cognitive and intellectual development occur through the increasing ability to use complex cognitive skills to analyze issues, manage changing circumstances, integrate multiple points of view, and make sound decisions independently (Perry, 1970). Individuals progress through stages of cognitive development, from seeing knowledge as finite and themselves as absorbers or memorizers of it, to viewing knowledge as relative and themselves as critical thinkers and lifelong learners. Such changes in worldview, similar to any type of growth, occur as a result of disequilibrium. When one's usual way of thinking is found to be lacking, one experiences disequilibrium and is challenged to think in new ways, ask new questions, and develop new strategies. The chaos and disequilibrium with which nurses in practice are challenged, therefore, can be viewed as a stimulus for growth and development. Nurses need to rethink their role in health care, the kind of leadership needed in this arena, and their responsibility to provide such leadership.

Erik Erikson, a developmental theorist, stated that physical, emotional, and social factors have an effect on an individual's development (Erikson, 1963). He asserted that development is a mixture of maturation (the potential growth a person has inherited) and learning (knowledge to be gained). Most nurses are working in a rigidly structured health-care system and, without leadership, may not move out of adolescence or young adulthood stages, where one of the tasks is to master involvement with others. Mastery of these developmental tasks results in intimacy and solidarity, whereas failure results in isolation. Because the new leadership is based on relationships, it is paramount that nurses accomplish the task of young adulthood so that they can be highly effective health-care team members. The accomplishment of the generativity task (Erickson, 1963) for those more advanced in life leads to productive and creative work. For nurses to experience this generativity, they need to have acquired leadership skills.

Just as our lives can be viewed developmentally, so too can our organizational systems. Only organizational structures that continue to be flexible and change will be able to support the development of people in the organization. Sometimes, it is only when a person is pushed, as happens in a chaotic job setting or in severe conflict with one's peers to accomplish tasks, that he or she actually develops and grows. Hence, developmental theory also suggests that disequilibrium is not a negative situation, but rather a positive experience that enhances growth.

Complexity theory describes the way life is ordered and emphasizes that life is based on the principles of emergence more than it is predetermined by other variables. McDaniel and Driebe (2005) explore how unpredictability and surprise affect our world both individually and through our various group classifications. The ideas of how complexity science influences everything we do, including leading, are explained by West (2006), who gives multiple examples of how emergence, self-organization, and pattern formation underlie the science of complexity. Crowell (2011) suggests a complexity leadership model that includes a transformational, collaborative, reflective, relationship-based leadership style. She recommends the use of a multidimensional lens to study the current complex health-care organizations nurses work in today. Using complexity science, nurses can view all quantitative and qualitative data, noting relationships and connections among the data. This leads to establishing new patterns of collaboration in contrast to the linear organizational structure in which authority controls the next level and blocks the feedback mechanisms that can lead the organization to grow. The complexity leadership model can help organizations adapt to change and uncertainty and propel the organizations' leaders to succeed.

Fawcett (1995) explained that "each nurse, as well as the healthcare system itself, requires time to evolve from the use of individual, implicit frames of reference for nursing practice to an explicit model" (p. 532). The process that occurs during this period of growth, when an individual has not clearly defined a frame of reference for nursing practice to a specific conceptual model, is perspective transformation. This growth depends on the experiences one has had in school or in the work setting. Fawcett's (1995, pp. 533–534) explanation of perspective transformation depicts how leaders can assist nurses to identify their own ability to lead and hence grow in these chaotic times.

> **Stage 1:** *Stability* reflects what many nurses are currently experiencing in their workplaces. Nurses easily maintain the status quo because many were never encouraged to think of themselves as leaders.
>
> **Stage 2:** *Dissonance* moves one toward the revelation that all nurses can be leaders. It generally means the beginning of a reawakening to one's situation. Nurses experiencing dissonance are aware of the very chaotic times they are in and know they need to start doing something. They may share their feelings with peers and start speaking out when serious staffing problems or unsafe situations occur.
>
> **Stage 3:** *Confusion* occurs when individuals gain courage from others who validate what they are feeling, speak openly about things not being right, and decide not to "put up with it anymore!"

Stage 4: *Dealing with uncertainty* is when individuals speak out, but they do so sporadically because they may believe that they do not have the ability or strength to change things.

Stage 5: *Saturation* occurs when people feel confident they have collected the right information and spoken to the right people about a new way of doing things or delivering care.

Stage 6: *Synthesis* heralds the organization of information to formulate a plan to change an unacceptable situation . . . a plan put into place because individuals care enough to make a change.

Stage 7: *Resolution* indicates that the problems are being solved with the changes that were put into place.

Stage 8: *Reconceptualization* occurs when those who initiated the change continue to "work out some of the kinks" in the system and empower others to continue to support and pursue new ways of doing things.

Stage 9: *Return to stability* indicates that the change has now become a part of the milieu and is no longer being evaluated and scrutinized extensively.

This framework provides an additional basis for arguing why we need to rethink the need for leadership. It depicts a change from nurses practicing in a private way to an entire nursing staff using a shared model of practice. This is a good example of how something positive can come from living or working in chaos. Perspective transformation is a helpful process to use in assisting nurses to practice more autonomously. It could also facilitate nursing receiving a greater portion of the health-care dollar because it should assist in measuring tangible patient outcomes, which are a direct result of nursing care.

CONCLUSION

We need to change our thinking about what leadership is if we are to survive and thrive during the tumultuous changes in health care. Complexity and chaos theory will assist us in understanding how the disorder and confusion we are feeling in our work settings today are equivalent to what happens in nature. The fact that the natural world we live in can automatically order itself after such turmoil is incredible. We have to realize that adapting the new science of leadership, with its focus on empowering followers and alleviating the bureaucratic organizational structure, will assist us in developing new ideas and new ways of working.

The transformation in health-care delivery that nurses are participating in is certainly disorienting and chaotic, but it is necessary to continue to reframe the hierarchical medical model on which the U.S. health-care system has been based. This major paradigm shift has the potential to improve the quality of health care and not merely reduce costs. That will happen, however, only if we have capable nurse leaders willing to take the risks needed to produce such positive outcomes. Quantum theory, cognitive theory, developmental theory, complexity theory, and perspective transformation frameworks provide evidence that chaos and disequilibrium can be positive instigators for growth and improvement. This new way of thinking about leading will help nurses provide a more collaborative and holistic approach to practice and help us achieve our visions for the profession.

CRITICAL THINKING EXERCISES

Explain how the new way of thinking about leadership described in this chapter can affect the way we conceptualize the role of the nurse today. How could you assist others in adapting this perspective?

_____

_____

Think about the environment in which you practice. Would you describe it as chaotic? Why or why not? What contributes to the chaos or relative "calm"? What have been the negative ways that you and others have dealt with chaos in your environment? What positive strategies have been used? What patterns do you see in the midst of all this chaos?

_____

_____

Listen to a jazz musical selection with an extended improvisational piece. Despite the seemingly chaotic notes and chords, do you hear or feel any patterns or synchrony? How did you identify such patterns? (This same exercise can be done by viewing a Picasso painting or even watching a soccer game.)

_____

_____

Who do you think of as leaders where you practice? What characteristics of the new science of leadership do these people portray?

_____

_____

Develop a list of behaviors that you use when you approach various situations regarding certainty or uncertainty. Describe how your work environment (the people and the structure) influences your certainty.

_____

_____

References

Aiken, L., Clarke, S., Sloane, D., Sochalski, J., & Siber, J. (2002). Hospital staffing and patient mortality, nurse burnout, and job dissatisfaction. *Journal of the American Medical Association, 288,* 1987–1993.

Aspden, P., Corrigan, J., Wolcott, J., & Erickson, S. (Eds.). (2004). *Patient safety: Achieving a new standard for care.* Washington, DC: National Academy of Sciences.

Bennis, W., & Nanus, B. (1997). *Leadership: The strategies for taking charge* (2nd ed.). New York, NY: Harper & Row.

Buerhaus, P., Donelan, K., DesRoches, C., & Hess, R. (2009). Still making progress to improve the hospital workplace environment. Results from the 2008 National Survey of Registered Nurses. *Nursing Economic$, 27*(5), 289–301.

Capra, F. (2002). *The hidden connections.* New York, NY: Doubleday.

Covey, S. (2004). *The 8th habit: From effectiveness to greatness.* New York, NY: Free Press.

Crowell, D. M. (2011). *Complexity leadership: Nursing's role in health care delivery.* Philadelphia, PA: F. A. Davis.

Eadie, D. (2009). *Extraordinary board leadership: The keys to high-impact governing* (2nd ed.). Sudbury, MA: Jones & Bartlett.

Erikson, E. (1963). *Childhood and society* (2nd ed.). New York, NY: W. W. Norton.

Fawcett, J. (1995). *Analysis and evaluation of conceptual models of nursing* (3rd ed.). Philadelphia, PA: F. A. Davis.

Grossman, S. (2007) Assisting critical care nurses in acquiring leadership skills: Development of a leadership & management competency checklist. *Dimensions of Critical Care Nursing, 26*(2), 57–65.

Hassmiller, S. (2010). Editorial. An "action-oriented blueprint" for the future of nursing. *American Journal of Nursing, 110*(12), 7.

Institute for Healthcare Improvement. (2007). *100K lives campaign.* Retrieved from http://www.ihi.org/IHI/Programs/Campaign

Institute of Medicine. (2001). *Crossing the quality chasm: New health system for the 21st century.* Washington, DC: National Academies Press.

Institute of Medicine. (2002). *Unequal treatment: Confronting racial and ethnic disparities in healthcare.* Washington, DC: National Academies Press.

Institute of Medicine. (2010). The future of nursing: Leading change, advancing health. Retrieved from http://www.iom.edu/Reports/2010/The-Future-of-Nursing-Leading-Change-Advancing-Health/Report-Release.aspx

Kouzes, J., & Posner, B. (2007). *The leadership challenge* (4th ed.). San Francisco, CA: Jossey-Bass.

Malloch, K., & Porter-O'Grady, T. (2009). *The quantum leader: Applications for the new world of work* (2nd ed.). Sudbury, MA: Jones & Bartlett.

Manfredi, C., & Valiga, T. (1990). How are we preparing nurse leaders? A study of baccalaureate curriculum. *Journal of Nursing Education, 29*(1), 4–9.

McBride, A. B. (2010). *The growth and development of nurse leaders.* New York, NY: Springer.

McDaniel, R., & Driebe, D. (Eds.). (2005). *Uncertainty and surprise in complex systems.* New York, NY: Springer.

Needleman, J., Buerhaus, P., Stewart, M., Zelevinsky, K., & Matke, S. (2006). Is there a business case for quality? *Health Affairs, 25*(1), 204–211.

Needleman, J., Kurtzman, E. T. & Kizer, K. W. (2007). Performance measurement of nursing care: State of the science and the current consensus. *Medical Care Research Reviews, 64,* 10S–43S.

Perry, W. (1970). *Forms of intellectual and ethical development in the college years: A scheme.* New York, NY: Holt, Rinehart, & Winston.

Porter-O'Grady, T., & Malloch, K. (2011). *Quantum leadership: Advancing innovation, transforming health care* (3rd ed.). Sudbury, MA: Jones & Bartlett.

Quality and safety education for nurses. (2010). Project overview. Retrieved from http://www.qsen.org/overview.php.

Sorensen R., Iedema R., Severinsson E. (2008). Beyond profession: Nursing leadership in contemporary healthcare. *Journal of Nursing Management, 16*(5), 535–544.

The Joint Commission. (2008). Hospitals, language, and culture. Retrieved January 15, 2011, from http://www.jointcommission.org/PatientSafety/HLC/HLC_Develop_Culturally Competent_Pt_Centered_Stds.htm

West, B. (2006). *Where medicine went wrong: Rediscovering the path to complexity.* Hackensack, NJ: World Scientific Publishing.

Wheatley, M. (2005). *Finding our way: Leadership for an uncertain time.* San Francisco: Berrett-Koehler Publishers.

Wheatley, M. (2006). *Leadership and the new science: Discovering order in a chaotic world* (3rd ed.). San Francisco: Berrett-Koehler Publishers.

CHAPTER 3

Followership and Empowerment

LEARNING OBJECTIVES

- Examine the differences and similarities between leaders and followers.
- Articulate the interdependence between leaders and followers.
- Describe sources of power.
- Examine how power can be used to empower oneself and others.
- Formulate strategies to develop oneself as an effective follower.

INTRODUCTION

With the kind of organizational environments described in this book, it is clear that leaders will need to work collaboratively with followers if any group or organization is to succeed. Indeed, "any organization is a triad consisting of leaders and followers joined in a common purpose. . . . Followers and leaders orbit around the purpose; followers do not orbit around the leader" (Chaleff, 2009, p. 11) (Fig. 3–1). Despite this need for collaboration, however, we know very little about followers and followership even though we are coming to know more and more about leaders and leadership.

> In today's socio-technical organizations, the culture is collective ("team"), the expectation is involvement and investment, and the style of implementation is facilitative and integrative —Porter-O'Grady, 1993, p.53

Old Conceptualization of Leader-Follower Interactions

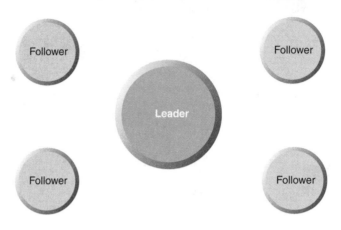

Contemporary Conceptualizations of Leader-Follower Interactions

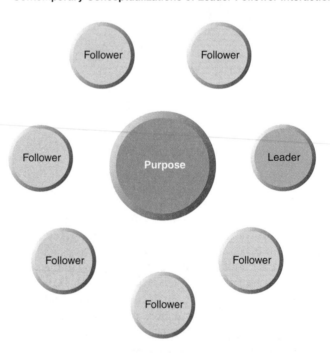

FIGURE 3-1 • Old and contemporary conceptualizations of leader-follower interactions.

Leadership and followership are two separate concepts, two separate roles that are complementary or reciprocal, not competitive (Barwick, 2007; Yukl, 2010). They are synergistic, "a dialectic . . . depend[ing] on each other for existence and meaning" (Kelley, 1992, p. 45). In other words, just as "up" has little meaning were it not for "down," the word "leader" has little meaning without the word "follower," and vice versa. In fact, *"there can be no leaders without followers"* (Goffee & Jones, 2006, p. 127), *and there can be no followers without leaders.*

No one person can know the best strategy, have the clearest vision, or identify the most effective approaches to solve problems. Additionally, "all leaders have weaknesses as well as strengths" (Yukl, 2010, p. 140), and "none of us is as smart as all of us" (Bennis, 2006, p. 136). Thus, "all participants [need to be] recognized as full partners in the organizational venture . . . [and they need to be] co-leaders in the enterprise" (Sullivan, 1998, p. 469).

As a duality relationship, leaders must understand that people seek, admire, respect, and follow those who let them know they are important and significant, who create a sense of community, and who create environments that produce a "buzzing feeling" (Goffee & Jones, 2006, p. 128), characterized by excitement, challenge, and a sense of engagement, where people feel they are part of something larger or more important than themselves. Organizations of today and the future need "a new, more democratic vision [that] . . . creates dynamic partnerships, combining the best of what we are collectively while empowering us as individuals" (Dreher, 1996, p. xiii), particularly because the "freedom to uncover new ideas and create an environment that encourages followers to share their best thinking with their leaders is essential to innovation and change" (Potter & Rosenbach, 2006, p. 143).

The leadership expert, Warren Bennis, once noted that the longer he studied effective leaders, the more he was convinced of the underappreciated importance of effective followers. He also claims that "in our society leadership is too often seen as an inherently individual phenomenon" (Bennis, 2006, p. 130) but acknowledges that "no change can occur without willing and committed followers" (p. 133). Thus, both leaders and followers are increasingly important (Fig. 3–2).

> *The secret of leadership is . . . the ability to inspire others with faith in their own high potential.*
> —J. Donald Walters

As many have noted, *leaders can be leaders only if they have followers.* Indeed, one might say that what defines leaders is that others embrace their vision and want to see it realized. Despite these assertions, however, the concept of followership is rarely addressed to the same extent as the concept of leadership.

Although "the investment in leadership education and development [primarily in the corporate world] was said to approximate some $50 billion" just a few years ago, "the concept of followership languished" (Kellerman, 2008, p. xvii). No conferences

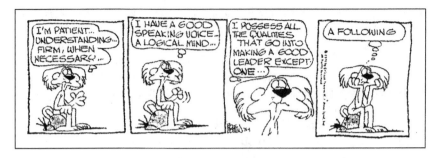

FIGURE 3-2 · Leaders need followers.

are held about followership. Individuals do not seek consultation on how to be an effective follower. There is little, if any, content in educational programs on effective followership, and little has been written on the concept. Why does such a significant role receive so little attention? Does our emphasis on leadership "compensate for something in our culture or our organizations that fills us with an exaggerated need to promote leadership and to silence whatever haunts us about the notion of followership?" (Berg, 1998, p. 28).

> *The final test of a leader is that he leaves behind him in other men the conviction and the will to carry on.* —*Walter Lippman*

Few would argue that followership is a neglected topic. Although some general books on leadership (e.g., Yukl, 2010) devote serious discussion of the concept of followership, a review of recent textbooks on nursing leadership and management (Anderson, 1999; Finkelman, 2011; Sullivan & Decker, 2008; Yoder-Wise, 2010) revealed no mention of the concept in two of the books and one brief chapter on "leading, managing, following" in each of the other two. It is worth noting, however, that chapters such as these were not included at all in nursing books published in earlier years, so perhaps the field is beginning to give recognition to the concept. Interestingly, in a seminal book titled *Strategies for the Future of Nursing* (O'Neil & Coffman, 1998), little mention is made of leadership and none of followership.

In one nursing leadership and management book, the word "follower" was used only as an example of a role someone in a group often takes to build and maintain the group. Follower was defined as "a group member who accepts the other group members' ideas and listens to their discussion and decisions" (Swansburg & Swansburg, 1999, p. 402). In this same book, the authors wrote about the mutual influence of leaders and those they lead; however, the authors chose to use the word "constituent" instead of "follower." Although they did not provide the reader with a reason for the choice of words, one might assume it has something to do with the negative connotations the word "follower" often carries.

> *In today's flatter, leaner environment, organizations and leaders cannot succeed without committed, contributing followers* —Kelley, 1992, p. 200

In her review of her own path to leadership as the president of the American Nurses Association, Dr. Lucille Joel (1999) said she was an "extraordinary follower . . . [who] learned the rules well and followed them exactly . . . [who was] too intimidated to question authority . . . [and who] lacked confidence" (p. 17). Joel concluded that she was, in essence, invisible.

One might conclude from these brief examples that there is something about the word "follower" or the notion of followership that is negative, demeaning, and unattractive. In reality, however, the follower role is a powerful one because it is the follower who truly makes the leader-follower relationship work. In fact, "as the result of changes now converging, followers are more important than ever before" (Kellerman, 2008, p. xxi).

THE CONCEPT OF FOLLOWERSHIP

Being a "good" follower takes special talents, just as being a "good" leader does. Indeed, the qualities of leaders and followers (e.g., being willing to take risks and challenge the status quo and being passionate about a goal) are very similar. Thus, conscious attention must be given to the development of followers, and followership must be cultivated . . . just as leadership development and the cultivation of leadership are important. If we fail to remember that followership is voluntary, fail to convey the importance of followership, and fail to cultivate effective followers, leaders will be left without the support needed to realize visions, make change, and create a preferred future. In essence, when the cry goes out to "follow the leader," few will know who to follow or how to follow, and little will be accomplished. Worse yet, the masses will not be prepared to identify the worthy leader and may follow the person with the loudest voice or the most charisma, as was the case with the Hitler Youth; the Jim Jones Guyana community; and the Waco, Texas commune. Indeed, Kellerman (2008, p. 14) notes, "It took genocide to get scholars systematically to consider this question: Why do followers follow their leaders?" She noted that as scholars studied the Nazi regime, it became "glaringly apparent perhaps for the first time that those who obey orders play as important a role in human affairs as those who issue them" (p. 15).

Being willing to follow is not about blindly accepting some leader's authority, or about abdicating all responsibility for progress, waiting passively for answers to be provided by the leader, or about sitting back and hoping to enjoy the ride. Effective followers are much more active and involved than this.

Followership is an art—a skill that can be learned, cultivated, and consciously developed and exercised. Followers need to be "self-directing, actively participating, practicing experts [who work] on behalf of the organization and the mutually agreed upon vision and goals" (Sullivan, 1998, p. 469). They need to trust others and be trustworthy themselves. They need to see themselves as a community, think and act as a team, and invest energy in team building by focusing on the common goal and drawing on the strengths and talents of each member of the team. Followers need to know their own strengths and what their unique contributions to the effort can be. They must complement each other's and the leader's specialties, strengths, and areas of expertise. They need to seek information so that they have the "bigger picture," which allows them to participate fully and provide significant feedback.

Followers should not invest their energy merely in their own or others' individual or personal agendas. They also should not ally themselves with group members whose goals are out of alignment with those of the rest of the team. They need to be counted on to "provide input that focuses on finding solutions, not just on articulating problems" (Sullivan, 1998, p. 478). They are expected to support the leader by asking questions, giving thoughtful feedback, working to achieve group goals, and providing encouragement when the leader takes a risk on behalf of the group. Leaders, in return, are expected to support followers by seeking their input, using their talents fully, and encouraging them to grow continually. Leaders and followers must "fuse to move together toward a common goal" (Joel, 1999, p. 30) because they are "inextricably enmeshed, each defined by and dependent on the other" (Kellerman, 2008, p. 9). Indeed, "better followers beget better leaders" (Kellerman, 2008, p. xxii).

> *The secret of leadership is . . . never to ask of others what you would not willingly do yourself.* —J. Donald Walters

Followership also involves knowing when and how to assume the role of leader when necessary. "The organization is essentially a community of many leaders and many followers, frequently changing places depending on the particular activity that is occurring" (Sullivan, 1998, p. 477). "We all have the capacity to become either leaders or followers and both are necessary. There are no leaders without followers, and no matter how high you climb the leadership ladder, there is always the requirement to follow some of the time . . . These roles are not in competition, but rather natural compliments [*sic*] to one another's success" (Joel, 1999, p. 29).

It has been asserted that followers, simply by being in the presence of a leader and feeling how that individual does what she or he does, will take on the necessary abilities to move toward realization of the vision (Goldsmith, 2007). Thus, leaders need to step aside and allow followers to take the lead in the group when their abilities, passions, and perspectives are more appropriate to the situation (Salacuse, 2005).

A follower is an individual who takes another as a role model and who acts in accordance with, imitates, supports, and advocates the ideas and opinions of another (Brown, 1980). In fact, the author of a recent article focusing on success in business (Shenkar, 2010) asserts that imitation is valuable, difficult, and "requires intelligence and imagination" (p. 28). Although Shenkar is talking about imitating the products and ideas of another company to advance one's own business, the idea can be extended to the concept of followership. He notes that, like followership, "imitation [often] is done in the dark without the strategic and operational attention it deserves" (p. 29) perhaps because "we've been socialized from a young age to treat imitation as undignified and objectionable" (p. 29). Is this not similar to how we are socialized to think of follower-ship as a passive role, a role we rarely discuss? Yet a follower who imitates an effective leader can become more effective in the former role and evolve into the latter role.

> *Followership is a discipline of supporting leaders and helping them to lead well. It is not submission, but the wise and good care of leaders, done out of a sense of gratitude for their willingness to take on the responsibilities of leadership, and a sense of hope and faith in their abilities and potential.* —Reverend Paul Beedle

Without both leaders and followers, "there can be no unity, no successful goal-directed activity, and no true . . . achievement" (Brown, 1980, p. 357). But "taking another as a role model," "imitating," and "acting in accordance with another" do not mean that followers are passive, unthinking individuals who have no ideas of their own. On the contrary, "supporting and advocating the ideas and opinions of another" demand that the follower think critically about those ideas and opinions, have the skills to advocate for those ideas, and take an active role in providing support to the leader as the ideas are fully developed and advanced. The following case study illustrates the powerful role followers play.

TYPES OF FOLLOWERS

Despite the vital role that followers actually play in effecting change and realizing visions, many still see the role as passive, dependent, unthinking, and lacking in status. Such negative perceptions of followers and followership are common, but they suggest that there is only one type of follower. Kelley (1992, 1998), on the other hand, suggests

Case Study

Helen is a staff RN in a long-term care facility that's resident population averages 80 years of age. She has read research showing that increased family involvement in the care of elderly people helps decrease their confusion and increase their participation in self-care activities. For the past month, Helen has provided leadership among her colleagues to find more ways to increase family involvement, and positive results are being observed. Although Helen feels encouraged by those outcomes and takes pride in knowing they are the result of her vision and leadership efforts, she is disappointed that only a few residents are benefiting. Knowing that more residents could benefit from the intervention, Helen encourages other staff to brainstorm about how to increase the involvement of more families. Several CNAs who have worked closely with the residents over time offer perspectives that Helen had not considered and suggest changes in the ideas Helen had proposed initially. Colleagues in dietary, physical therapy, and social services support these new ideas and add to them. Helen appreciates the value of these suggestions from those whom had been following her lead, and together, the team designs a "menu" of ways in which actual or surrogate family members can participate more actively in the care of all residents on the unit.

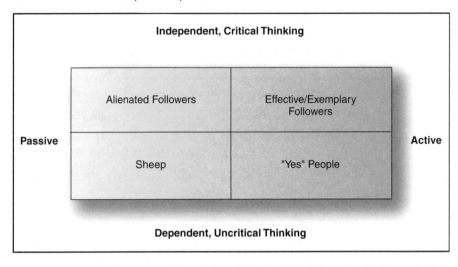

Independent, Critical Thinking

Alienated Followers	Effective/Exemplary Followers
Sheep	"Yes" People

Passive   **Active**

Dependent, Uncritical Thinking

FIGURE 3-3 · Types of followers. (Adapted from Kelley, R.E. [1998]. In praise of followers. In W. E. Rosenbach & R. L. Taylor [Eds.], *Contemporary issues in leadership* [4th ed., p. 98]. Boulder, CO: Westview Press; and Kelley, R. [1992]. *The power of followership: How to create leaders people want to follow and followers who lead themselves* [p. 97]. New York, NY: Doubleday Currency.)

that there are several types of followers, ranging from those who are vital to the success of the group or organization to those who are passive and unthinking. Using an active/passive dimension and one of dependence/independence (Fig. 3–3), Kelley defines four types of followers:

- *Effective or exemplary followers:* These individuals function independently, think critically about ideas that are proposed or directions that are suggested, and are actively involved. They challenge the ideas of the leader, suggest alternative courses of action, and invest time and energy to arrive at the best possible solution for the group.
- *Alienated followers:* These individuals think critically about what the leader or other members of the group are suggesting, but they remain passive and perhaps even somewhat hostile. They may complain about "the way things are being done," are unhappy, and seem disengaged at times. Alienated followers rarely invest time or energy to suggest alternative solutions or other approaches.
- *Yes people:* These are the conformists who are actively involved in the work of the group and enthusiastically support the leader. They are eager to take orders, defer to the leader, yield to the leader's views and opinions, and please the leader. They enjoy a great deal of structure, order, and predictability. "Yes" people are uncomfortable with having to make and live with decisions, and they find freedom almost terrifying. They do not initiate ideas, think for themselves, raise questions, critique the ideas of others, or challenge the group.

- ***Sheep:*** These are the passive individuals who are dependent and uncritical, going along with whatever the leader tells them to do. They are easily led and manipulated, lack initiative, require a great deal of direction, and never go beyond their given assignment. "Sheep" are not particularly committed to the goals of the group and do not invest themselves to any great extent to see that the group continues to move forward.

Types of followers, or followership styles, have also been described by Pittman, Rosenbach, and Potter (1998), who used the dimensions of "performance initiative" and "relationship initiative" to define four followership styles (Fig. 3–4).

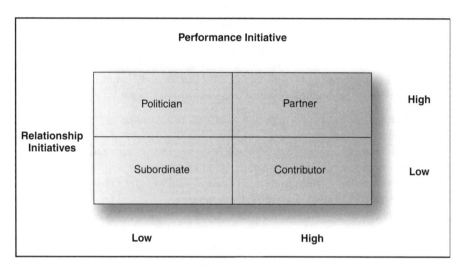

FIGURE 3-4 • Followership styles. (Copyright © 2006 William E. Rosenbach, Robert L. Taylor. Reprinted by permission of Westview Press, a member of the Perseus Books Group.)

Performance initiatives relate to the follower's performance—how his or her assigned job gets done, how good the person is at what he or she does, the standards the person sets for himself or herself, how well the person works with others, and how valuable the person is to the organization. *Relationship initiatives* concern the follower's relationship to the leader—how much the person understands the leader's perspective, the person's willingness to give negative feedback or disagree with the leader, and how the person demonstrates his or her reliability and trustworthiness. Each of the four followership styles reflects extensive or limited activity in these dimensions:

- ***Partner:*** This follower is committed to high performance and building a positive, reciprocal relationship with the leader. The partner may be thought of as a "leader-in-waiting" (Pittman, Rosenbach, & Potter, 1998, p. 118).
- ***Contributor:*** This person does the job very well, is effective with coworkers, embraces change, and successfully balances work and other aspects of life. The contributor does not, however, try to understand the leader's

perspective or promote the leader's vision, nor does he or she negotiate differences maturely, communicate courageously, share her or his expertise and knowledge, or take initiative.

- *Politician:* This individual is highly sensitive to and skilled with inter-personal relationships. The person is willing to give honest feedback and supports the leader; however, he or she may neglect the job and have poor performance levels.
- *Subordinate:* This type of follower may be competent at assigned tasks and do what he or she is told, but there is no commitment to excellence in his or her performance. In addition, the subordinate is not particu-larly sensitive to relationships, does not make an effort to support the leader, is disaffected, and is not interested in giving anything extra.

In a more recent analysis, Kellerman (2008) outlined a typology of followers based solely on one metric: level of engagement. She outlined a continuum that ranges from "feeling and doing absolutely nothing to being passionately committed and deeply involved" (p. 85). The descriptors used along that continuum are as follows:

- *Isolates* . . . completely detached, alienated, uninterested, uninformed, and do nothing.
- *Bystanders* . . . aware, but deliberately disengaged, choosing to stand by and watch, rather than stepping up and participating.
- *Participants* . . . invest some time, energy, or talent to try to have an impact, but do not "go overboard" in doing so.
- *Activists* . . . eager, energetic, and engaged, working hard on behalf of leaders (or to undermine them).
- *Diehards* . . . deeply devoted to the leader (or ready to remove them) and prepared to do anything for the cause.

Regardless of the model used to think about types of followers, each type often can be identified by the behaviors exhibited (Potter & Rosenbach, 2006). Consider the follower's active efforts to do a good job, including actual performance, effectiveness in working with others, serving as a resource for others, and the extent to which change is embraced. One also can examine the follower's working relationship with the leader, including the extent to which one identifies with the leader, active attempts to strengthen the relationship, efforts to build and sustain trust, the ability to negotiate differences, and the willingness to engage in "courageous conversations" (Potter & Rosenbach, 2006, p. 152) during which the follower is honest, may disagree with the leader, and takes risks.

An excellent example of effective followers was presented by Chade-Meng Tan (2010), an engineer at Google. Tan describes several initiatives undertaken by Google employees that were aligned with the corporation's mission and helped solve problems in local and global communities. He describes Google as a compassionate company that creates an inspiring workforce. Employees mutually inspire each other toward greater good, which creates a vibrant, energetic community in which people admire and respect each other. Surely such employees—followers?—are not passive or alienated. They are inspired, engaged, and effective. They take the initiative to do something, others join in, and the project often gains enough support to become official. New initiatives at Google, according to Tan, almost always starts from the bottom up. Such is the power of followers.

Blindly following some leader without question or taking a passive role in one's work setting, community, or professional organization will do little to advance the profession, promote individual growth, and achieve quality patient care. What nursing needs as we participate in and, indeed, work to shape today's health-care arena are effective or exemplary followers, partners, or activists. We need people who can support even small changes in practice that then become the new norm, a process referred to as the "normalization of deviation" (Kohn, Corrigan, & Donaldson, 2000, p. 55).

Nursing needs followers who have characteristics that are similar to those of leaders: a willingness to serve, assertiveness, determination, a willingness to challenge ideas, courage, an ability to act as a change agent, and an openness to new ideas and perspectives. Indeed, followers and leaders must complement each other (Corona, 1986), as noted in Table 3–1, and leading effective followers can, in essence, be thought of as "getting leaders to follow" (Clarke, 2005, p. 46). Leading people who are "very talented, very independent, and over whom [the leader does not] have that much authority" (Clarke, 2005, p. 47) is a challenge like that of "herding cats," as is the title of her article, but it is not hard to imagine how far a group or organization can go toward realizing the vision when the followers are like leaders. This may be particularly relevant for nursing because "many people in complex hierarchical organizations are both leaders and followers" (Keohane, 2010, p. 51).

The interrelation between leaders and followers—and the similar characteristics of individuals who are effective in each role—led James McGregor Burns (2004) to pose what he called "the Burns paradox:" If leadership and followership are so intertwined and fluid, how do we distinguish conceptually between leaders and followers?" (p. 171).

TABLE 3-1 Traits of Leaders and Followers

LEADERS	FOLLOWERS
Study and create new ideas	Test new ideas
Make decisions	Challenge decisions as needed
Assign appropriate responsibilities	Know when to accept responsibility and do so
Create environments of trust, resulting in freedom	Use freedom responsibly
Take risks	Risk following
Are reliable	Are trustworthy and respectful
Are loyal to the followers	Are loyal to the leader
Are self-confident	Know themselves
Assume the leadership position	Follow when appropriate

Perhaps we would do well to accept the similarities, give more credence to the significance of the follower role, and focus less on trying to make such distinctions and more on developing effective or exemplary followers.

CHARACTERISTICS OF EFFECTIVE OR EXEMPLARY FOLLOWERS

Although the term "follower" often "conjures up images of docility, conformity, weakness, and failure to excel" (Chaleff, 2009, p. 3), effective or exemplary followers possess many of the same characteristics as individuals who exercise leadership. Each of us may do well to reflect on the extent to which we are characterized by the following:

- Strength and independence
- Critical thinking
- Ability and willingness to think for ourselves
- Ability to give honest feedback and constructive criticism, particularly in a timely fashion
- Willingness to be our own person
- Innovativeness and creativity
- Active engagement in all we do
- Cooperativeness and collaborativeness
- Being a self-starter
- "Going above and beyond the call of duty"—beyond our job assignments
- Willingness to assume ownership
- Taking initiative
- Positive sense of self-worth
- "Can do" aura (Kelley, 1992, p. 143)
- Attentiveness to what is happening around us
- "Holding up our end of the bargain"
- Being energized by our work and organizations

Through his work with workshop participants, Berg (1998) identified additional characteristics of exemplary followers. He described these individuals as "interesting characters" (p. 40) who were bold and colorful—not passive or bland—loyal, and supportive. They possessed their own distinctive voices that leaders typically heeded well. Exemplary followers openly expressed their own ideas, concerns, perspectives, and even conflicting views; and effective leaders paid attention to these voices. A nurse who proposes to the nurse manager and colleagues how family members can be more involved in planning and, indeed, coordinating or directing the care of patients with serious illnesses—when that is not the norm on the unit—is being bold, not passive, and expressing conflicting views. The colleagues who take this suggestion seriously and consider changing the practice standards on the unit are enriched by this nurse's proposal, and the ultimate goal toward which they are all working—quality patient and family care—is more likely to be realized.

> *Followers are more important to leaders than leaders are to followers." —Barbara Kellerman*

Berg (1998) also found that an emotional connection exists between leaders and exemplary followers, a relation he suggested may be needed so that each can reassure the other "during those times when each must show his or her limits and weaknesses to the other" (p. 41). For example, the nurse manager who has been unsuccessful in securing additional staff positions so that nurses can attend valuable in-service programs and participate in grand rounds needs to be able to express that frustration. Likewise, staff need to be able to acknowledge when they do not have the knowledge or skill to care for a particular patient. Showing one's limitations and weaknesses requires a mutual trust, a bond, and an emotional connection between the leader and the followers.

Effective followers stimulate and inspire leaders, challenge their creativity, collaborate with them, complement them, give them feedback, and support them. Leaders may inspire vision, but it is the followers who supply much of the energy to achieve that vision. Indeed, followership is "the important phenomenon to study if we are to understand why organizations succeed or fail" (Kelley, 1992, p. 5).

Followers assume such an active role, however, only when they get what they expect from leaders, and what they expect is credibility (Kouzes & Posner, 2011). Followers want leaders who are *honest*—individuals who are consistent, ethical, and principled. They want leaders who are *competent*—who know their field of endeavor and know the work that needs to be done. They want leaders who are *inspiring*—individuals who are enthusiastic, contagious, visionary, and effective in communicating a dream. And, they want leaders who are *forward looking*—oriented toward the "big picture" and able to help followers see their important place in that picture. We might think of these factors in terms of a formula for successful leadership and effective leader-follower relations:

Honesty + Competence + Inspiration + Vision = Credibility

Leaders and followers are interdependent. Theirs is a reciprocal relationship, and they reinforce each other. Indeed, the qualities of leaders and followers are so closely aligned that one could assume that the same people who are seen by their peers as desirable leaders would also be seen as desirable followers. Individuals often move back and forth between leader and follower roles, depending on the situation. They draw on the same skills to be effective in either role. Both have power, but where does that power come from, and how do leaders and followers use it to empower themselves and others?

SOURCES OF POWER

Leadership has sometimes been referred to as a power relationship, and Bass (2008) asserted that one cannot lead without power. Thus, part of the leadership process is the ability to use power, not control, to influence the direction of the group and realization of the vision.

Power wins, not by being used, but by being there. —Anonymous

Often, we think of power negatively, conjuring up images of exploitation and manipulation. Those in authority may abuse the power of their positions when allowing personal feelings for or against a staff member, for example, to influence staffing assignments, performance evaluations, or the awarding of "perks" or benefits (e.g., time off to attend a conference, serving as a preceptor). Power, however, does not derive only from one's position of authority.

In 1960, French and Raven published a seminal work in which they identified five sources of power:

> **Legitimate power** comes from one's title or position, or role in a family or culture.
> **Coercive power** comes from the ability to penalize others. For example, in his discourses on freedom in the first century A.D., Epictetus said, "No one is afraid of Caesar himself, but he is afraid of death, loss of property, prison, [and] disengagement."
> **Reward power** comes from the ability to help and get things (e.g., money, praise) for others.
> **Expert power** comes from one's knowledge or competence.
> **Referent power** comes from followers' respect for and their desire to be liked and admired by the leader. As Reed (2004) notes, "There is inherently more power and leverage in serving your [followers] versus them attempting to simply serve you."

> *Power and influence can be wielded with grace and authority, even when results must be delivered without fail.* —Nancy Austin

In addition to these sources of power, one gains power by having information that she or he can control; from the people one knows and can call on; and from a strong sense of self, knowing one's values, being self-confident, being able and willing to take risks, and standing up for that in which one believes. To increase one's power base, leaders and effective followers alike would do well to know themselves, develop a strong self-concept, develop and use good communication skills, establish support groups and networks, develop and show their expertise (i.e., market themselves), be willing to take risks, build coalitions, eliminate unnecessary dependence, understand "the system" and how it works, and be politically astute and active. Perhaps completing a tool like the "Power Perception Profile," developed by Hersey and Natemeyer (n.d.) (http://www.ncsu.edu/csleps/leadership/eac301_word_documents/POWER_PERCEPTION_ PROFILE.doc), may help leaders and followers appreciate their sources of power and how effectively they use power.

Another perspective on power has been proposed by a leader in nursing, Rosemarie Rizzo Parse (2009). Her humanbecoming leading-following model emphasizes that although power may lie in one's position, it is the power that lies within the person that is more effective. She quotes her own earlier work to explain that "power with person is the force emanating from the core of a person who commands the respect of others without the authority or responsibility of a position" (p. 369), thus allowing for both "leaders" and "followers" to have power in various situations.

In a very thoughtful book entitled, *The Power Tactics of Jesus Christ*, Haley (1989) summarizes what he believes were the strategies Jesus used to realize his vision: He spoke whenever and wherever an audience would listen. He said what was unorthodox. He spoke openly about existing problems or injustices, consistently, publicly, and cleverly. He chose others to join in the "movement." He did not ask more of others than He was willing to give Himself. He articulated long-range plans. He used a flexible strategy, and He put His hope in the young, those who had not yet become entrenched in established ways. Through strategies such as these, Haley claimed, Jesus Christ came to be a powerful force for change.

> *The world is moved not only by the mighty shoves of heroes, but also by the aggregate of the tiny pushes of each honest worker.—Helen Keller*

Nurses, too, can be powerful forces for change in complex health-care settings. That power comes from their knowledge, the intimate and substantive relationships they develop with patients and families, the holistic perspective they bring to care, and their sheer numbers. Such power is retained by keeping current with best practices, involving the patient and family as part of the health-care team, serving as an advocate for patients and for quality care, not allowing oneself to become too narrowly focused or specialized, and collaborating with nursing and other health-team colleagues to promote excellence in care. Nurses strengthen their power base by speaking up in a knowledgeable, informed manner, calling on networks of colleagues who have the expertise that may be needed in a particular situation, and constantly learning.

EMPOWERING SELF AND OTHERS

As noted earlier, leaders engage in several tasks (Gardner, 1989) that help define them as leaders. Among those tasks are several that, in reality, can be thought of as means to empower oneself and one's followers. By *affirming values*, leaders help followers reflect on and perhaps challenge their values and the values of others. This helps followers become more powerful, as they come to know clearly what it is they believe and are willing to invest in. By *motivating followers*, leaders unlock or channel motives, promote positive attitudes, and encourage creativity, all of which empower followers to believe in themselves and take action. By striving to a*chieve a workable unity*, leaders establish trust, cohesion, and mutual tolerance, circumstances that empower followers to focus on the "big picture" and move out of their own "little corner of the world." *Explaining* helps followers understand the vision, why they are being asked to do certain things, and how they can and do contribute to achieving the group's goals. Followers are thereby empowered by information and understanding. By *serving as a* *symbol,* a risk taker who acts as the group's source of unity, voice of anger, collective identity, and source of hope, the leader helps followers seize the power that comes from debate, honest expression of feelings, and sharing in a struggle with others. Finally, through the process of *renewing,* both leaders and followers are empowered to break routines, habits, fixed attitudes, perceptions, assumptions, and unwritten rules, thereby allowing them to grow.

> *Each time a man stands up for an idea, or acts to improve the lot of others, or strikes out against injustice, he sends forth a tiny ripple of hope, and crossing each other from a million different centers of energy and daring, those ripples build a current that can sweep down the mightiest walls of oppression and resistance. Few are willing to brave the disapproval of their fellows, the censure of their colleagues, the wrath of their society. Moral courage is a rarer commodity than bravery in battle or greater intelligence. Yet it is the one essential, vital quality for those who seek to change a world that yields most painfully to change.* —Robert Kennedy

When leaders empower followers—and when followers feel empowered—many benefits emerge. Citing the research of scholars in the field, Yukl (2010, p. 114) outlines the following potential benefits from empowerment: "(1) stronger task commitment, (2) greater initiative in carrying out role responsibilities, (3) greater persistence in the face of obstacles and temporary setbacks, (4) more innovation and learning, and stronger optimism about the eventual success of the work, (5) higher job satisfaction, (6) stronger organizational commitment, and (7) less turnover." With benefits such as these, leaders would be wise to engage followers so that they are empowered, and followers would be wise to function effectively so that they feel and act in a powerful way.

Gladwell (2000) notes that "there are exceptional people out there who are capable of starting epidemics" (p. 132). These are the "tempered radicals" (Meyerson, 2001) who "want to rock the boat, and [at the same time] stay in it" (p. xi). What underlies successful epidemics or revolutions "is a bedrock belief that change is possible [and] that people can radically transform their behavior or beliefs" (Gladwell, 2000, p. 258). Followers can be helped to believe that change is possible, transform their behavior or beliefs, and start epidemics or revolutions, if leaders use the power they have to continually move the group toward the vision and to empower followers. Empowered followers do not materialize simply because a leader has acted to empower them. They can and do engage in activities that will enhance their followership skills.

DEVELOPING EFFECTIVE FOLLOWERSHIP SKILLS

Although there are many opportunities to assume the role of leader, each of us also will have countless opportunities to function as a follower. We need to consciously develop the skills of followership and cultivate and appreciate that role so that we can draw on those skills to assume the mantle of leadership when it becomes necessary.

In fact, we need to be willing to be the first follower, as pointed out by Sivers (2010) in a short presentation on "How to Start a Movement." Among the points made by Sivers that have relevance for this discussion are the following:

- A leader needs guts to stand out and be ridiculed.
- The first follower is a crucial role, an underestimated form of leadership.
  - He is embraced by the leader as an equal, and it becomes apparent that it is not about the leader but about them and about the movement.
  - He shows others how to follow.
- New followers emulate the follower, not the leader.
- More followers join in, there is a tipping point, and a movement is born.
- As more join in, it is less risky to be a follower, and the movement can take off.
- Leadership is overglorified . . . If you really care about starting a movement, have the courage to follow and show others how to follow as well.

In a commentary on heroes and brave men, Barnum (1987) noted that "sometimes a field, any field, needs a hero or a bunch of heroes, an elite to set its course, to chart new lands, to brave new waters" (p. 5); the hero clears the way and "blazes the trail." Yet the only trails today's leaders can suggest, according to Barnum, "are slippery, fraught with rock slides, and inevitably lead up steep mountain sides" (p. 5), making it difficult for even the best of followers. Despite this challenge, however, in the contemporary world—and even more so in the future—the heroes may have the easier job and the followers the more difficult one.

> *From Gandhi to Mandela, from the American patriot to the Polish shipbuilders, the makers of revolutions have not come from the top.* —Gary Hamel

Barnum asserted that "never before has the action of the masses had such potential to influence the direction of our profession" (1987, p. 5), an assertion that is as true today as it was nearly 25 years ago. It is the nurses practicing at the bedside who demonstrate quality patient care, not the administrator who writes standards of care. It is the nurse working in the community who can influence local legislators with personalized human stories about the pain and suffering associated with polluted environments, lack of food, inadequate shelter, and poor prenatal care, not the statisticians who merely cite numbers and trends without providing a human dimension. The student experiencing the curriculum and the teacher/student relationships can best speak to the quality and effectiveness of the learning environment that exists in a school, not the faculty who design experiences but do not "live" them. In other words, followers have the most significant effect on the future of our profession and the world, an idea supported by Vaclav Havel, the dissident, poet, and ex-president of the Czech Republic who advocated solidarity in Communist Czechoslovakia and asserted and demonstrated that "followers hold significant power, even in totalitarian states, . . . if they act on it" (Kelley, 1992, p. 235).

If it is true that the future of our profession and the world will be most significantly affected by the actions of followers, then each of us needs to develop effective skills of followership. This notion has been expressed by many (Chaleff, 1998, 2009; DiRienzo, 1994; Guidera & Gilmore, 1988; Kelley, 1992, 1998; Litzinger & Schaefer, 1984; Lundy, 1993; Meyerson, 2001; Pittman et al., 1998), but how can we develop such skills? According to Chaleff (1998, p. 89), "follower skills are learned informally, like street fighting," but they are, nevertheless, learned.

In her book on "paths to leadership," Andersen (1999) did not talk about followers or followership, per se. She and the various contributing authors talked about how students can chart a course toward assuming leadership positions in nursing. Inherent in those discussions was an implication that one develops as a leader by being an effective follower, a strategy Kelley (1992) refers to as "apprenticeship." Indeed, Aristotle, Plato, Homer, and Hegel, among others, insisted that mastering followership is a necessary part of becoming an effective leader (Kelley, 1992; Rosenbach & Taylor, 1998).

Thus, nurses who aspire to effective followership and leadership should apprentice themselves as followers by assuming that role, thinking about what it means, reflecting on how they are contributing to their organization and the nursing profession by fulfilling that role, and *being the best they can be*. In addition, such nurses would do well to study and implement many of the strategies that are suggested (later in this text and elsewhere) for developing leaders because the roles of leader and follower are so complementary. Among the strategies to help you be a more effective or exemplary follower are the following, which have been grouped into three major categories:

Know Yourself and Your Organization, and Continue to Grow as a Person and a Professional

- Continue your education, both formal and informal. Knowledge is power and will serve you well as a follower.
- Be committed to something other than your own career development. Find your passion in life and be passionate about what you do.
- Know your organization.
- Know your values and hold on to them.
- Set high standards. Others will model that.
- Seek mentors or accept an offer of mentoring if it is made.
- Develop your professional networks—within and outside your organization —and use them.
- Remain fully accountable for your actions.
- Share information rather than hoard it.

- Help colleagues grow and do their job well. Help them develop the skills of giving needed feedback.
- Be reflective.
- Have a sense of humor and laugh at your own mistakes.
- Develop positive relationships with colleagues, rely on each other, and be responsible to each other. Be a good team player.
- Continue to develop a wide array of skills in communication, assertiveness, clinical practice, decision making, and writing.
- Analyze your performance by asking others for feedback and being honest in your own self-appraisal. Do you engage in gossip? Do you use language that suggests you are not as important as other people, or your ideas and suggestions are not as valuable as theirs? Do you allow yourself to be subservient? Are you cynical? Do you allow the leader or others to show disrespect for your coworkers' ideas or views? Are you willing to take risks? Are you destructive when you offer criticism?
- Give credit where it is due.
- Follow through on your commitments. Be credible.
- Know your job and do it well. Be competent, demonstrate your value to the group, and make a difference to the organization.
- Be enthusiastic and spread that enthusiasm to others.
- Know yourself, and be honest with yourself.
- Be comfortable with uncertainty and ambiguity. Resist the understandable fear of the unknown.
- Seek wise counsel.
- Develop self-confidence. Believe in and have faith in yourself.
- Remain calm. Do not be hostile.
- "Discover or create opportunities to fulfill [your] potential and maximize [your] value to the organization" (Chaleff, 2009, p. 6).
- Develop a record of successes.
- Do deep-breathing or other relaxation exercises before having a conversation with an authority figure.
- Do not give in to peer pressure.
- Ask for feedback.
- Set personal goals and take responsibility to meet them.
- "Learn the ropes," "pay your dues," and prove yourself in the follower role.
- Be dependable and reliable.
- Be creative.

Be Involved and Speak Up
- Be involved in your practice setting. Have a sense of ownership and stewardship; do not be merely a spectator.
- Be involved in professional organizations.
- Feel free to criticize because thoughtful feedback helps a leader make good decisions; but do not just complain and walk away.

- Contribute as an equal partner.
- Figure out the steps needed for the group to achieve its goals, then be sure to be an integral part of those steps rather than on the periphery of "the action."
- Be cooperative with, rather than adversarial to, the leader.
- Appreciate the needs, goals, and constraints placed on the leader.
- Play devil's advocate because effective leaders encourage and benefit from healthy dissent.
- Exercise a "courageous conscience . . . the ability to judge right from wrong and the fortitude to take affirmative steps toward what [you] believe is right" (Kelley, 1992, p. 168).
- Understand the importance of speaking out . . . and do it!
- Speak up so others can benefit from your views. Speak the truth and be willing to "stand up, to stand out, to risk rejection, to initiate conflict" (Chaleff, 2009, p. 7).
- Provide opportunities for the leader to talk about his or her vulnerabilities and concerns, as well as his or her strengths and vision.
- Help sacred cows be "gently led to pasture" (Chaleff, 2009, p. 89) so that all subjects are open to discussion and all options are possible. Do not discard what may seem like wild ideas before considering them carefully.
- Express skepticism about ideas, proposals, and "pronouncements," but do so in a respectful way.

Be Active
- Take initiative. Take action without being told to do so.
- When they impede progress, be willing to "bend, circumvent, or break the rules to get things done" (Chaleff, 2009, p. 47).
- Accept a place at the table where decisions are made, or if such a place is not offered, create such a place for yourself. For example, agree to serve on a committee when invited to do so or volunteer to revise the admission data form if the one currently being used focuses too much on patient weaknesses and limitations and does not adequately address patient strengths and abilities.
- Be proactive. Advocate and be a catalyst for change.
- Independently think up and champion new ideas.
- Try to solve difficult problems rather than expecting the leader to do it all.
- Present your position in a forthright manner. Develop excellence in communication by using a variety of channels.
- Stand up for and support your leader when he or she needs to make difficult decisions.
- Ask a great deal of the leader, but do not expect perfection from him or her.

It is obvious that there are many ways in which you can be an effective or exemplary follower. It also is obvious that it is only with concerted personal effort that you will develop the skills of effective followership. These "keys to effective followership" may be summarized as follows:

- Be a critical thinker, not a "yes" person.
- Be consistent and dependable.
- Be humble and patient.
- Be able to receive and offer constructive criticism.
- Be a tireless worker.
- Be a disciplined student of study and work (theory and practice).
- Be persistent and consistent at developing leadership (and followership) skills.

CONCLUSION

Followers have more power than they may realize. They confer the leadership role, and "the responsibility for making the leader-follower relationship work remains with the 'follower'" (Berg, 1998, p. 33). Indeed, followers can create a "conspiracy" (Bennis, 1989) that, although largely unconscious, can prevent leaders from leading, keeping them from "taking charge and making changes" (p. xii). "We are a nation of followers" (Kelley, 1992, p. 24), where "the spirit of American democracy elevates and celebrates the role of the follower" (p. 24). In such a society, the masses actually create history, and because "healthy followership is a conscious act of free will" (Chaleff, 2009, p.151), the masses allow certain individuals to exert leadership. Leaders, then, are accountable to followers, and followers play a significant role.

All of us are both leaders and followers, and most of us are followers more than we are leaders. That, however, is not anything for which we should apologize or anything about which we should feel badly.

"Thinking leadership without thinking followership is not merely misleading, it is mistaken" (Kellerman, 2008, p. 23). "Leaders cannot function without the eyes and ears and minds and hearts of followers" (DePree, 1992, p. 200), and they "only really accomplish something by permission of the followers" (p. 201). "The mark of a great leader is the development and growth of followers. The mark of a great follower is the growth of leaders" (Chaleff, 2009, p. 27). Therefore, when we find ourselves in the follower role, we should rejoice!

CRITICAL THINKING EXERCISES

What is appealing about being in the follower role? What is unattractive about being in that role?

_____

_____

Review the characteristics of effective followers. How would you describe yourself in the follower role? How effective have you been in that role?

_____

_____

Talk to your nursing colleagues about followership. What are their views on the concept? Was the concept ever addressed in their educational programs? Do they rate themselves as effective followers? How did they develop the abilities to be effective in that role? Whom do they identify as the most effective followers among their work group? What is the basis for that rating? Are these the same individuals they identify as leaders (or potential leaders) among the group?

_____

_____

How do your colleagues' opinions on followership and its development compare with your own views? How are nurses' views similar to or different from those outside health care or those outside a predominantly female field?

_____

_____

Should we focus more on developing effective and exemplary followers in nursing than on developing leaders all around us?

_____

_____

Read Chaleff's (2009, pp. 177–178) "Meditation on Followership." Are these principles by which you could live and that could guide your practice as a follower? This meditation may be something to review regularly as you implement your role as a professional nurse.

_____

_____

CRITICAL THINKING
EXERCISES—cont'd

Meditation on Followership

I am a steward of this group and share responsibility for its success.
I am responsible for adhering to the highest values I can envision.
I am responsible for my successes and failures and for continuing to learn from them.
I am responsible for the attractive and unattractive parts of who I am.
I can empathize with others who are also imperfect.
As an adult, I can relate on a peer basis to other adults who are the group's formal leaders.
I can support leaders and counsel them, and receive support and counsel from them.
Our common purpose is our best guide.
I have the power to help leaders use their power wisely and effectively.
If leaders abuse power, I can help them change their behavior.
If I abuse power, I can learn from others and change my behavior.
If abusive leaders do not change their behavior, I can and will withdraw my support.
By staying true to my values, I can serve others well and fulfill my potential.
Thousands of courageous acts by followers can, one by one, improve the world.
Courage always exists in the present. What can I do today?
—I. Chaleff

Complete the Followership Style Test that follows. What did you learn about yourself by taking this test? What did you learn about followership and the relationship between followers and leaders?

_____

_____

FOLLOWERSHIP STYLE TEST

This questionnaire includes statements about the type of boss you prefer. Imagine yourself to be in a subordinate position of some kind and use your responses to indicate your preference for the way in which a leader might relate with you.

The format includes a five-point scale: "Strongly Agree" (SA), "Agree" (A), "Mixed Feelings" (MF), "Disagree" (D), and "Strongly Disagree" (SD). Select one point on each scale and mark it as you read the 16 statements relating to followership.

	STATEMENT	SA	A	MF	D	SD
1.	I expect my job to be very explicitly outlined for me.	1	2	3	4	5
2.	When the boss says to do something, I do it. After all, he or she is the boss.	1	2	3	4	5
3.	Rigid rules and regulations usually cause me to become frustrated and inefficient.	5	4	3	2	1
4.	I am ultimately responsible for and capable of self-discipline based on my contacts with the people around me.	5	4	3	2	1
5.	My job should be made as short in duration as possible so that I can achieve efficiency through repetition.	1	2	3	4	5
6.	Within reasonable limits, I will try to accommodate requests from persons who are not my boss because these requests are typically in the best interests of the company anyway.	5	4	3	2	1
7.	When the boss tells me to do something that is the wrong thing to do, it is his or her fault, not mine, when I do it.	1	2	3	4	5
8.	It is up to my boss to provide a set of rules by which I can measure my performance.	1	2	3	4	5
9.	The boss is the boss. The fact of the promotion suggests that he or she has something on the ball.	1	2	3	4	5
10.	I accept orders only from my boss.	1	2	3	4	5
11.	I would prefer my boss to give me general objectives and guidelines then allow me to do the job my way.	5	4	3	2	1
12.	If I do something that is not right, it is my own fault, even if my boss told me to do it.	5	4	3	2	1
13.	I prefer jobs that are not repetitious, the kind of task that is new and different each time.	5	4	3	2	1

	STATEMENT	SA	A	MF	D	SD
14.	My boss is in no way superior to me by virtue of positions. He or she does a different kind of job, one that includes a lot of managing and coordinating.	5	4	3	2	1
15.	I expect my boss to give me disciplinary guidelines.	1	2	3	4	5
16.	I prefer to tell my boss what I will, or at least should, be doing. I am ultimately responsible for my own work.	5	4	3	2	1

Scoring

Score your followership style by simply averaging the numbers for your answers to the individual items. For example, if you scored item number one "Strongly Agree," you will find the point value of "1" for that answer. To obtain your overall followership style, add all the numerical values associated with the 16 followership items and divide by 16. The resulting average is your followership style.

SCORE	DESCRIPTION	FOLLOWERSHIP STYLE
Less than 2.0	Very autocratic	Cannot function well without programs and procedures; needs feedback
2.0–2.4	Moderately autocratic	Needs solid structure and feedback but can also carry on independently
2.5–3.4	Mixed	Mixture of above and below
3.5–4.0	Moderately participative	Independent worker; does not need close supervision, just a bit of feedback
More than 4.0	Very democratic	Self-starter, likes a challenge and likes to try new things by himself or herself

Source: Adapted from Douglas, L. M. (1992). The effective nurse leader and manager (4th ed., pp. 25–28). St. Louis: Mosby.

References

Anderson, C. F. (1999). *Nursing student to nursing leader: The critical path to leadership development*. Albany, NY: Delmar.

Barnum, B. (1987). The need for heros [*sic*] and the need for brave men. *Courier (Newsletter of the Teachers College, Columbia University Nursing Education Alumni Association)*, *54*, 5.

Barwick, J. (2007). Following the leader and leading the followers. In J. F. Wergin (Ed.), *Leadership in place: How academic professionals can find their leadership voice* (pp. 88–99). Bolton, MA: Anker Publishing.

Bass, B. M. (2008). *The Bass handbook of leadership: Theory, research, and managerial applications* (4th ed.). New York, NY: Free Press.

Bennis, W. (1989). *Why leaders can't lead: The unconscious conspiracy continues.* San Francisco, CA: Jossey-Bass.

Bennis, W. (2006). The end of leadership: Exemplary leadership is impossible without full inclusion, initiatives, and cooperation of followers. In W. E. Rosenbach & R. L. Taylor (Eds.), *Contemporary issues in leadership* (6th ed., pp. 129–142). Boulder, CO: Westview Press.

Berg, D. N. (1998). Resurrecting the muse: Followership in organizations. In E. B. Klein, F. Gabelnick, & P. Herr (Eds.), *The psychodynamics of leadership* (pp. 27–52). Madison, CT: Psychosocial Press.

Brown, B. (1980). Follow the leader. *Nursing Outlook, 28*(6), 357–359.

Burns, J.M. (2004). *Transforming leadership: A new pursuit of happiness.* New York, NY: Grove Press.

Chaleff, I. (1998). Learn the art of followership. In W. E. Rosenbach & R. L. Taylor (Eds.), *Contemporary issues in leadership* (4th ed., pp. 89–91). Boulder, CO: Westview Press.

Chaleff, I. (2009). *The courageous follower. Standing up to and for our leaders* (3rd ed.). San Francisco, CA: Berrett-Koehler.

Clarke, K. (2005). Herding cats: The art of getting leaders to follow. *Associations Now,* (November), 46–51.

Corona, D. (1986). Followership: The indispensable corollary to leadership. In E. C. Hein & M. J. Nicholson (Eds.), *Contemporary leadership behavior: Selected readings* (2nd ed., pp. 87–91). Boston, MA: Little, Brown.

DePree, M. (1992). *Leadership jazz.* New York, NY: Doubleday Currency.

DiRienzo, S. M. (1994). A challenge to nursing: Promoting followers as well as leaders. *Holistic Nursing Practice, 9*(1), 26–30.

Dreher, D. (1996). *The Tao of personal leadership.* New York, NY: HarperBusiness.

Finkelman, A. (2011). *Leadership and management for nurses* (2nd ed.). Upper Saddle River, NJ: Prentice Hall.

French, J. P., Jr., & Raven, B. (1960). The bases of social power. In D. Cartwright & A. Zander (Eds.), *Group dynamics* (pp. 607–623). New York, NY: Harper and Row.

Gardner, J. W. (1989). The tasks of leadership. In W. E. Rosenbach & R. L. Taylor (Eds.), *Contemporary issues in leadership* (2nd ed., pp. 24–33). Boulder, CO: Westview Press.

Gladwell, M. (2000). *The tipping point: How little things can make a big difference.* Boston, MA: Little, Brown.

Goffee, R., & Jones, G. (2006). Followership: It's personal, too. In W. E. Rosenbach & R. L. Taylor (Eds.), *Contemporary issues in leadership* (6th ed., pp. 127–128). Boulder, CO: Westview Press.

Goldsmith, B. (2007). Finding the great leader within. *Association Executive* (January/February), 24–25.

Guidera, M. K., & Gilmore, C. (1988). In defense of followership. *American Journal of Nursing, 88*(7), 1017.

Haley, J. (1989). *The power tactics of Jesus Christ.* New York, NY: W. W. Norton.

Joel, L. A. (1999). Life review of an ANA President: The path of leadership. In C. A. Andersen (Ed.), *Nursing student to nursing leader: The critical path to leadership development* (pp. 17–32). Albany, NY: Delmar.

Kellerman, B. (2008). *Followership: How followers are creating change and changing leaders.* Boston, MA: Harvard Business Press.

Kelley, R. (1992). *The power of followership: How to create leaders people want to follow and followers who lead themselves.* New York, NY: Doubleday Currency.

Kelley, R. E. (1998). In praise of followers. In W. E. Rosenbach & R. L. Taylor (Eds.), *Contemporary issues in leadership* (4th ed., pp. 96–106). Boulder, CO: Westview Press.

Keohane, N. O. (2010). *Thinking about leadership.* Princeton, NJ: Princeton University Press.

Kohn, L. T., Corrigan, J. M., & Donaldson, M. S. (Eds.). (2000). *To err is human: Building a safer health system.* Washington, DC: National Academy Press.

Kouzes, J. M., & Posner, B. Z. (2011). *Credibility: How leaders gain and lose it, why people demand it* (2nd ed.). San Francisco, CA: Jossey-Bass.

Litzinger, W., & Schaefer, T. (1984). Leadership through followership. In W. E. Rosenbach & R. L. Taylor (Eds.), *Contemporary issues in leadership* (pp. 138–143). Boulder, CO: Westview Press.

Lundy, J. L. (1993). *Lead, follow, or get out of the way: Invaluable insights into leadership styles.* San Diego, CA: Pfeiffer & Co.

Meyerson, D. E. (2001). *Tempered radicals: How people use difference to inspire change at work.* Boston, MA: Harvard Business School Press.

O'Neil, E., & Coffman, J. (Eds.). (1998). *Strategies for the future of nursing: Changing roles, responsibilities, and employment patterns of registered nurses.* San Francisco, CA: Jossey-Bass.

Parse, R. R. (2009). The humanbecoming leading-following model. *Nursing Science Quarterly, 21*(4), 369–375.

Pittman, T. S., Rosenbach, W. E., & Potter, E. H., III. (1998). Followers as partners: Taking the initiative for action. In W. E. Rosenbach & R. L. Taylor (Eds.), *Contemporary issues in leadership* (4th ed., pp. 107–120). Boulder, CO: Westview Press.

Porter-O'Grady, T. (1993). Of mythspinners and mapmakers: 21st century managers. *Nursing Management, 24*(4), 52–55.

Potter, E. H., III, & Rosenbach, W. E. (2006). Followers as partners: The spirit of leadership. In W. E. Rosenbach & R. L. Taylor (Eds.), *Contemporary issues in leadership* (6th ed., pp. 143–153). Boulder, CO: Westview Press.

Reed, M. (2004, August 26). Transformational servant leadership. Webinar sponsored by Encounter Collaborative.

Rosenbach, W. E., & Taylor, R. L. (1998). Followership: The underappreciated dimension. In W. E. Rosenbach & R. L. Taylor (Eds.), *Contemporary issues in leadership* (4th ed., pp. 85–88). Boulder, CO: Westview Press.

Salacuse, J. (2005). *Leading leaders: How to manage smart, talented, rich, and powerful people.* Boston, MA: AMACOM.

Shenkar, O. (2010). Imitation is more valuable than innovation. *Harvard Business Review, 88*(4), 28–29.

Sivers, D. (2010, February). How to start a movement (TED Talks). Retrieved from http://www.ted.com/talks/derek_sivers_how_to_start_a_movement.html?utm_source=newsletter_weekly_2010-04-06&utm_campaign=newsletter_weekly&utm_medium=email

Staub, R. E., II. (1996). *The heart of leadership: 12 practices of courageous leaders.* Provo, UT: Executive Excellence Publishing.

Sullivan, E. J., & Decker, P. J. (2008). *Effective leadership and management in nursing* (7th ed.). Upper Saddle River, NJ: Prentice Hall.

Sullivan, T. J. (1998). *Collaboration: A health care imperative.* New York: McGraw-Hill.

Swansburg, R. C., & Swansburg, R. J. (1999). *Introductory management and leadership for nurses* (2nd ed.). Sudbury, MA: Jones & Bartlett.

Tan, Chade-Meng. (2010, November). Everyday compassion at Google (TED Talks). Retrieved from http://www.ted.com/talks/chade_meng_tan_everyday_compassion_at_google.html

Yoder-Wise, P. S. (2010). *Leading and managing in nursing* (5th ed.). St. Louis: Mosby.

Yukl, G. (2010). *Leadership in organizations* (7th ed.). Upper Saddle River, NJ: Prentice Hall.

CHAPTER 4

Leadership as an Integral Component of a Professional Role

LEARNING OBJECTIVES

- Identify characteristics of transformational and transactional leaders.
- Compare and contrast the leader–follower relationship in a transformational environment and a transactional environment.
- Explain how transformational leadership generates growth in an individual, an organization, and a group.
- Describe how the four components of principle-centered leadership can assist an individual's personal and professional leadership ability to grow.
- Describe how Maslow's hierarchy of needs relates to leadership development.
- Explain how leadership ability is enhanced by emotional competence.
- Explain how leadership is an integral component of being a nurse professional.

INTRODUCTION

Professional nurses can no longer think of themselves as "just nurses." Nurses are increasingly expected to provide leadership, whether they hold staff positions or are vice presidents, nurse practitioners, or nurse educators. Nurses must be competent if they are to provide leadership. Grossman (2007) developed a Leadership and Management Competency Checklist to assist critical care nurses in obtaining experiences and gaining competency in leading and managing. Based on Kolb's Experiential Model

(1984), this checklist is recommended for nurses who precept to guide the new orientee staff nurses or student nurses in practicing leadership and management skills. The idea is that individuals learn more if they can integrate what they pick up from an experience with an expert, ideally receive some constructive feedback on their performance, and then have time to process the new learning and reflect on how to improve the next time they are faced with a similar experience. Box 4–1 identifies the major behaviors that nurses need to acquire in order to be competent in leading and managing. Individuals with these strengths will be able to exert leadership in making decisions, facilitate partnerships with other health-care agencies and health-care workers, accomplish goals, and reach stated visions.

Nurse leaders know what needs to happen to achieve quality patient care and excellence in nursing education. By following a framework such as checklist in the Box 4-1, nurses can assist themselves and other nurses in gaining the knowledge they need to lead and manage the people in their unit so that it will become a positive and exciting place to work. Individuals will generally feel more collaborative and less competitive if they are empowered with knowledge and are feeling competent themselves. This is what Covey (1991) calls principle-centered leadership; he suggests that an individual needs to be trustworthy in order to gain trust from others and be able to empower those he leads. Without the followers perceiving competence and trust in the leader, there will be no staff empowerment or organizational alignment. Eventually, if principle-centered leadership is embraced by all levels of the organization's structure, the work culture will evolve into a more caring environment where new ideas will be welcomed and used by everyone. It stands to reason that when people are feeling good about their family or personal lives, they can be more effective in their work setting. A healthy work environment (HWE) is crucial to morale, patient safety, patient satisfaction, and nurse retention (Ritter, 2011; Lavoie-Tremblay, Wright, Desforges, Gelinas, Marchionni, & Drevniok, 2008). Similar to Covey's tenets of principle-centered leadership, a healthy work environment has been described by the American Association of Critical Care Nurses (Gilmore, 2007) as including effective communication, interdisciplinary collaboration, an evidence-based practice environment, the potential for professional advancement, and an atmosphere of empowerment that allows all members of the HWE to feel confident and competent.

BOX 4-1 **Components of a Leadership and Management Competency Checklist**

Communication: oral and written
Collaboration and networking: interprofessionally and intraprofessionally
Decision making, problem solving, and troubleshooting: using nursing models
Unit vision and research development: structure, culture, and quality improvement
Risk management: legally and ethically
Professional role development and image: authority, power, and confidence
Unit management regarding care delivery: care patterns and patient safety
Team building and empowerment: leadership, followership, and group dynamics
Personal and unit specialty skill development: skills geared to specialty unit

Nurses who are just beginning their careers can be excellent leaders and make a great contribution to the profession while at the same time jump-starting their career. It is important that new nurses become part of the HWE transformation so that they feel comfortable and empowered in their work setting (Lavoie-Tremblay et al, 2008). A review of the Institute of Medicine and the Robert Wood Johnson Foundation initiative, *The Future of Nursing: Leading Change, Advancing Health,* makes it apparent that staff nurses must lead (2010). As nurses increase their skills to achieve these goals, the profession will become stronger and more productive. Also, the profession's image will be more transparent and visible to the public. Now is the time for such action.

When thinking about the leadership that is exercised in a nursing group or organization, it must be realized that every individual, not just the nurse manager, dean, or committee chair, has the potential and the responsibility to assume the role of leader and work with others to fulfill the goals of the group or organization. The individual who happens to be in the appointed, authoritative role (e.g., the nurse manager) may or may not be the person who actually fulfills the role of the leader. As discussed earlier, effective followers have skills comparable to those of leaders, and the effectiveness of the leadership that any individual provides depends largely on the followers. Gardner (1990) said, "Leadership can be distributed among members, and the leader must recognize the needs of the followers, help them see how these needs can be met, and give them confidence that they can accomplish results through their efforts" (p. 149). So, leaders must be able to lead others as well as themselves. If there is a determined and powerful followership, leaders and followers can be successful. The leader and followers should also be cognizant of the unique characteristics and talents of each of the multigenerational nurses and health-care workers on their unit (Twenge, 2009). Perhaps a creative leader or follower will institute some social networking processes as a mechanism of connecting all these players with their diverse interests and needs (Shih, 2011).

It is common, however, for nurses to fail to be effective followers or leaders. For example, instead of acting as leaders or effective followers, nurses criticize their managers, the institution, the director, the physician, or other people occupying positions of leadership. Instead of suggesting solutions or assuming leadership positions, nurses blame other nurses, failing to collaborate with each other. Nurses fail to challenge the "orders" of a physician, are often scared to try anything that differs from the "way things have always been," do not have the confidence to capitalize on their extensive knowledge or experience, or claim to be "only a nurse" when talking to a physician or a patient. These examples point to low self-esteem. If nurses are to increase their level of responsibility and if the profession is to survive and thrive, all nurses must exercise their leadership ability. Clinical nursing leadership is a competency that all nurses need to acquire and continue to improve just as they do with their clinical specialty area content and expertise. Educators need to integrate this clinical leadership into all of the clinical practice area courses. The *Clinical Nursing Leadership Cognitive Model* developed by Pepin, Dubois, Girard, Tardif, and Ha (2011) takes the learner through different learning stages that would be helpful for educators to integrate into each clinical rotation or with staff nurses on the unit. These stages are awareness of clinical leadership in nursing, integration of clinical leadership in actions, active leadership with patients/families, active leadership with health-care team, and ability to lead at the organizational level.

Nurse leaders also need to be authentic leaders, that is, they need to be true to themselves. Authenticity can only be recognized by others, not by the nurse; the staff perceive that the leader is "real, sincere, and defined by honesty and integrity that means the leader is authentic" (Kerfoot, 2006, p. 319). Goffee and Jones (2006) refer to a leader as someone with vision, energy, and purpose who works on being oneself more, with skill. Each individual identifies and portrays his or her own style of leadership. Being able to identify what makes a good leader as well as to use those skills that demonstrate good leadership would seem to inherently improve oneself. It is important to adapt a specific leadership style and to practice that type of leadership, but it is difficult to be effective when the challenges and stresses of the environment become overwhelming. In these cases, a different style using other leadership skills might be more beneficial for both the leader and the followers involved. A strategy that may assist the leader to become more effective and to remain true to oneself is to be mindful at work and to pay attention to one's well-being and performance. The skill of mindfulness is the ability to be nonjudgmental, to focus on the present reality, and, at the same time, to foster more effective use of resources for the organization (Marianetti & Passmore, 2008).

Individuals are not born leaders; rather, leaders emerge and continue to evolve as a result of experiences, purposeful self-development, and interactions with a variety of people. All nurses need to practice their leadership and encourage others to get involved, either as effective followers or as leaders. By creating a vision, strategizing how to accomplish the vision, seeking creative ways to implement change, and effectively leading or following in a collaborative manner, nurses exercise the leadership skills that will assist the entire health-care team in accomplishing the goal of quality patient care. In other words, a more positive and passionate outlook must prevail in nurses' work environments. Burston and Stichler (2010) studied how nurse caring was identified as the key motivational factor influencing nurse retention and recruitment. McCormack and McCance (2006) developed a person-centered nursing model to use when changing the culture of a work setting. This framework includes prerequisite traits and skills the nurse needs to have, the care environment, the patient-centered processes routinely used in care delivery, and the expected outcomes a unit is looking to achieve. To transform a work setting into a caring environment, one could apply the above-mentioned model and use the Nursing Context Index to measure how well the adaptation is processing (Slater, McCormack, & Bunting, 2009). This is an excellent example of how a unit or practice setting could change their HWE to encompass more caring interprofessionally and intraprofessionally as well as with patients and families. The added benefits would be to actually measure whether there was a change to becoming a more caring milieu and, if so, to work together to strengthen the change. Or, if the evaluation demonstrated little to no change, the group could collaborate to determine what behaviors in the evaluation were identified as not contributing to a caring HWE. Staff could determine and implement strategies to improve their work environment.

TYPES OF LEADERSHIP

In a classic work that still has relevance more than 40 years later, Burns (1978) described two types of leadership that are used to make change and create new futures: transactional leadership and transformational leadership.

Transactional Leadership

Transactional leadership involves an exchange in which both the leader and the followers "get something." The leader gets the job completed or the goal achieved, and the followers get promotions, money, or other benefits. The focus of this type of leadership system is the accomplishment of a task, and it is the type often seen in health-care organizations. Some even argue that nurses too often focus on tasks and rewards.

Transactional leaders focus on getting the job done and see task completion as the "bottom line." Bass and Riggio (2006) described transactional leaders as more self-concerned and outcome focused. Verbal praise, recognition for successful employees, and financial incentives are very visible in organizations that consider transactional leadership an important style of leading their employees (Northouse, 2010). Although there may be some type of "connection" between these leaders and their followers, this connection often is something other than a common purpose or a shared vision. With such a relationship, both leaders and followers may perceive their work only as a job, and not invest in it as a career. As such, this philosophical approach, as has been seen in all too many hospital settings, is limiting.

Transformational Leadership

In contrast, transformational leadership is a process in which "leaders and followers raise one another to higher levels of motivation and morality" (Burns, 1978, p. 20). This motivation energizes people to perform beyond expectations by creating a sense of ownership in reaching the vision. And, it is not to say the employees do not have financial incentives and recognition for accomplishments. Bass (1985, pp. 62, 67) compared transformational leadership with inspirational leadership that arouses motivation of followers. He cited examples of transformational leadership from a Reserve Officers Training Corps (ROTC) study, including the following:

- Instilling pride in all
- Building morale through "pep talks"
- Acting as a positive role model
- Building the confidence of others through personal encouragement
- Complimenting individuals' performances and contributions as a way to instill pride in the group

Bass (1985) characterized transformational leaders as charismatic, able to instill motivation in others, and able to give individualized consideration. Burns (1978) described them as individuals who heighten followers' awareness of what must be done to accomplish the shared goal. Bennis and Nanus (1997) defined transformational leaders as individuals who follow through with getting people to act, assist others to lead, and ultimately facilitate change.

All great leaders have had one characteristic in common: it was the willingness to confront unequivocally the major anxiety of their people in their time. —John Kenneth Galbraith

Several strategies have been identified (Bennis & Nanus, 1997) to assist leaders to be more transformational: attention through vision, meaning through communication, trust through positioning, and deployment of self through positive self-regard and optimism about a desired outcome. But one merely has to look around and know that although most people can develop into transformational leaders if they choose to, some individuals may be more or less successful. In fact, some support that one's genes predispose an individual to develop certain personality characteristics, temperaments, and cognitive styles (Shane, 2010).

Transformational leaders emphasize the importance of following a vision and assisting others to participate in making it a reality; they communicate their values and beliefs to others so that they can achieve a common meaning in their work and realize the vision toward which all are striving; they trust others, are honest, and act responsibly; and finally, they use their talents and expertise as a way to express their desire for and commitment to a vision. To realize a vision for a unit, department or practice, nurses must have an interdisciplinary collaboration with the other health-care members involved (Bainbridge, Nasmith, Orchard, & Wood, 2010). Nurses can be particularly savvy with interdisciplinary collaboration because they are the professionals who spend the most time with the patient and assumedly would have the opportunity to obtain the most knowledge about the patient. This information would be helpful for every member on the patient's professional team. Stakeholders, such as the hospital's governing Board, the surrounding community, and regulatory agencies, are also very much a part of achieving a successful vision. If nurses are to be transformational leaders, they must follow their dreams, communicate in an articulate manner, be concerned with their own growth as well as the growth of their followers, establish trusting relationships, and identify their strengths and limitations. They also need to readily accept change and constantly seek new ways of doing things despite the risk (Bass, 1985).

Bass (1985) and Burns (1978) believed that transformational leaders have strong personal value systems and that by sharing these values, they are able to affect and even change followers' beliefs, even without needing to negotiate "what's in it for the follower." In essence, transformational leaders have a spirit that creates special leader–follower relationships and promotes individual and group growth. In fact, this spirit, this feeling of mutual involvement, is of greater significance than any isolated task accomplishment. This excitement about a vision or idea that is worthwhile attracts others to follow.

Transformational Leadership and Nursing Practice

An example of how transformational leadership affects patient care through increased nurse job satisfaction is described by Allen and Vitale-Nolen (2005). The implementation of a new patient care delivery model, namely the Relationship Based Nursing Model at New Hampshire Hospital, improved nurse job satisfaction significantly with a 14% increase ($N = 70$). By redefining nursing care that encourages empowerment and consideration of both professional and personal values, this hospital's nurse leadership group generated a change in how nurses made decisions and validated that it is the nurse "who knows what to do [and how] to choose how to do it" (p. 281). Simply put, this creates an empowered environment "where nurses feel they make a difference" (p. 277).

Casido and Parker (2011) studied self-reports of 278 staff nurses working with nurse managers who practiced transactional and transformational leadership. They found that nurses using transformational leadership—defined as visionary, charismatic, and promoting out-of-the-box thinking—were successful in predicting positive leadership outcomes. Additionally, nurses identified that having mentors and role models using transformational leadership assisted in facilitating their success.

Sashkin and Sashkin (2003) demonstrated in their research that many aspects of transformational leadership can be developed. Being able to recognize colleagues' feelings, motivate others, and manage one's own emotions well in relationships serves to foster an environment that facilitates transformational leadership. For example, with the multifaceted problems health-care organizations face today, there are numerous crises that demand the entire staff, ranging from the maintenance crew to the chief executive officer, to be able to communicate to the public in a positive and nonthreatening manner. How to convey the organization and unit's mission in caring for patients using appropriate wording and emotion with the ever-changing technology of communications is part of everyone's responsibility (Fearn-Banks, 2007). In fact, with the competitiveness in today's market, where one obtains health care is something that cannot be left up to chance. Being part of a health-care organization's system for primary and wellness care is beneficial to patients when they need acute or emergency care.

EMOTIONAL COMPETENCE

Goleman (1998) suggested that one of the most important attributes of leadership is emotional intelligence, which is quite different from one's intelligence quotient (IQ). He defined emotional intelligence as a group of competencies (self-awareness, self-management, social awareness, and relationship management) that influence the ability to respond to others and manage one's own feelings. Currently, most refer to this concept as emotional competence instead of intelligence (Harrison & Fopma-Loy, 2010; Wilson, & Carryer, 2008; Yiu, Mak, Ho, & Chui, 2010). Goleman's research indicates that emotional intelligence is nearly twice as significant as IQ in becoming a leader. People are born with certain cognitive abilities, or IQ, and that is not likely to change dramatically throughout one's life, but emotional intelligence is something one can acquire and, basically, transfer into improving one's professional behavior. It is essential for nurses to realize the power they have in making positive change on their units, in their agencies, and in the health policy arena. Currently, in America, nurses are perceived to be among the most honest workers. This, coupled with having high emotional intelligence and becoming confident with managing oneself in a highly stressful setting, puts nurses in a position to affect the status quo.

Goleman, Boyatzis, and McKee (2002) recommended that leaders need the following skills: self-awareness, self-regulation, motivation, empathy, and social skills. Using these skills, all leaders can inspire others by effecting change, being creative, articulating visions, helping visions become reality, managing conflict, taking risks, networking, and adapting to new initiatives. Nurse followers and leaders can use their emotional competence to create a work culture that fosters collaboration for their units (Yiu et al, 2010). Leaders can maximize their successes as well as facilitate others' achievements by fostering an environment more conducive to using emotional competence, such as

Case Study

The following is a case study about how emotionally competent nurses can affect their job satisfaction as well as their patients' care.

Cynthia came from one of the urban acute trauma centers to the community hospital to be the nurse manager of the inpatient Orthopedic Unit and outpatient Orthopedic Center. She decided to work as a staff nurse 1 day per week on the unit and 1 half-day in the outpatient Orthopedic Surgery and Rehabilitation Center. She quickly established rapport with the patients, staff, and physicians in both areas. Her clinical competency with new orthopedic technology and her charismatic manner of leadership were highly respected by the staff. She collaborated with the physicians and members of the units' staff to determine whether the hospital could purchase more equipment in order to expand their services. This was determined to be a definite "yes."

Data showed that most orthopedic patients were waiting up to 3 months for surgery, so some were going to other hospitals far from their homes. The units in both the hospital and outpatient clinics were expanded for surgical procedures, and additional staff was hired to manage the workload. Cynthia felt it would be more cost-effective and satisfying for the nurses and technicians in each area to be able to rotate (similar to the physicians) through the different settings with the new expansion. She set up a committee to explore this option. The committee, under her leadership, found that 90% of the nurses, assistants, and technicians were supportive of the rotations, although 10% preferred to stay in their current position. The units had a meeting to discuss these findings, and they unanimously decided that the 10% who did not want to rotate would not have to. The nurses were quite excited about the idea of having a new and expanded scope of practice. Cynthia assisted the committee in setting up in-services, orientations, and precepting for each individual so that they would be prepared for this rotating unit schedule. Nurses volunteered to present the in-services and orientations as well as to precept for each other. Once the scheduling was set up and piloted, the staff was able to anticipate potential problems and deal with them. Schedules were tweaked, and staff worked in a cohesive way.

One year later, job and patient satisfaction were at the highest level ever obtained. Length of stay was the lowest ever measured, and the cost of managing the units was down. Nurses were excited to learn new aspects of orthopedics and were joining the Orthopedic Nursing Society, becoming certified by the American Nursing Credentialing Center, attending conferences and reporting findings back, and conducting two evidence-based practice studies. The nurse manager asked for feedback from her staff every 6 months and found that the staff was overwhelmingly supportive of her leadership. Using the skills of emotional competence, Cynthia was successful in turning her unit into a cost-generating unit in which staff morale and retention increased.

by sponsoring staff recognition days, publishing accomplishments in a unit or agency newsletter, and having peer-evaluated employee-of-the-month designations. Increasing self-awareness, which is an important aspect of emotional competence, will most likely help build high self–esteem.

SELF-ESTEEM AND LEADERSHIP IMAGE

Barker, Sullivan, and Emery (2006) believed that the most significant tool for transformational leaders to be effective is oneself, particularly one's self-awareness, self-development, and trust of followers. They called this positive self-regard, which is very similar to how Bennis and Nanus (1997) described transformational leaders. Barker and colleagues (2006) and Burns (1978) suggested that Maslow's (1970) concept of self-esteem would be enhanced if it included the concept of positive self-regard. Self-esteem includes the need for achievement, mastery, competence, confidence, independence, and freedom to act. Satisfying one's self-esteem needs tends to result in higher self-confidence and eventually self-actualization (Maslow, 1998). These abilities are congruent with those that define transformational leaders and effective followers, and because individuals who have high self-esteem are able to develop and grow, followers can become leaders.

Nurses must be self-motivated to change or improve their personal and professional lives. Individuals who are not motivated to change will most likely maintain the status quo and fail to provide leadership to or facilitate others' growth. However, one should not expect success simply because one feels that he or she has worked very hard. A good example of this entitlement issue is depicted in the story (Box 4–2) of an aspiring pre-Olympian who would not likely be a transformational leader to her teammates because she is so self-oriented (Campbell, 1996, p. 9).

Many nurses have the attitude that they deserve more simply because they have seniority or have "paid their dues." When they don't get more, they perceive themselves to be victims of the system. Circumstances do not change just because people think they deserve special favors (i.e., treatment that ignores system constraints). This idea that experienced nurses have paid their dues only propagates more unhappiness and victimization for the nurses. Kouzes and Posner (2007) note that the unprecedented instability in today's world calls for strong leadership. They recommend that leaders engage in practices that transform followers and help realize visionary goals, such as the following:

- Challenge the status quo.
- Inspire a shared vision.
- Enable others to act, rather than to react.
- Be role models.
- Encourage the heart.

The first four practices are self-explanatory. The last practice, encourage the heart, highlights the importance of leaders caring deeply about the vision and working hard to accomplish it. It also suggests that people who perform well will be self-satisfied. Kouzes

---

BOX 4-2 Expect Success Through Self-Confidence, Not Entitlement

"One young lady had listed everything she had done to get into the finals, all of her exercising, her nutritional plans, her workouts, all of the sweat and pain and exertion and self-denial that she had gone through, and then she had written, 'DESERVE a place on the Olympic team!' I [as her coach] had to take her aside and give her a short lecture about that kind of thinking.

"Look," I said, "You don't deserve squat. Every other person in these trials has done exactly what you have done— they have exercised, they have sweated, they have gone through pain, they have given up other pleasures, they are just as deserving as you are. Saying that you deserve something special puts you in the role of potential victim, so that you can later say, 'Poor me, life has failed me'."

I told her, "You can say I EXPECT to earn a place on the Olympic team. That's okay, that's an expression of self-confidence, a stance from where you can perform better because you expect to be among the best, but let's not have any more of these victimizing statements."

and Posner (2007) strongly recommended that leaders celebrate accomplishments of the people working in the department. Leaders need to feel good about themselves and focus on themselves but also to appreciate their followers' accomplishments. Therefore, it is crucial that leaders enhance their own initiative, self-esteem, assertiveness, and positive self-regard if they are to provide leadership in and advance the nursing profession.

WOULD-BE LEADERS BECOME LEADERS

Nurses need to reinvent themselves, much as others have done. Bennis (1993) explains the process of reinventing himself "to avoid accepting roles [which he] was brought up to play" (p. xv). He further describes the significance of being able to invent and reinvent himself so that he would not have to be "content with borrowed postures, secondhand ideas, [or] fitting in instead of standing out" (p. xv). His warning not to accept stereotypical perceptions offers a lesson for nurses and non-nurses alike: Do not accept stereotypes of nursing. By reinventing oneself, nurses "do not accept the roles we were brought up to play" (Bennis, 1993, p. 2). If nurses reinvented themselves and used their entrepreneurial spirit to focus on larger issues rather than merely the tasks of the day and tried new delivery patterns, it would be a very different world! Nurses who wish to develop their entrepreneurial spirit must have courage, vision, and the ability to communicate effectively as well as be open to new ideas (Elange, Hunter, & Winchell, 2007).

Another strategy is to use a more global perspective of connecting with others who are pursuing new initiatives, experiencing similar problems, or have resources that can be shared with other organizations. Shih (2011) shares multiple strategies for forming social bonds and community networks in her book, *The Facebook Era: Tapping Online Social Networks to Market, Sell, and Innovate.*

It is imperative to appreciate that nurses complement, but are not subservient to, other health-care providers, and this perspective develops as one learns to be a nurse. Therefore, nurse educators need to foster leadership in their students, help students integrate leadership as an integral component of their role, and focus as much on the development of leadership skills as on the acquisition of clinical skills. Development of leadership skills must be a part of the student's professional as well as personal journey in life. These skills need to be introduced from birth and reinforced by family, friends, and the community as well as by the individual's school and faculty long before post-secondary education.

Bolman and Deal (2001) describe one such journey of an adult as he acquired the ability to lead with heart. The main character in this book, Steve, was tired of leading for the "bottom line" and shares how he had a deep self-reflection of what he felt to be most important to him to portray as a leader. Bolman and Deal (2001) discuss the love, power, and significance of the bond between leaders like Steve and the followers he interacted with and how spirituality and one's work connect.

LEADERSHIP AS AN INTEGRAL COMPONENT OF EACH NURSE'S ROLE

Nurses are increasingly expected to assume the roles of advocate, teacher, caregiver, disseminator of knowledge, manager, contributor to public health policy development, and leader. Nurses are also expected to be heavily involved in partnering with other nurses and members of other health-care disciplines to achieve quality patient care. Nurses, therefore, are expected to play a major role in evoking change in health care and ensuring their significant role in the restructured system of managed care.

Nurses must acquire principle-centered leadership to be effective in the new health-care system. Principle-centered leadership involves "keeping promises, developing virtues, changing bad habits, being faithful to vows, exercising courage, and being genuinely considerate of others" (Covey, 1991, p. 18). These principles are similar to compasses in that they always point the way and keep us from becoming lost amid conflicting ideas and values. Covey (1991) says principles constantly apply, and they surface in the form of "ideas, norms, values, and teachings which uplift, fulfill, empower, and inspire people" (p. 19). Characteristics that exemplify principle-centered leaders include continually learning, having a service orientation, having positive energy, believing in others, leading a balanced life, viewing life as an adventure, being synergistic, and having the ability to self-renew.

Leaders must also possess exceptional communication skills. Nurses, therefore, must be consistent, assertive, and knowledgeable speakers about their role, the state of the health-care system, and their patients' care. Likewise, nurses would be more effective leaders if they possessed sophisticated interpersonal relationship skills to use with patients, families, communities, other health-care providers, and the public.

Credibility is another important characteristic that admired leaders possess. Kouzes and Posner (2005) studied people's reasons for respecting, trusting, and being willing to be influenced by others and found the following behaviors as indicative of credibility: supporting, having the courage to do the right thing, challenging, developing and acting as a mentor to others, listening, celebrating good work, following through on commitments, trusting others, empowering others, making time for people, sharing the vision, opening doors, overcoming personal hardships, admitting mistakes, advising others, solving problems creatively, and teaching well. These behaviors reflect the characteristics of a credible, transformational leader. The four components that correlated highest with being credible included honesty, competency, inspiration, and being forward-looking (Kouzes & Posner, 2005).

> *To achieve all that is possible, we must attempt the impossible . . . to be as much as we can be, we must dream of being more.* —Gale Baker Stanton

Nurses must be morally fit leaders, capable of using good, ethical judgment in making decisions about delivering quality care to all patients. They must be patient advocates and representatives of their patients' needs. Each has obligations of promoting ethical leadership, which is composed of communication, quality, and collaboration (Rhode, 2006). Today's corporate scandals emphasize the need for nurses to lead ethically and morally.

Taking a risk to try something new, taking time to dream and imagine how one could make a difference, joining a professional organization and becoming actively involved, and taking courses for personal gain (e.g., public speaking) or to complete a degree or certificate are all activities that nurses should consider as part of their self-renewal. By self-evaluating or using peer evaluation effectively, one can identify strengths and weaknesses, nurture one's strengths, and either work on or work around one's limitations. Nurses also need to become comfortable with trying new things and realizing competency will be achieved. Nurses need to take risks and try something they have never done before if they are interested in a change. For example, just as becoming a per diem or cross-trained in another clinical area will expand one's growth, so will taking on a leadership position or participating in a new organizational initiative. There are multiple resources, and hopefully role models, to assist one in developing competency as one meets the challenges of a nursing leadership position (MacMillan-Finlayson, 2010). As leaders in the health-care arena today, nurses must embody the qualities mentioned here for nursing services to be accessible to patients, for nurses to be involved in multidisciplinary collaboration, and for nursing care to be identified as the reason for positive and cost-effective patient outcomes. Nurses can and must be leaders.

CONCLUSION

One does not have to be in nursing management to be a "true" nursing leader; there are unlimited opportunities for nurses to exercise leadership. For many, that may require much self-reflection and reinvention. As Bennis (1993, p. 1) recommended, "People who cannot reinvent themselves must be content with borrowed postures, second-hand ideas, and fitting-in instead of standing out."

Nurses are increasingly "standing out" and providing leadership as they begin new roles in promoting health in inner-city homeless centers and school-based health clinics and in taking health-care vans to the most needy of people. Nurses are starting satellite outpatient dialysis and chemotherapy centers, cardiac rehabilitation centers, and pre-operative learning clinics to assist people in restoring their health. Nurses in acute care areas are developing new nurse-driven protocols; collaborating with other health-care disciplines in creating critical pathways that focus patient care on meeting outcomes; and participating in teaching smoking cessation, cholesterol lowering, and alternative nonpharmacological programs.

Many nursing leaders are making a difference in patient outcomes and using their leadership potential to meet their own expectations of self. The profession needs more nurses like this. Nursing educators must revise curricula to provide students with opportunities to practice leadership as well as clinical roles. Nurse administrators need to create environments that encourage and support open dialogue, peer feedback, innovation, and change. Nurses need to mentor each other and call on the strengths of one another, much like geese who fly in a "V" formation (Box 4–3). When each nurse sees leadership as an integral component of her or his professional role, nurses will be able to transform health care.

BOX 4-3 Learning Lessons From Geese

Although we may know that geese fly in a "V" formation, what we may not know is that as each bird flaps its wings, it creates an uplift for the bird following. By flying in formation, the whole flock adds 71% more to the flying range than if each bird flew alone.

A second fact about geese is that when the lead goose gets tired, it moves back into the formation, and another goose flies the point position.

Third, if a goose falls out of the formation, it feels the drag and resistance of trying to fly alone and quickly gets back into formation to take advantage of the power of the bird it follows.

What are the lessons here for leadership? First, leadership must be shared. We all must take our turn doing the work that will help our profession evolve, our organizations grow, and ourselves continue to develop. Second, every member of the group has the potential to "fly the point position" and serve as the leader; we should not limit our expectations of the potential within each of us. Finally, the work we do can stimulate and excite others in our group to also perform better and achieve a level of excellence perhaps previously unexpected. There is much we can learn about leaders and leadership from geese. We need only to pay attention and be open to new ideas, perspectives, and possibilities.

CRITICAL THINKING EXERCISES

Describe how you could reinvent yourself, personally and professionally, so as not to merely "live the status quo."

_____

_____

How would you describe individuals you think of as leaders? Individuals you do not consider to be leaders? What are some of the differences between these two groups of individuals in terms of a "leadership image"?

_____

_____

How would you describe the image you convey? Look at the way you dress, things you have written, presentations you have made, your participation on committees or in class, and so on. Is this the image you want to convey? If not, what aspects are unsatisfactory to you, and how could you change them?

_____

_____

Watch the film _Jerry McGuire_ and describe how the leaders have a sense of moral courage and the desire to speak up when something is not right. List some of the issues that you feel were "not right" and suggest leadership behaviors that you would use to do things "right."

_____

_____

Continued

CRITICAL THINKING
EXERCISES—cont'd

Compare the "leadership image" of nurses in various roles: staff nurse, advanced practice nurse, nurse educator, nurse advocate, nursing service administrator, and so on. How are they alike? How are they different? What kinds of things can a nurse do to convey a strong image?

_____

_____

What can aspiring nurse leaders do to overcome negative stereotypes of nurses and nursing, create a genuinely positive leadership image, and project that image to achieve desired goals?

_____

_____

Develop a Facebook site for your business or educational program so that you can readily obtain other's feedback regarding your initiatives. By being more knowledgeable about what other nurses or health-care workers want from your business or educational program, you can be more productive and offer optimal services.

_____

_____

References

Allen, D., & Vitale-Nolen, R. (2005). Patient care delivery model improves nurse job satisfaction. *Journal of Continuing Education in Nursing, 36*(6), 277–282.

Bainbridge, L., Nasmith, L., Orchard, C., & Wood, V. (2010). Competencies for interprofessional collaboration. *Journal of Physical Therapy Education, 24*(1), 6–11.

Barker, A., Sullivan, D., & Emery, M. (2006). *Leadership competencies for clinical managers: The renaissance of transformational leadership.* Sudbury, MA: Jones & Bartlett.

Bass, B. (1985). *Leadership and performance beyond expectations.* New York: Macmillan.

Bass, B. M., & Riggio, R. E. (2006). *Transformation leadership* (2nd ed.). Mahwah, NJ: Laurence Earlbaum.

Bennis, W. (1993). *An invented life: Reflections on leadership and change.* Reading, MA: Addison-Wesley.

Bennis, W., & Nanus, B. (1997). *Leadership: The strategies for taking charge* (2nd ed.). New York: Harper & Row.

Bolman, L., & Deal, T. (2001). *Leading with soul: An uncommon journey of spirit* (2nd ed.). San Francisco: Jossey-Bass.

Burns, J. (1978). *Leadership*. New York: Harper & Row.

Burston, P. L., & Stichler, J. F. (2010). Nursing work environment and nurse caring: Relationship among motivational factors. *Journal of Advanced Nursing, 66*(8), 1819–1831.

Campbell, D. (1996). Inklings. *Issues & Observations, 16*(1), 9.

Casido, J., & Parker, J. (2011). Staff nurse perceptions of nurse manager leadership styles and outcomes. *Journal of Nursing Management, 19*(4), 478–486.

Covey, S. (1991). *Principle-centered leadership*. New York: Summit Books.

Elange, B., Hunter, G., & Winchell, M. (2007). Barriers to nurse entrepreneurship: A study of the process model of entrepreneurship. *Journal of American Academy of Nurse Practitioners, 19*(4), 198–204.

Fearn-Banks, K. (2007). *Crisis communications: A casebook approach* (3rd ed.). Mahwah, NJ: Lawrence Erlbaum Associates.

Gardner, J. (1990). *On leadership*. New York: Free Press.

Gilmore, J. (2007). Healthy work environments. *Nephrology Nursing, 34*(1), 11.

Goffee, R., & Jones, G. (2006). *Why should anyone be led by you? What it takes to be an authentic leader*. Boston: Harvard Business School Publishing.

Goleman, D. (1998). *Working with emotional intelligence*. New York: Bantam Books.

Goleman, D., Boyatzis, R., & McKee, A. (2002). *Primal leadership: Realizing the power of emotional intelligence*. Boston: Harvard Business School Press.

Grossman, S. (2007). Assisting critical care nurses in acquiring leadership skills: Development of a leadership and management competency checklist. *Dimensions of Critical Care Nursing, 26*(2), 57–65.

Harrison, P. R., Fopma-Loy, J. L. (2010). Reflective journal prompts: A vehicle for simulating emotional competence in nursing. *Journal of Nursing Education, 49*(11), 644–652.

Institute of Medicine and Robert Wood Johnson Foundation (2010). *The future of nursing: Leading change, advancing health*. Retrieved June 22, 2011, from http://www.iom.edu/Reports/2010/The-Future-of-Nursing-Leading-Change-Advancing-Health.aspx.

Kerfoot, K. (2006). Authentic leadership. *MEDSURG Nursing, 15*(5), 319–320.

Kolb, D. A. (1984). *Experiential learning: Experiences as the source of learning and development*. Englewood Cliffs, NJ: Prentice Hall.

Kouzes, J., & Posner, B. (2005). *Credibility: How leaders gain and lose it, why people demand it* (2nd ed.). San Francisco: Jossey-Bass.

Kouzes, J., & Posner, B. (2007). *The leadership challenge: How to keep getting extraordinary things done in organizations* (4th ed.). San Francisco: Jossey-Bass.

Lavoie-Tremblay, M., Wright, D., Desforges, N., Gelinas, C., Marchionni, C., & Drevniok, U. (2008). Creating a healthy workplace for new generation nurses. *Journal of Nursing Scholarship, 40*(3), 290–297.

MacMillan-Finlayson, S. (2010). Competency development for nurse executives: Meeting the challenge. *Journal of Nursing Administration, 40*(6), 254–257.

Marianetti, O., & Passmore, J. (2008). Mindfulness at work: Paying attention to enhance well-being and performance (pp. 189–200). In P. A. Linley (Ed.), *Oxford handbook of positive psychology and work*. New York: Oxford University Press.

Maslow, A. (1970). *Motivation and personality* (2nd ed.). New York: Harper & Row.

Maslow, A. (1998). *Maslow on management*. New York: John Wiley.

McCormack, B., & McCance, T. V. (2006). The person centered nursing conceptual framework. *Journal of Advanced Nursing, 56*(5) 472–479.

Northouse, P. G. (2010). *Leadership theory and practice* (5th ed.). Los Angeles: Sage.

Pepin, J., Dubois, S., Girard, F., Tardif, J., & Ha, L. (2011). A cognitive learning model of clinical nursing leadership. *Nurse Education Today, 31*(3), 268–273.

Rhode, D. (Ed.). (2006). *Moral leadership: The theory and practice of power, judgment, and policy*. San Francisco: Jossey-Bass.

Ritter, D. (2011). The relationship between healthy work environments and retention of nurses in a hospital setting. *Journal of Nursing Management, 19*(1), 27–32.

Sashkin, M., & Sashkin, M. (2003). *Leadership that matters: The critical factors for making a difference in people's lives and organizations' success*. San Francisco: Berrett-Koehler.

Shane, S. (2010). *Born entrepreneurs, born leaders: How your genes affect your work life*. New York: Oxford University Press.

Shih, C. (2011). *The Facebook era: Tapping online social networks to market, sell, and innovate*. Upper Saddle River, NJ: Prentice Hall.

Slater, P., McCormack, B., & Bunting, B. (2009). The development and pilot testing of an instrument to measure nurses' working environment: The nursing context index. *World Views on Evidence Based Nursing, 6*(3), 173–182.

Twenge, J. M. (2009). Generational changes and their impact in the classroom: Teaching generation me. *Medical Education, 43*(5), 398–405.

Wilson, S. C., & Carryer, J. (2008). Emotional competence and nursing education: New Zealand study. *Nursing Praxis in New Zealand, 24*(1), 36–47.

Yiu, J. W., Mak, W. W., Ho, W. S., & Chui, Y. Y. (2010). Effectiveness of a knowledge-contact program in improving nursing students' attitudes and emotional competence in serving people living with HIV/AIDS. *Social Science & Medicine, 71*(1), 38–44.

CHAPTER 5

Vision and Creativity

- Define the concept of vision as it relates to leadership.
- Describe how a nurse leader, follower, and group can facilitate the identification, articulation, and communication of a personal vision.
- Identify strategies that would be effective in making one's personal vision become a reality.
- Formulate a personal vision for the profession or one's particular area of practice.
- Identify characteristics of nursing and non-nursing leaders who are viewed as visionary.
- Describe characteristics of creative persons, processes, and environments.
- Project potential outcomes of using creativity as a nurse leader or follower.
- Identify how the new science of leadership fosters creativity in order to improve leadership and followership.
- Examine how the incorporation of vision and creativity into one's professional role can help vitalize and energize a nurse.

INTRODUCTION

One of the most significant characteristics of a leader is to have a vision of a "better world." Words such as "vision," "impact," "empowerment," and "facilitation" are common in everyday conversation. The time has come to stop repeating the words and begin to take action.

Having a vision, as well as being able to energize followers to join in the effort of making that vision a reality, involves credibility, communication skills, an ability to maintain momentum, and creativity. Nurses typically are skilled in communication, have high energy levels, and are seen as credible. They often do not think of themselves as creative and have difficulty sustaining and capitalizing on the momentum of a group. The mere idea of being creative may seem foreign to nurses who are accustomed to following fairly strict protocols for delivering patient care. Everyone should participate in creating a vision for the organization, not just the leader (Kouzes & Posner, 2007). In addition, the expectation that nurses have and can articulate a vision also may seem unusual if one has been socialized to expect that only the chief nursing officer (CNO) or vice president has the right or responsibility to have a vision. Being able to incorporate a new philosophy of leadership into one's professional role, accepting responsibility for articulating a vision, and allowing oneself to be creative are all essential.

Leaders do many extraordinary things, but one of their greatest contributions is having a focus or a purpose that emerges from their knowledge and experience, emotional intelligence/competence, and passion. This purpose then underpins their idea of what would facilitate the work of the group in question. Visionary leadership involves identifying the focus of the organization, department, or group; a plan that allows for that focus to become reality and be sustained; and an outcome evaluation mechanism that encourages frequent communication among all involved as to whether that focus is to continue or be changed. In order to lead, one must have a vision (Bennis, 2009). Leadership is essentially about outcomes or deliverables that can be measured; according to Goffee and Jones, leaders must have meaningful performance, not just performance, and it is their vision, as well as how they are able to attract followers to work with them, that makes them true leaders (2006).

THE CONCEPT OF VISION

What is vision? A vision is a dream or idea that is "specific enough to provide guidance to people, yet vague enough to encourage initiative and to remain relevant under a variety of conditions" (Kotter, 1990, p. 36). A vision for many nurses involves creating a work setting that offers all nurses the opportunity to develop their potential for leadership and to collaborate with each other. Creating a culture of innovation in nursing education is a vision for some educators; for example, one institution renamed their College of Nursing to the College of Nursing and Health Innovation, Arizona State University, and created a PhD program called Leadership in Healthcare Innovation (Melnyk & Davidson, 2009). Most educational and clinical leaders realize that the nursing profession needs to have a shared vision for nursing education and practice as well as have nurses lead the multidisciplinary health-care team. This echoes the Institute of Medicine and the Robert Wood Johnson Foundation Initiative on the Future of Nursing (2010), which recommends that each nurse, at every level of the profession, be assisted to increase his or her ability and skills to do more leading. The report includes recommendations such as, "nurses should practice at the full extent of their education and training and nurses should be full partners with physicians and other health care professionals in redesigning the health care delivery system" (see http://www.iom.edu for further details of the report). Certainly, all nurses need more opportunities to practice leadership skills while in their educational programs and also during on-the-job training. Nurses can become more involved in health policy changes, formally advocate for their patients' rights, run their professional organizations, initiate change on their unit or department, and mentor both colleagues and student nurses. Taking on more responsibilities such as these can assist nurses to become more involved in their organization's mission and to accomplish their own and their agency's vision. Quite simply, it is time that nurses are more visible in the health-care delivery system, and as McBride (2010) suggests, nurses are the ones that need to transform the health-care delivery system. All nurses need to create their own opportunities instead of waiting for someone else to offer them challenging opportunities.

Kouzes and Posner (2007) report that multiple leaders of large organizations identified vision as a key strategy for their organization's success. They describe vision as a reason to be, something to exemplify one's life mission, a purpose, a legacy, a personal agenda, and a dream (pp. 104–105). The authors also ask, if one does not have a vision for the future, why take the lead? A vision overlaps a variety of ideas and values in an organization or group. A vision may begin with an internal orientation and a narrow perspective, then grow into a more external direction with a broader perspective. For example, developing nurse and certified nurse assistant teams may be a step toward realizing the vision to "refocus care to the patient." A nursing unit or clinic may begin by developing or implementing new ways of care delivery by nurses, physicians, and other interdisciplinary staff. As this idea takes hold among all the health-care providers, word about the positive patient outcomes and cost-effective results of using the new assignment technique spreads to other departments in the organization (e.g., accounting, human resources, staffing). Consumer representatives who had served on the committees to institute the redesign start sharing outcomes outside of the hospital, and soon there is more external community and consumer interest in the patient-centered rather than provider-centered care.

PURPOSE AND DEVELOPMENT OF A VISION

One can have both personal and professional visions. Personal vision gives one a purpose in life, and professional vision helps one accomplish work ideas and the mission of an organization, group, or profession. Sometimes it takes a new idea heard from someone else to inspire one to think of "how things could be" before actually investing time to create a personal vision. Too many times, one only thinks of career and work life when asked, "What is your vision?"

Developing a Vision

Some conversation starters (e.g., "What might be one of your professional goals?" "I have always had some idealistic dreams about what I was looking for in my work setting, do you find yourself dreaming about what might be?" or "Even though I know my ideas are not what others may aspire to accomplish, I think if more than one person works on a project one can maximize his or her own ideas in ways one may not have thought of before") may assist individuals in connecting with others to develop visions and create solutions to barriers that may block their dreams and any plans to accomplish them. Wheatley (2002) suggests that one should reach out to others with a few connector phrases (e.g., "I liked how you expressed your goals with illustrations and would enjoy sharing some of my ideas with you" "Perhaps you could help me illustrate them like you did yours" "My idea about care delivery seems to be similar to your proposed safety practice regarding patient discharge. Do you think we could possibly combine our ideas and develop a policy for the safety aspect of patient care?" or "I am at a loss for wording to explain my rationale for cost reduction on the intravenous tubing connectors. Do you think you could assist me in coming up with a procedure so less intravenous tubing connectors would be needed?"). Wheatley also warns that not much will change if one does not reach out, and therefore, one undoubtedly will not accomplish his or her dreams (2002, p. 54). Also, nurses can improve their practice through reflective techniques, such as reviewing how they managed a similar problem in the past and determining whether they should handle it differently; asking others for feedback on what they perceive would be the best response to a problem and using those ideas; obtaining more information regarding an action they plan to take that will affect other staff and patients; and understanding the importance of taking time to think about ideas and actions in multiple ways,.

Using the Clinical Judgment Model (Tanner, 2006), which includes four stages (noticing, interpreting, responding, and reflecting), nurses can learn more about how to lead just as they do regarding clinical decision making. The Clinical Judgment Model can be used in developing one's vision in a department, unit, clinic, or professional organization as well as one's personal vision. During the noticing phase, the nurse is continually assessing the situation, gathering data, and identifying patterns of what is happening or should be happening. By reflecting on their own experiences and observing other effective and noneffective leaders, nurses can compare experiences and know what is actually occurring. While in the interpreting stage, the leader can prioritize what should be included and determine the actual vision. During the responding stage, the nurse can implement the vision, making sure to use good communication skills and listening to the group's perceptions of what should be included in the vision. Finally, during the reflecting stage, the nurse thinks about what went right and what went wrong and plans for improvement for the future regarding the vision.

The term "co-missioning," created by Covey (2004), merges an individual's personal goals and the organization's vision. He describes this process as "the key to unleashing the power of the workforce" (p. 224). Co-missioning is defined as a way of linking mission and vision of a workplace so that there are similarities with the employee's needs.

One must be able to identify opportunities to clarify one's vision and act on incorporating new strategies that will facilitate implementation of that vision. One also must be cognizant of the potential for "roadblocks" that may interfere with the vision becoming a reality, although roadblocks may, in the long run, actually assist in mobilizing people to change and accept a new plan or vision. For example, the advanced practice nurses (APNs) at a new inner-city nurse-run clinic felt "blocked" by their medical director, who insisted that all new prescription orders be co-signed by a physician before the medication could be dispensed. Concurrently, the clinic administrator was negotiating with the director of the adjacent detention center regarding servicing the inmates. One of the detention center's primary needs was immediate service, including prescriptions for a very transient, mobile clientele who might be at the jail for only 1 to 2 hours per day. A contract with the detention center would generate a large amount of work and a positive image for the clinic; however, this agreement could not be made if the APNs could not independently dispense medications. The roadblock put up by the medical director (e.g., not allowing nurse practitioners to autonomously prescribe new medications) was overturned. The medical director attended a meeting to discuss the role of the APNs and the state's APN practice act. This meeting resulted in a better understanding of the APN role overall and an expanded mission for the nurse practitioner–run clinic, outcomes that never would have been achieved had it not been for the roadblock regarding autonomous prescription writing.

Thus, it is important for each nurse to think positively, speak in possibilities, and not give up. Each and every nurse must work toward accomplishing an organization's vision and being part of the change initiative in order for a successful outcome to be realized. Evidence suggests that much leadership development of individuals occurs on-the-job through everyday relationships and typical daily assignments (Van Velsor, McCauley, & Ruderman, 2010). Additionally, one must be totally imaginative when developing a vision and "think big" because this first vision must be seen as something in process that will evolve into a new vision or expand to include more ideas as time goes by. It seems essential that nurses realize that their most promising possibility of accomplishing a vision is to find ways to encourage many people to fit this vision into their own trajectory. These people will then have a reason to "buy into" the vision and totally invest their energy and resources to work toward obtaining it. Additionally, nurses can see that the ultimate success falls to all who were invested in the work it took to implement the vision and that now each and every individual nurse must activate her or his own possibilities generated by the main vision (McCloughton, O'Brien, & Jackson, 2010).

> *The secret of leadership is . . . far-sightedness: gazing beyond the visible to the potential on the horizon.*
> —J. Donald Walters

Actualizing a Vision

Many leaders have demonstrated the importance of being flexible or being able to accept some unforeseen change in plans in order to actualize one's vision. When Bill Gates and Paul Allen founded Microsoft Corporation in 1975, their vision was to have a computer in every home, office, and school. Gates was a college student at the time, but he was able to visualize a new role for computers in our personal lives. He took a leave from his undergraduate program at Harvard to follow his dream, and he took risks, used his creative talent, convinced others, and kept pursuing his dream. Today, Gates is in his early 40s, and his company is the leading worldwide provider of personal computer software with revenues of $11 billion annually. If he had not left school and risked pursuing his vision with Paul Allen, Bill Gates may have never actualized his dream, and computers would not have as dramatically changed the world as we have witnessed in recent years. Such is the power of dreams—of visions (Manes & Andrews, 1993).

Mother Teresa, winner of a Nobel Peace Prize in 1979, founded the Missionaries of Charity in Calcutta, India. She had to make a difficult decision to leave the order of nuns to which she belonged at the time in order to follow her vision—"helping the poorest of the poor while living among them" (LeJoly, 1983, p. 26). Mother Teresa worked from morning to night helping the poor and guiding the nuns who joined her to fulfill her vision. She was not satisfied with her purpose on Earth as a nun in her original order, which felt like the status quo for her, so she took risks, used her creative talent, convinced others, and kept pursuing her dream, even without any funding. Mother Teresa founded a whole new order of sisters, provided exquisite care to the world's poor, and made the world more conscious of the needs of millions of fellow human beings. Such is the power of dreams—of visions.

Kouzes and Posner (2007) describe leaders who can "envision the future as being people who can 1. Find a common purpose, and 2. Imagine the possibilities" (pp. 105–106). Parse (2009) says that with "innovative visionary leadership and a plan to advance the nursing profession there is no need to have a practice research gap" (p. 198). By using nursing theory, guided research, and practice, nurses can practice consistently with current evidence-based guidelines. Many (Conger, 1989; Kotter, 1990; Kotter, 2008) believe that a leader's most significant function is to produce a change that cannot actually be identified as it transpires step by step but is more of a feeling that people grab onto, attempt to implement, and then share serendipitously! This perspective is most congruent with the new leadership, which suggests it would be nonproductive to be too orderly and attempt to implement a vision in a step-by-step fashion because it is unlikely that no change would occur with such a linear approach.

> *Vision without action is merely a dream. Action without vision passes the time. Vision and action can change the world.* —Joel Barker

Porter-O'Grady and Malloch (2011) believe the pace of change in and the advancement of an organization or group strongly correlate to the underlying vision that guides it. Although these authors hesitate to recommend short-term goal setting because they are proponents of the new science of leadership, they do advocate that managers become leaders and break down the barriers of the bureaucratic organizational structure that is so prevalent. Perhaps then, and only then, will leaders and followers be successful in owning a vision that does not suggest a lockstep approach to achievement, but rather suggests an approach that is open to possibilities and creative decision making. Conger (1989) suggested that one positive advantage of having a vision is that it brings people a "sense of contribution to themselves, to an industry, or to a society," and "draws workers together as a team" (p. 43). To share the same vision, the leader must inspire followers, and the leader must value the followers' contributions (Kotter, 1990). Recognition for an extraordinary job in the form of an award, public announcement, or financial reimbursement may assist the follower to connect better to the overall vision.

An excellent example of a leader who had a dream, motivated others, and made followers feel as if they owned the dream was Dr. Martin Luther King, Jr. His "I Have a Dream" speech, delivered on August 28, 1963, at the Lincoln Memorial in Washington, DC, is a testament to the power of a vision and how it can energize people toward action (see http://www.americanrhetoric.com/speeches/mlkihaveadream.htm).

Dr. King's dream was clearly articulated, and the way he conveyed his vision showed his passion and enthusiasm and how they reflected his inner being. Whether a nurse works in administration, in teaching, or in a clinical role in schools, homes, hospitals, or clinics—or is a student—each has a reason for choosing to become a nurse. That reason may have been to help others, to champion the "underdog," to care for others in need, or to develop health-care programs for all. Perhaps some nurses need to reflect on that original dream and think about how what they are currently doing relates to why they wanted to be nurses in the first place. It is possible that the motivation to enter nursing is still important and drives the nurse to enjoy his or her present work; but it also is possible that the nurse is stuck in a "dead end" or a "rut" and feels unfulfilled. For those who get up day after day without thinking about why, it may be time for a change. Perhaps we need to revitalize ourselves.

By formulating a vision, one can take risks, use creative talents, convince others, and keep pursuing dreams. One can be energized and can make a difference. One may have ideas about how the staffing mix could be more effective, how nurses could better collaborate with other members of the health-care team, or how technology can be used to better improve patient outcomes. Any of these ideas could be the groundwork for a vision or a dream. Sometimes, an idea that starts out as one person's "pet peeve" or "personal agenda"—a computer in every home or school, helping the poorest of the poor, or achieving racial equality—can, if communicated effectively, become a group's quest. However one looks at it, one person's dream can excite others to follow or to envision their own separate piece of a larger vision. It seems that people who have dreams want to make a difference and are willing to do whatever it takes to fulfill those dreams. They believe that it is better to risk potential chaos or even failure than to accept the status quo. In other words, they are leaders in the fullest sense of the term.

Kouzes and Posner (2007, pp. 123–127) suggest that potential leaders use the following framework when clarifying a vision:

- What are some ways to change things for yourself and organization?
- What exactly do you think you want regarding how you go down in history?
- If people could plan their future, how would you do this for yourself and organization?
- What is your passion in life?
- What is the most significant aspect of your work?
- What are your talents?
- Are you enthralled by any issues?
- Do you have a dream?
- What do you foresee occurring in 10 years regarding this dream?
- What is your personal overall plan?

For example, a graduate student in nursing decides to apply for a scholarship. The application asks for the usual information about previous work, grade point average, memberships in professional organizations, and so forth. It then requests that applicants share why they think they should be awarded a scholarship. Using Kouzes and Posner's (2007) framework, this student might focus her application on the following points, emphasizing how obtaining a graduate degree will assist her to grow and make a bigger difference in advocating for health care for all. Her work as a staff nurse is described in terms of tangible patient outcomes, and it is clear that she has made a difference. She notes the creative teams of which she was a member or that she led. She describes research with which she assisted and the protocols she helped develop to create improved patient care. She articulates clearly her reasons for pursuing the role and for which this particular graduate program will prepare her, specifically relating those goals to what she currently does in practice, what topics she will be studying, and what issues in health policy she will be researching that will assist her to accomplish her goals. She describes how she believes the advanced degree will prepare her to work on her passion, which is health policy. She integrates this information into a short vision statement of how this graduate program will prepare her for her ideal dream job. She shares her insights about the health-care system and explains how she thinks she can really make a difference, using examples to maximize her viewpoints. She concludes by writing her goals upon graduation and her expectations for 1, 3, and 5 years after graduation and for her future and the future of nursing. Such an application—with a clearly articulated vision—is likely to be reviewed quite positively by the scholarship selection committee as well as serve as a professional guide for this nurse during the next few years of working on her graduate degree.

What Happens If There Is No Vision?

When people wander aimlessly through their professional and personal lives, they tend not to accomplish the same results as those who are more focused. They may not take advantage of opportunities for professional growth because they were unaware of such opportunities, they did not think they could "measure up" and be successful, and they chose to fulfill a short-term goal instead (e.g., a "vacation of a lifetime") or did not wish to invest the time and energy needed to succeed.

Manfredi (1995) described what she called the art of legendary leadership by telling a story that depicts what can happen if one does not have a vision. Many years ago when the long-term mayor of a village passed away, the town elders gathered to select a successor. They asked for volunteers, and after a short time, three candidates were found. There were no job descriptions or selection criteria, so the elders decided to test the candidates' leadership by placing each in charge of the village for 1 month. The most successful candidate would become the mayor. One candidate believed he should keep the village stable and espoused the motto, "No need to grow, support the status quo." The town was so bored, they let this candidate go. The second candidate believed one must create structure in order to lead, so he developed many rules and regulations to be followed by the people (but not by their leader). Not agreeing with this perspective, the elders had a bonfire and burned all 700 volumes of rules that this candidate had developed. The third candidate believed leaders know what is best for the people and the villagers cannot be trusted to make decisions or develop ideas, so he made all the decisions and never consulted anyone. After 1 month of such rule, the elders decided this candidate also was not suitable. But what to do? All three candidates were rejected. The elders could not come to an agreement about exactly what the role of a leader should be, so they went off and discussed this for awhile. They finally came up with five roles for a leader to possess: "Leaders create visions, leaders create climates, leaders create conflict, leaders create change, and leaders create leaders" (p. 62). Basically, if a person or group does not have a vision, he or she cannot create a climate for conflict, change, and growth. Without conflict, change, and growth, new leaders will not be able to emerge from the group to inspire further conflict, change, and growth, and "the status quo will be perpetuated" by the leader who "knows best for the group" and creates many "rules and regulations."

Who Should Participate in Vision Development?

Bennis (2009) believed that one can learn how to develop a vision, and Manfredi (1995) made the point that anyone, not only the leader, can initiate an idea that is visionary. Everyone needs to integrate her or his individual goals to create an overall vision for a group or organization. For example, a unit with nurses who are attempting to create more evidence-based protocols, use research-based data, and improve care quality can form an Evidence-Based Practice Committee that meets monthly and an active online communication forum to facilitate participation by all staff in accomplishing the vision of providing evidence-based practice.

It is the idea that sparks a vision that is the most significant part of developing a vision, and we all have had creative ideas that have been of great interest to others. Sometimes one individual will express a thought, someone else will add to it, and another person will expand it even more. Soon the entire group is involved in creating the idea. When this happens, change is likely to occur quickly or with minimal barriers. This process can occur when nurses want to develop a new approach to staffing, a philosophy of patient care, or a new nursing-driven protocol. For example, a group of staff nurses are discussing the challenges presented by maintaining the intravenous lines of patients with hard-to-stick veins. One nurse says how difficult she finds having to insert a new line every 4 hours, hurt the patient, and explain to the patient and family over and over again why a restick is necessary. Another nurse suggests that perhaps nurses should have a voice in determining which patients receive routine intravenous access and which receive a more invasive line. Someone else then asserts that nurses should insert the peripherally inserted central catheter (PICC) and manage the patients who have these more invasive lines. The entire group then goes on to talk about quality patient care in general. Thus, the idea of providing nurses with more independence regarding intravenous fluid and medication administration served as the starting point for the even bigger dream of having significantly more nurse-driven protocols so that higher-quality, more cost-effective care can be delivered. In nursing, the direct care providers typically are most aware of what is best for the patient and what would improve the way care is delivered. Such nurses have ideas, dreams, and visions. Sadly, however, they often fail to do anything significant about them. Although it generally falls to the leader to implement a vision, everyone in the group needs to be involved to achieve success.

In a classic article on leaders and vision, Zaleznik (1989) suggests two ways to influence people: (1) help them realize that the proposed change will advance their interests, and (2) influence them to want to succeed for the group or organization, not just for self-recognition and promotion. Both the leader and the followers, therefore, need to be immersed in the process of formulating the vision and integrating it into the day-to-day work of the group. Throughout this process, the leader needs to be available to followers to help them clarify the vision, see how their efforts contribute to the vision, and be passionate about working toward the vision.

Strategies to Assist People With Vision Development

Having positive experiences with trying new things, being involved in new opportunities, and being encouraged to take risks will assist with vision development. In 1991, Sarah Weddington, past counsel for *Roe v. Wade,* delivered a keynote address at the National League for Nursing Annual Convention in which she shared several ideas on how to gain practice in leading. The major focus of her presentation was that a leader must be passionate about what he or she does and must always strive to accomplish his or her dream. The dream must be a product of the ideal and what would have the most positive impact for the future. This perspective clarifies that to be effective, a vision must encompass many perspectives, and it also must be future oriented. Leaders, therefore, must be proactive and not shy away from change. Rather, they need to take time to try different ways, think in a new fashion, and have the confidence to encourage others to share the dream.

Koestenbaum (2002) offers an analysis of what he thinks it takes for people to be successful leaders and how to achieve specific goals. His book, in essence, is a compilation of how to create environments and societies that will facilitate the achievement of goals. Koestenbaum describes his Leadership Diamond Model, which revolves around the concepts of time, democracy, motivation, teamwork, and salesmanship. When analyzing one's leadership ability or contemplating developing new visions, using these concepts to visualize the plan is helpful.

Cohen (2004) emphasizes the importance of being aware of environmental influences and how it sometimes is necessary to change strategy or components of a strategy in order to fulfill goals. He also reminds us that the success of strategy depends on the "judgment and leadership qualities of the individual responsible for the undertaking" (p. vii). He offers 10 essential principles that are helpful when developing and carrying out one's vision:

- Commit fully to a goal. . . . Always invest fully in what you have identified as a goal.
- Seize the initiative and keep it. . . . Grab the opportunity to share your thoughts and maintain the idea's visibility.
- Economize to best use your resources. . . . Think twice before spending so you will have enough resources to fill your needs.
- Use strategic positioning. . . . Think carefully how your new idea or change will affect everyone and how it interacts with every part of the system.
- Do the unexpected. . . . A surprise change (if the change is something that has to occur) is sometimes seen more positively than one that is carefully planned.
- Keep things simple. . . . Always best to follow basic policies when introducing a new initiative.

- Prepare multiple, simultaneous alternatives . . . . Allowing for participant flexibility will increase buy-in by all.
- Take the indirect route to your objective . . . Demonstrate how your goal can be accomplished along with several others.
- Practice timing and sequencing. . . . As one says: timing is everything!
- Exploit your success. . . . Be transparent with successful outcomes so that all participants will see the fruits of their efforts.

Cohen describes realistic examples of strategizing both successfully and unsuccessfully and offers reasonable ideas of how to examine one's plan and make changes both midstream and in crises so that success is the most potential outcome.

> *Harry Truman was right, it's the leaders who shape history. There would have been no United States without Thomas Jefferson, no Third Reich without Adolph Hitler. But no man or woman becomes a leader unless he or she wants to. They've got to have a burning need to get there.* —Robert Ludlum (in The Icarus Agenda, p. 264)

One can learn how to communicate a vision in an articulate and persuasive manner. Conger (1989) suggests that the leader use metaphors and analogies to excite others and that the leader stimulate multiple senses (intellect, emotions, values, and imagination) simultaneously. Abraham Lincoln's powerful words in the Gettysburg Address— "government of the people, for the people, and by the people"—had a much greater impact than if he had said, "government of, for, and by the people" (Conger, 1989, p. 169). Franklin Delano Roosevelt tended to use folk imagery to share his ideas with the citizenry, and he used sports analogies in his fireside chats (Conger, 1989, p. 81); both were concepts with which people could easily relate. Another example of someone who related well at the grassroots level and established trust is Lee Iacocca, former CEO of Chrysler. Iacocca expressed his dream to rebuild the car company and his willingness to give everything it would take when he announced that he would accept a $1.00 salary for the whole year. Such a strategy created a strong identification between Iacocca and the average Chrysler employee, and it demonstrated an extraordinary level of personal commitment to a vision (Conger, 1989, pp. 73–74). In fact, more and more leaders are appreciating the importance of having commitment and passion for work and are "re-infusing passion, zest, and spirit into the workplace" (Bolman & Deal, 2001, p. 6) so that over time a bottom-line focus does not take a toll on employees' motivation, loyalty, and performance.

Although some leaders may be inclined to try to convince others with impressive numbers, Conger (1989) asserts that statistical summaries are uninformative and lack impact because they are colorless. He suggested brief face-to-face comments as being most substantial in getting people to buy into an idea, pursue a vision, or make a change.

Other speech techniques, such as repetition, rhythm, and alliteration, are effective in helping articulate one's vision, as is evident in Martin Luther King, Jr.'s "I Have a Dream" speech. Conger also suggests that one use a loud volume, some body movements, and complete sentences with few pauses between them. It also is helpful to avoid "I think," "I guess," "please," and "thank you." Focusing on the basic message portrays the leader as confident, effective, and someone others would want to follow. In essence, leaders must be able to communicate their vision effectively, a skill that many believe is the most important characteristic of being a leader (Bennis & Nanus, 1997; Nanus, 1992).

Nurses today are knowledgeable and sophisticated. Therefore, nurse leaders must be able to communicate a clear vision but be open to the team's ideas regarding how the vision can be realized. A framework of skills is needed to be successful in articulating, communicating, and propelling a vision. Senge (2006) says that a leader, particularly one in the health-care arena, must be a systems thinker, have shared visioning, facilitate team learning, and have personal mastery. Champy (1995) agrees with Senge's list of competencies for health-care leaders and adds the skills of association, collaboration, communication, and mobilizing others. Drucker (1989) reaffirmed these descriptions of a leader when he articulated the skills of envisioning, coaching, knowing technology, and facilitating. All three of these organizational behaviorists agree on the necessity of a leader having and being able to clearly and effectively communicate the dream, the vision.

Look before you leap ... or you'll find yourself behind.
—Benjamin Franklin

An analogy serves to summarize these ideas about vision. A sailor is returning to port in the middle of a thunderstorm with barely 3 feet of visibility. The best thing the sailor can do is to concentrate on the ultimate destination, not on every foot of sea between him and land. This metaphor can be used in describing the journey a group, organization, or professional takes in reaching a dream. One must constantly look forward even if it takes a long time and a great deal of work and energy to get there. To "keep on track," the leader must help all members of the group feel a sense of ownership and be creative throughout the process of moving toward the vision.

THE PROCESS OF CREATIVITY

The essence of creativity is having the ability to play (Bennis, 2009). Creativity "demands intuition, uncertainty, unconventionality, and individual expression" (Conger, 1989, p. 17). Creativity, as it relates to leaders, occurs when leaders review their experiences to create new ideas (Valiga & Bruderle, 1997). Leadership is about living an entirely new way and changing the status quo type of philosophy that so many people embrace (Kouzes & Posner, 2003). If chaos describes our current reality, as many experts claim, then creativity is one skill we will need to appreciate, develop, and incorporate to successfully navigate this whitewater turbulence. When unexpected events happen, leaders need to use them as learning experiences and not block learning by perceiving surprises as always negative happenings (McDaniel, Jordan, & Fleeman, 2003).

Creativity involves believing that "there is no one answer that is right but many answers that might work" (Wheatley & Kellner-Rogers, 1996, p. 16). Nurses must reframe how they think about their work so that they are more creative, open to a variety of possibilities, and open to options that might lead to successful outcomes. It is always conceivable that some of our options may not work the way we visualize them, but after observing new methods of providing care and determining they are not feasible, we will discover new options that, with some work and feedback from the team, will be even "better" options. These new ideas would never have been created if trying different options was not attempted.

There are multiple Creativity Tests that can be accessed from the Internet. Most give some type of psychometrics on the tool and are free and easily accessible. An example is the *Right Brain vs Left Brain Creativity Test* developed by the Art Institute of Vancouver (2010), which is a multiple-choice screening test containing 54 questions. By taking a Creativity Screening, one can review what kind of traits are considered "creative," and perhaps this knowledge will facilitate some individuals to modify their behaviour so that they take their time to try to use their creativity and not follow the "same ole way everyday."

Perhaps nurses need to become more involved in developing programs for outpatients to attend, writing grants to obtain funding for health promotion programs, educating larger groups of patients, trying different staff mix patterns, being more flexible with time schedules to include 9- or 7-hour shifts depending on unit as well as nurse's needs, developing health-care policies, serving on political action boards, and any number of other activities that will improve health care for people. In other words, nurses will have to become more comfortable with ambiguity and uncertainty so that they can see "new forms take shape, new ideas develop, and new goals fulfilled" (Valiga & Bruderle, 1997, p. 234). Most probably, it is easier to increase creativity by changing conditions in the work setting or home atmosphere than by influencing people to think in a more creative fashion (Csikszentmihalyl, 1996). In other words, it may be easier and more effective to focus on providing a creative ambiance in schools, day-care centers, homes, churches, and work settings than to focus on the process of thinking creatively.

Using reflective practice opens up multidimensional ways of thinking about experiences one has had or will anticipate having. Experts (Bulman & Schutz, 2008; Freshwater, Taylor, & Sherwood, 2008) suggest that reflective practice can influence the way one learns and thinks—and perhaps reflective practice can change people's level of creativity and generally improve their leadership ability. By using reflective practice in a consistent fashion, one should be able to use more creative methods of communication and be more successful in making decisions regarding work-related issues, patient care, and even personal ambitions. Schon (1983) found that individuals tend to make decisions based on their experiences more so than on technical rationality. Types of reflective practice have been defined: "reflecting-in-action," means being able to think intuitively when the time presents, and "reflecting-on-action" being able to retrospectively review how one performed in a previous situation (Schon, 1983). By using reflective practice, individuals can begin to think differently and perhaps in a more creative way. Asking more questions of one's performance, analyzing situations in more depth, applying evidence-based interventions, and conducting more self-evaluation after encounters with colleagues lead to accomplishing the following goals of consistently reflecting on one's practice:

- Think about creating a nursing based theory
- Integrate theory consistently and holistically
- Focus on increasing one's flexibility and confidence
- Create new ways of delivering health that augment patient outcomes (Freshwater et al., 2008)

Reflective practice is a result of having more mindful awareness. The underlying neurophysiology behind this process explains that repetitive use of reflective practice techniques will expand emotional circuits in the brain and further develop an individual's prefrontal cortex (Siegel, 2007). Those who go on to achieve increased mindfulness will augment their resilience, flexibility, and emotional balance. This will undoubtedly influence their ability to be more creative. The more we can increase our neural circuits with reflective practice, the more neuroplasticity or reorganization of neural pathways occurs (Siegel, 2007). This increased neuroplasticity causes expanded passion and knowledge about our work. More often than not, leaders are made, not born, and they accept that the growth process includes making mistakes (Bennis, 2009). This has relevance for the individual nurse who is a leader or an effective follower. It is no longer acceptable for nurses to deal only with the here and now of a specific patient assignment in the hospital or home setting. Nurse leaders need to partner with the patient and form alliances with family members, community groups, and other health-care professionals to provide health teaching, promote self-competence for the patient, and gather relevant data to determine whether desired outcomes are being realized. It is time to change the belief that what is known is all there is, and it is time to change the belief that how things are done has to be the way things continue to be done. Wheatley and Kellner-Rogers (1996, pp. 13–14) challenge us with the following beliefs about life creating itself:

> *Everything is in a constant process of discovery and creating. Everything is changing all of the time: individuals, systems, environments, the rules, and the processes of evolution. Even change changes. Every organism reinterprets the rules, creates exceptions for itself, and creates new rules.*
>
> *Life uses messes to get to well-ordered solutions. Life doesn't seem to share our desires for efficiency or neatness. It uses redundancy, fuzziness, dense webs of relationships, and unending trials and errors to find what works.*
>
> *Life is intent on finding what works, not what's right. It is the ability to keep finding solutions that are important; any one solution is temporary. There are no permanently right answers. The capacity to keep changing, to find what works now, is what keeps any organism alive.*
>
> *Life creates more possibilities as it engages with opportunities. There are no "windows of opportunity," narrow openings in the fabric of space-time that soon disappear forever. Possibilities beget more possibilities; they are infinite.*

Life is attracted to order. It experiments until it discovers how to form a system that can support diverse members. Individuals search out a wide range of possible relationships to discover whether they can organize into a life-sustaining system. ese explorations continue until a system is discovered. This system then provides stability for its members, so that individuals are less buffered by change.

Life organizes around identity. Every living thing acts to develop and preserve itself. Identity is the filter that every organism or system uses to make sense of the world. New information, new relationships, changing environments—all are interpreted through a sense of self. This tendency toward self-creation is so strong that it creates a seeming paradox. An organism will change to maintain its identity.

Everything participates in the creation and evolution of its neighbors. There are no unaffected outsiders. No one system dictates conditions to another. All participate together in creating the conditions of their interdependence.

There is no one right answer to most situations. There is no way anyone can plan for all of the potential problems that might occur when attempting to institute creative and innovative approaches to reach a vision, and there is no room for an "everything has to be right" attitude. It makes no sense waiting for everything to be "just right" before we act because things will continue to change and some sort of acceptable order will emerge.

Perhaps as nurses we should develop our right-brain skills more so that we can be more intuitive, conceptual, and artistic instead of being dominated by the left side of the brain with our logical planning, to-do lists, and conservative perspective. Bennis (2009) suggests we become whole-brain thinkers, using both concrete and abstract ideas. For example, the mindmap of creativity (Fig. 5–1) depicts various actions that a creative person uses. Mindmapping is a method of note taking that could be effective in stimulating our creativity and developing our right-brain skills, as well as stimulating the flow of ideas from our more concrete-thinking left brain. This exercise of illustrating what one reads or sees may be helpful in developing

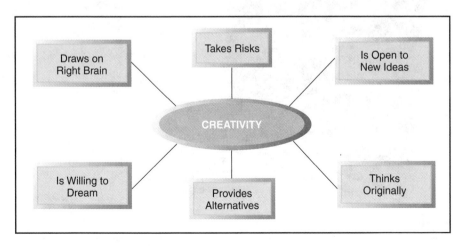

FIGURE 5-1 • Mindmap of creativity.

the whole brain. For example, a nurse may want to show his or her colleagues on the evening staff how they can be more creative in care delivery so that they can actually sit down for a half-hour dinner period. By using Figure 5–1, the nurse can ask each person to write on a whiteboard what they think Creative Care Delivery is. They could then each describe their ideas to the other members of the evening shift. This could spark a dynamic discussion, with a Creative Care Delivery Model evolving that would be more time efficient for their evening work

Think back to when you were in first grade. How do you think your teacher would have reacted if you gave an answer such as the one shown in Figure 5-2? For most of us, the teacher probably would have scolded us for being too right-brained! Nurse educators can assist the profession by designing learning experiences that allow for student creativity and the use of skills governed by both the right and left sides of the brain. In this way, nursing will achieve a better balance of task-oriented left-brain thinkers and creative right-brain thinkers.

Nurses also must focus less energy on and worry less about an unknown future; instead, they should focus more on the opportunities before them today and the possibilities awaiting them tomorrow. Thinking more openly, being more aware of possibilities, and being less structured and more creative will take them a long way. "If we believe that the world is self-organizing, then we don't have to be the organizers; in fact, we don't have to struggle to create networks, affiliations, or teams, . . . groups will just happen" (Wheatley & Kellner-Rogers, 1996, p. 35). The following case study illustrates this point.

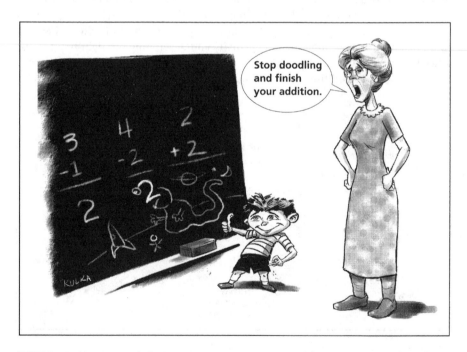

FIGURE 5-2 • Using our right brain.

Case Study

This case depicts how nurses were able to use their creative abilities and energize themselves and colleagues by following their dream.

There was much unhappiness and low morale on the trauma unit where a group of nurses were employed. It was related to strictly enforced role limitations for RNs. Because of the multiple residents rotating through their unit, it was difficult to gain new skills, communicate with physicians, and collaborate with the Intensivists about the challenging cases. The nurse manager was not interested in having an Acute Care Nurse Practitioner and constantly blocked any ideas to hire one. The unit was fairly noncollaborative with the physicians. Nurses took orders from the doctors and were not encouraged to discuss their perceptions or share their knowledge about individual patients.

Three nurses on the unit were interested in becoming Acute Care Nurse Practitioners so that they could achieve more autonomy in their practice. They were matriculated in the same master's program and beginning their clinical component. The hospital's policy was that staff should not do their student rotations at their place of employment, if possible, so the students were assigned to the other level 1 trauma hospital in the city. The three nurse practitioner students observed that the RNs at this other institution had a larger practice scope than the RNs at their original hospital. Because the RNs' role was expanded, their student nurse practitioner role was also expanded and created opportunities for growth that they had never expected. The three students developed and communicated a new vision for their unit with their colleagues, which allowed for an upgrading of the RN role and empowered the RN staff to dispel the "handmaiden mentality."

The staff, led by the three nurse practitioner students, generated multiple changes and soon had an impact on the culture of the unit to such a degree that the nurse manager transferred to another position out of the critical care area. One of the students applied and was promoted to the nurse manager position and led the nurses in creating goals, accomplishing them, gaining new skills and responsibilities, creating new Acute Care Nurse Practitioner roles, and restructuring the unit to become a collaborative practice model. This unit's progress was a result of a team effort, which created a new vision and empowered staff to step up to a new role that eventually involved the entire unit. This is an example of how three nurses' efforts encouraged a whole unit to have ownership in the change process by being energetic, excited, and enthusiastic.

In health care today, the mergers, affiliations, and partnering are necessarily not a bad thing but a natural force—a bringing together of talent; resources; and, one hopes, better patient outcomes. Nurses' ability to be creative and use networking will ultimately allow nurses to survive. Nurses must foster rethinking, discovery, and curiosity as they support change. This is the new way of thinking about leadership, and nurses have to change their way of thinking about their responsibilities.

> *In a self-organizing system, people do for themselves most of what in the past has been done to them. Self-organizing systems create their own structures, patterns of behavior, and processes for accomplishing their work. [These systems are designed to allow what is necessary for the nurses] to do the work. The [participants] agree on behaviors and relationships that make sense to them. Those not directly involved in the doing of their work can give up fussing about designs, believing that our timelines make things happen, or that our training programs change the behavior of the organization.* (Wheatley & Kellner-Rogers, 1996, p. 38)

Nurses can support and trust one another and create possibilities or dreams never thought of before, if they can give up the need to organize every tiny detail, allow themselves to be creative, use their ingenuity, and collaborate with others to maximize creativity.

The Significance of Creativity

Creativity is necessary if nurses are to effectively manage the multitude of changes occurring in health care today and expected to continue well into the future. "Partnering" is a buzzword that to most nurses means a change in responsibilities or a loss of job. Perhaps if more nurses were entrepreneurs, our profession could undergo some serious growth despite the current environment. Being willing to try new things, challenge traditional ways of thinking and behaving, and being open to new ways of thinking will broaden our visions. We cannot let ourselves accept that all "flowers are red [and] green leaves are green" (Chapin, 1978). The words to Harry Chapin's song, "Flowers Are Red," illustrate what can happen when individuals are not allowed to think creatively. Creativity allows one to accomplish his or her visions with excitement and enthusiasm. One gets a resurgence of energy when something new and exciting occurs, or when one has an "a-ha" insight. This energy also comes from change itself, and when that change relates to one's work and what one does, he or she can experience phenomenal growth. "Work comes from the inside out, work is an expression of our soul, our inner being. It's unique to the individual, it's creative" (Fox, 1994, p. 49). Work, therefore, should not be boring, repetitive, tiring, and frustrating. Instead, it should be and can be energizing, challenging, rewarding, and growth producing.

Using Creativity

Nurses have the capacity to use their creative talents to staff units in new ways, research new protocols, administer medications and treatments differently, communicate patient information to other professionals more powerfully, develop materials to market nurses' skills for patients at home, implement support groups for inpatients and outpatients, or build partnerships with clinics or school-based health-care providers. For too long, nurses have been accustomed to staying in the same environment (home, long-term care facility, school, clinic, or hospital) for their entire career. As new roles emerge and new settings provide opportunities for nurses, there is no need to feel stuck or to be stuck. Nurses are becoming more independent as they practice autonomously and in multiple environments. Today, nurses are vital members of multidisciplinary health-team efforts, willing to do things differently, revising protocols to be more patient-oriented, focusing more on measuring patient outcomes, and acting on their concerns about providing quality, cost-effective care.

Zander and Zander (2000) suggest that the way each person sees the world is an indication of whether we see through glasses of scarcity or possibility. If more nurses could use the half-full glass perspective rather than the half-empty glass one, they could serve as powerful role models for future nurses. One study (Grossman, 2004), in fact, demonstrated this very clearly. In a shadowing experience in which students were assigned to work alongside mentor nurses, the researcher found that if the mentor was positive in her thinking, creative in finding new ways to do things, and visionary and goal oriented, students reported having a productive and growth-producing clinical experience.

McCall (1989) suggests some interesting methods by which leaders can use creative strategies to clarify and achieve their visions. By being "feisty," leaders can deliberately create conflicts to spark new ideas between selected, key people and propel their ideas forward. Creative leaders also are "crafty" in that they are politically astute, know how to increase their power base, and can enlist broad support for creative, different pursuits. If creative leaders are to survive, they must be able to disassociate with failure and associate with success. Being creative puts a leader in a bit of danger because it involves taking risks. Using standards of excellence also characterizes a creative leader because one would have to be very demanding to help everyone involved with the new idea meet the highest, most impeccable standards. McCall (1989) also asserts that a creative leader has to act before thinking, rather than think before acting, and has to be inconsistent so that the leader can keep the system "open" for new ideas and changes. Finally, creative leaders must use intuition and hunches so that they do not miss a potentially new way to accomplish the vision. By using these strategies in any nursing role, it would be difficult to become bored with a job, to burn out, or to feel stuck.

Vision is the art of seeing things invisible. —Jonathan Swift

CONCLUSION

There is no doubt that leaders must be passionate about their visions, their dreams of making a significant difference or bettering the world. It is also crucial that leaders be able to persuade people to "grab on" to this vision and become involved in creating change. As Zaleznik (1989) noted, "One cannot be successful without using one's imagination and without being more comfortable with disorder and chaos. In other words, nurses need to avoid the 'If it ain't broke, don't fix it' way of thinking" (p. 62). Change will occur no matter what we do to maintain the existing order. If nurses have articulated worthy visions, become comfortable with the notion of creativity, and if they use creative strategies to achieve their vision, they will thrive from this change, grow personally, and be effective leaders who shape a better world.

CRITICAL THINKING EXERCISES

Read the story "Footprints." How does this relate to creativity? To leadership? To providing leadership and fostering creativity in nursing?

FOOTPRINTS

In a faraway land long ago, there was once a wise and good village chief who had a most exciting announcement. "Of utmost importance," he reminded his villagers, "is the ability to travel to the port to trade our jewelry for food. Until recently those traveling to the port simply left our village and wandered aimlessly until they either found the port or died. I am happy to announce that thanks to the efforts of our wise and most scientific medicine man we have captured the essence of travel. We have discovered that all travel is based on footprints. Follow footprints precisely and you will never get lost going to or from the port again."

"But what about trees?" asked one villager.

"Trees are not footprints, and trees should be ignored," replied the chief.

"May we consider the stars?" questioned another.

"Don't be foolish," commanded the chief. "What could be farther from footprints than stars? Have I not told you already? There is no travel without footprints. Footprints are the essence of travel. Understand footprints, and the concept of travel is yours forever. You will never be lost again."

That was many years ago. And since that time many villagers have come and gone from the port, never taking their eyes off the footprints. Some of the more scholarly villagers over the years have studied and refined footprintology, writing long, scholarly discourses on the many things that footprints show, and of the many truths to be found through scrutiny of footprints.

Over the years the methods of observing footprints have been refined to such an exact science that many years of studying with rigorous examinations are required to truly practice and teach footprintology. In fact, before each young man is able to leave the village he must be thoroughly educated in footprintology as the essence of travel, lest some day he look up at the trees or stars and lose sight of that essence that the wisest of wise know as travel.

Source: Bagley, D. (1979). Footprints (a parable about knowledge). *Journal of Creative Behavior, 13*(4), 286–287.

_____

_____

What is your vision for nursing in general? What is your vision for yourself in your current practice setting? What goals do you have for your own growth as a nurse and for the profession? Which of these goals can be achieved by nurses themselves, and which need external support or action? How can you use Wheatley's (2002) conversation starters to assist you in connecting with others to help you accomplish your vision?

_____

_____

CRITICAL THINKING
EXERCISES—cont'd

Envision your professional goals for the near future and for 3 years down the road. Imagine your long-term goals. Given the chaotic health-care system and changes the nursing profession is experiencing, think about how you need to design your career in order to realize these long-term goals by taking small steps now to lay the footprint for your overall vision.

_____

_____

Think about your current leadership abilities. How can you maximize these skills so that you will be able to accomplish your professional goals and increase your impact on the health-care system? Using reflective practice, describe an example of when you have recently succeeded in making a measurable difference on your unit or in the organization.

- Explain your plan, using at least four objectives, to promote and implement your professional vision.
- Validate your growth over the last 6 months regarding your leadership skills. Are you where you want to be? How can you facilitate more growth in promoting your vision?
- Describe your evaluation outcomes for use in determining whether your vision is successful.

_____

_____

_____

Using Martin Luther King, Jr.'s "I Have a Dream" speech (see http://www.americanrhetoric. com/speeches/mlkihaveadream.htm) or the speeches of other powerful orators (e.g., John F. Kennedy, Margaret Thatcher, Abraham Lincoln), identify communication methods you could use to articulate your dream clearly.

_____

_____

Compare and contrast an experience you've had professionally to Harry Chapin's song "Flowers Are Red." How could you use "every color" to prevent a recurrence? (see http://harrychapin.com/music/flowers.shtml).

_____

_____

Create a mind map of leadership.

_____

_____

References

Art Institute of Vancouver. (2010). Right brain vs left brain creativity test. Retrieved from http://www.wherecreativitygoestoschool.com.

Bagley, D. (1979). Footprints (a parable about knowledge). *Journal of Creative Behavior, 13*(4), 286–287.

Bennis, W. (2009). *On becoming a leader: Leadership classic—updated and expanded* (4th ed.). New York, NY: Perseus Book

Bennis, W., & Nanus, B. (1997). *Leader: Strategies for taking charge* (2nd ed.). New York, NY: Harper & Row.

Bolman, L., & Deal, T. (2001). *Leading with soul: An uncommon journey of spirit* (2nd ed.). San Francisco, CA: Jossey-Bass.

Bulman, C., & Schutz, S. (Eds.) (2008). *Reflective practice in nursing* (4th ed.). Oxford, UK: Wiley & Sons.

Champy, J. (1995). *Reengineering management.* New York, NY: Harper Business.

Chapin, H. (1978). Flowers are red. *Legends of the lost and found album.* The Harry Chapin Archive. Retrieved from http://harrychapin.com/music/flowers

Cohen, W. (2004). *The art of the strategist: 10 essential principles for leading your company to victory.* New York, NY: American Management Associates.

Conger, J. (1989). *The charismatic leader: Behind the mystique of exceptional leadership.* San Francisco, CA: Jossey-Bass.

Covey, S. (2004). *The 8th habit: From effectiveness to greatness.* New York, NY: Free Press.

Csikszentmihalyl, M. (1996). *Creativity flow and the psychology of discovery and intervention.* New York, NY: HarperCollins.

Drucker, P. (1989). *The new realities: In government and politics/in economics and business/in society and world view.* New York: HarperCollins.

Fox, M. (1994). *Reinvention of work: A new vision of livelihood for our time.* San Francisco, CA: Harper.

Freshwater, D., Taylor, B., & Sherwood, G. (2008). *International textbook of reflective practice in nursing.* Oxford, UK: Wiley & Sons.

Goffee, R., & Jones, G. (2006). *Why should anyone be led by you?* Boston, MA: Harvard Business School Press.

Grossman, S. (2004). Developing leadership through shadowing a leader in health care. In H. Feldman & M. Greenberg (Eds.), *Educating for leadership.* New York, NY: Springer.

Institute of Medicine (IOM). (2010). *The future of nursing: Leading change, advancing health.* Retrieved from http://www.IOM.edu/mursing.

King, M. (1963). I have a dream. Retrieved from http://www.americanrhetoric.com/speeches/mlkihaveadream.htm

Koestenbaum, P. (2002). *Leadership: The inner side of greatness.* San Francisco, CA: Jossey-Bass.

Kotter, J. (1990). *A force for change.* New York, NY: Free Press.

Kotter, J. (2008). *A sense of urgency.* Boston, MA: Harvard Business Press.

Kouzes, J., & Posner, B. (2003). *Credibility: How leaders gain and lose it, why people demand it* (2nd ed.). San Francisco, CA: Jossey-Bass.

Kouzes, J., & Posner, B. (2007). *The leadership challenge* (4th ed.). San Francisco, CA: Jossey-Bass.

LeJoly, E. (1983). *Mother Teresa of Calcutta.* New York, NY: Harper & Row.

Manes, S., & Andrews, P. (1993). *Gates: How Microsoft's mogul reinvented an industry and made himself the richest man in America.* New York, NY: Doubleday.

Manfredi, C. (1995). The art of legendary leadership: Lessons for new and aspiring leaders. *Nursing Leadership Forum, 1*(2), 62–64.

McBride, A. B. (2010). *The growth and development of nurse leaders.* New York, NY: Springer.

McCall, M. (1989). Conjecturing about creative leaders. In W. E. Rosenbach & R. L. Taylor (Eds.), *Contemporary issues in leadership* (2nd ed., pp. 111–120). Boulder, CO: Westview Press.

McCloughlin, A., O'Brien, L., & Jackson, D. (2010). More than vision: Imagination as an elemental characteristic of being a nurse leader-mentor. *Advances in Nursing Sciences, 33*(4), 285–296.

McDaniel, R., Jordan, M., & Fleeman, B. (2003). Surprise, surprise, surprise! A complexity science view of the unexpected. *Health Care Management Review, 28*(3), 266–278.

Melnyk, B. M., & Davidson, S. (2009). Creating a culture of innovation in nursing education via a shared vision, leadership, interdisciplinary partnerships, and positive deviance. *Nursing Administration Quarterly, 33*(4), 288–295.

Nanus, B. (1992). *Visionary leadership.* San Francisco, CA: Jossey-Bass.

Parse, R. R. (2009). Visionary leadership: Making a difference in health care through research. *Nursing Science Quarterly, 22*(3), 197–198.

Porter-O'Grady, T., & Malloch, K. (2011). *Quantum leadership: Advancing innovation, transforming health care* (3rd ed.). Sudbury, MA: Jones and Bartlett.

Schon, D. (1983). *The reflective practitioner: How practitioners think in action.* New York, NY: Basic Books.

Senge, P. (2006). *The fifth discipline: The art and practice of the learning organization* (2nd ed.). New York, NY: Doubleday Currency.

Siegel D. (2007). *The mindful brain.* New York, NY: W. W. Norton.

Tanner, C. (2006). Thinking like a nurse: A research based model of clinical judgment in nursing. *Journal of Nursing Education, 45*(6), 204–211.

Valiga, T., & Bruderle, E. (1997). *Using the arts and humanities to teach nursing: A creative approach.* New York, NY: Springer.

Van Velsor, E., McCauley, C. D., & Ruderman, M. N. (Eds). (2010). *The center for creative leadership handbook of leadership development* (3rd ed.). San Francisco, CA: Jossey-Bass.

Weddington, S. (1991). Leaders are made not born (the Novello Lecture). Presented at the National League for Nursing Convention, Nashville, TN, June 1991.

Wheatley, M. (2002). *Turning to one another: Simple conversations to restore hope to the future*. San Francisco, CA: Berrett-Koehler.

Wheatley, M., & Kellner-Rogers, M. (1996). *A simpler way*. San Francisco, CA: Berrett-Koehler.

Zaleznik, A. (1989). Why managers lack vision. *Business Month, 8,* 59–64.

Zander, R., & Zander, B. (2000). *The art of possibility*. Boston, MA: Harvard Business School Press.

CHAPTER 6

Gender Perspectives in Leadership

LEARNING OBJECTIVES

- Explore commonalities and differences between "feminine leadership" and "masculine leadership."
- Describe barriers women face when exercising leadership in organizations.
- Examine the concept of androgyny as it relates to leadership.
- Compare "web" organizations with "hierarchical" ones.
- Propose strategies that women and men can use to enhance their effectiveness as leaders in organizations.

INTRODUCTION

Most studies about leaders and leadership focus on men and the male perspective. Although this information is valuable, and much of what we know about leadership—the need to have a vision, the reciprocal relationship between leaders and followers, the willingness to take risks, and so on—has broad applicability, it still is rooted largely in a masculine framework. A growing body of literature, however, notes differences in the ways women lead (Austin, 2002; Babcock & Laschever, 2003; Felder, 1996; Gordon, 1991; Grunwald, 1992; Helgesen, 1990a; Kaufman & Grace, 2011; Keohane, 2010; Klenke, 1996; Kram & Hampton, 1998; Lambert & Gardner, 2009; Lipman-Blumen, 1992; Long, 1998; May, 2001; Melia & Lyttle, 1986; Paludi & Coates, 2011; Rosener, 1990; Salas-Lopez, Deitrick, Mahady, Gertner, & Sabino, 2011; Schein, 1989; Sylvia, Grund, Kimminau, Ahmed, Marr, & Cooper, 2010; Yukl, 2010). Because most nurses are women, understanding gender perspectives in leadership is an essential area of exploration.

109

This chapter explores some of the typical stereotypes about differences between men and women and how they translate into (1) differences in each gender's approach to leadership and (2) different types of organizational structures that best fit with each approach. This chapter also examines similarities in the way women and men lead, as well as ways in which the best of both gender perspectives can be combined to create a truly effective leader.

COMMON GENDER DIFFERENCES

Leaders reflect the values, norms, strengths, and weaknesses of their groups and, indeed, of the larger society. Although this is usually considered a strength and an advantage, it can present a challenge for a female leader functioning in "a man's world," who may be sent to "Bully Broad Boot Camp" if she is too aggressive (Austin, 2002).

"Maleness" often is associated with concepts such as dominance, independence, objectivity, rationality, competitiveness, aggressiveness, boldness, decisiveness, toughness, being logical, and being "thing-oriented." Because these terms are typically associated with leadership, masculine traits often are equated with effective leadership skills (Kellerman & Rhode, 2006; Stivers, 1991). "Femaleness," on the other hand, typically is associated with ideas that are not aligned with leadership, ideas such as compliance, dependence, emotionality, weakness, acceptance, passivity, nurturance, and being "people-oriented."

As noted by Yukl (2010), "leaders whose actions display humility, compassion, or conciliation are more likely to be viewed as weak and ineffective in a 'masculine' culture" (p. 444). And "most political philosophers and innumerable ordinary folk have simply assumed that women are incapable of leadership" (Keohane, 2010, p. 123). Comparisons such as those noted in Table 6–1 often are made in jest, but the basis of them is all too real for women in many arenas.

TABLE 6–1 A Businessman Versus a Businesswoman

BUSINESSMAN	BUSINESSWOMAN
A businessman is aggressive.	A businesswoman is pushy.
A well-dressed businessman is fashionable.	A well-dressed businesswomen is a "clotheshorse."
He loses his temper because he's so involved with his job.	She's "bitchy."
He's a man of the world.	She's "been around."
He's confident.	She's conceited.
He's enthusiastic.	She's emotional.
He's careful about details.	She's picky.
He's depressed , so everyone tiptoes past his office.	She's moody, so it must be "her time of the month."
He follows through.	She doesn't know when to quit.
He's firm.	She's stubborn.
He makes wise judgments.	She reveals her prejudices.
He isn't afraid to say what he thinks.	She's opinionated.
He exercises authority.	She's tyrannical.
He's discreet.	She's secretive.
He's a stern taskmaster.	She's difficult to work for.

The Gender Divide

Although it is no longer remarkable to find women in positions of authority, power, and leadership, many women in the workforce still are clustered at the bottom of the employment "heap" (e.g., clerical jobs and low-paying professional jobs). And although women often have influence, few, as noted by Keohane (2010, p. 125), "have exercised authority in institutional settings over men and women of comparable social and economic status." Most individuals with political influence are men, and organizational heads tend not to be women.

Women and men alike sometimes comment that women are taught and encouraged to master only a few skills rather than the broad range needed to function effectively in today's complex and ever-changing world. They then become limited in what they can do, the opportunities they can pursue, and the breadth or possibly even the significance of contributions they can make to an organization or to the attainment of a goal. Ultimately, their opportunities for advancement, personal growth, and leadership are limited.

About 15 years ago, women filled nearly one third of all management roles, most of which were positions with relatively little power and authority. And in health care, "as of 1999, women simply [were] not present in senior management positions to the extent that we would expect when 85 percent of U.S. healthcare workers are female" (Robinson-Walker, 1999, p. 3). More recently, Yukl (2010, p. 448) goes so far as to say that "widespread discrimination is clearly evident in the low number of women who hold important, high-level leadership positions in most types of organizations."

Some argue that this "gender divide" (Babcock & Laschever, 2003) is widening, but others claim that women are making significant strides in providing leadership in our society. Oprah Winfrey has influenced millions around the world, Vera Wang has changed the way we think about fashion, Condoleezza Rice and Hillary Rodham Clinton have demonstrated the ability to influence affairs of state, and women hold close to one third of the top management jobs at Xerox, including that of CEO. There is no doubt that women are exercising influence in many parts of the world, but those numbers are still relatively small.

Barriers to Female Leaders

Reasons why there have been a limited number of women exercising leadership are many. Society does not expect and value leadership in women, and they typically are not socialized as leaders. There are few women leader role models, and women who do try to exert strong leadership behaviors sometimes are discriminated against and not supported in those efforts. It also has been claimed that women fear success and that they are fearful of competition. Although women typically are quite expert at multitasking and managing successfully with limited resources, they often are afraid to ask for things they need (Babcock & Laschever, 2003) and often are willing to settle for what they are given.

Many of these reasons were borne out in a study undertaken by Salas-Lopez and colleagues (2011), who examined reasons for "the persistent lag of women as leaders" (p. 34). Using a case study method, they conducted semistructured interviews of seven women physicians to better understand the challenges they faced as they aspired to leadership positions in medicine (clinical environments) and academic medicine (medical school and clinical environments). The way these women identified core attributes of successful leaders was congruent with what is described in the literature—visionary, an ability to inspire others to follow, drive and perseverance, good communication skills, commitment to core values (e.g., integrity, honesty, and fairness), self-awareness, and courage—so they understood the phenomenon. But all believed they had to work harder than their male counterparts and continually "prove" themselves, that family responsibilities affected them differently than was the case for their male colleagues, and that having mentors was extremely beneficial, though mentors were sometimes difficult to find. The researchers conclude by acknowledging that women will "continue to pour into the American workforce and . . . their representation in leadership positions within medicine and academic medicine will become more prominent" (p. 41). Despite the challenges to exercising leadership in their fields, these researchers also noted that "the most optimistic scenario is that women in leadership positions will soon form a critical mass that will allow them to make the very bold changes needed for advancement" (p. 41).

In one study of women who participated in a grassroots organization's leadership training program, the researchers (Kaufman & Grace, 2011) found that these women believed gender-related obstacles were preventing them from being effective leaders. They reported facing persistent stereotypes and bias, feeling separated and isolated from male participants, being frustrated by the seemingly static and "clique-like" nature of the male-dominated board, and being frustrated by the unwillingness of the organization to change or appreciate the added value women and new voices could bring to the organization.

Frustrations regarding opportunities to exercise leadership or to do so in a different way do not arise solely from males, however. Women often make it difficult for one another, often through what has been referred to as the "Queen Bee syndrome," a term first used in 1973 (Staines, Travis, & Jayerante) to describe women in positions of authority who view or treat subordinates more critically if they are female and who have succeeded in their careers but refuse to help other women do the same. When this syndrome is operating, women who have "made it" or are "at the top" want to be only with men, want to keep other women down, and downplay the concerns expressed by women who are trying to succeed with comments such as, "I did it without much help; why can't you?"

Many women, however, have challenged the "system," overcome fears, fought vigorously for resources, dealt with the "Queen Bees," and obtained the education, training, and skills needed to compete effectively and move into positions of power and leadership. As a result, these hard-working, ambitious women may be seen as a threat to men and to other women, and have their "every move scrutinized, dissected, poured over, interpreted and reinterpreted" (Austin, 2002, p. 57). Therefore, they need to invest energy into dealing with all the stereotype issues (e.g., being perceived as threats or as not being "real" women), as well as dealing with the issues inherent in the job itself (e.g., improving the bottom line or producing a product before the competition does).

Socialization and Gender Differences

The challenges that women face in pursuing leadership roles are clearly related to early socialization as nurturers, caregivers, and team members, as well as assumptions made about what is appropriate for girls and boys (e.g., "boys don't cry or play with dolls," and "girls are emotional and prefer more isolated play activities rather than competitive team sports"). Relationships develop based on these assumptions; they become deeply ingrained over time through experiences such as school (American Association of University Women, 1992), and socialization along these lines continues throughout adulthood. It is the woman, for example, who is more likely to struggle to balance work, family responsibilities, and other commitments because—even though changes continue to be made toward greater sharing of responsibilities—our society continues to allow the male partner to emphasize the work or professional role while expecting the female partner to "do it all."

> *Women tend to stick it out too long and just try to work harder for recognition.* —Marie Wunsch

Women who attempt to break away from these stereotypes are often regarded as "deviant" (Vance, 1979). Deviance is thought to occur when an individual varies too widely from the norm and fails to obey group rules. It is considered essentially pathological and a symptom of social disorganization. Thus, women who assert themselves as leaders may be viewed negatively by the larger society.

Even women who *do* achieve high positions and exert significant influence may be viewed with less credibility and respect than their male counterparts, and male and female peers alike may criticize them. Women leaders also may be considered inferior and "second class." Despite these challenges, however, women bring a unique dimension to leadership roles.

Current research suggests that "it is not our genes or our hormones but our situation" (Keohane, 2010, p. 148) that influences how we act as leaders. How we are brought up as children and treated as adults—in other words, how we are socialized—has a profound influence on who we are as leaders. Perhaps our energies would be better spent by focusing on ways in which girls and boys learn together and play together so that the socialization of both is directed toward development as leaders, rather than "female leaders" or "male leaders."

WAYS OF LEADING

Distinctions between men and women often are outlined in a humorous way (as noted in Table 6–1). And there is validity in the warning that because "leadership is such a multifaceted, complex phenomenon that generalizations about *all* leaders or *all* women leaders [emphasis added] cannot survive scrutiny" (Keohane, 2010, p. 128). However, differences between the styles of men and women and the way they lead have been reported.

Alpha and Beta Leadership

For example, the "alpha" and "beta" types of leadership described in a classic work by Levenstein (1981) may be aligned with masculine and feminine leadership. According to this author, *alpha leadership* is analytical, relies heavily on rationale, is quantitative, relies on hierarchical relationships, and favors engineered solutions. It is a style that thrives on competitive challenges and sees power as a goal. In comparison, *beta leadership* is intuitive, qualitative, and concerned about growth. It relies on support relationships and is future-oriented. It is a style in which power is seen as a means to a goal that has relevance for the members of the group and those served by the group, rather than a goal in and of itself or a means to a goal that has relevance only for the leader. Alpha leadership might be more closely aligned with a male perspective, and beta leadership might be more reflective of female leadership.

> *Transformational leadership feels right to women because it's not asking anything that they haven't done.* —Jacquelyn M. Belcher

Robinson-Walker's (1999) study of nearly 100 women and men responsible for managing a significant portion of America's health care supported such findings. In addition, she reported on work done by the sociologist Neuhauser who noted in 1988 that "'tribal' membership profoundly affects values and behavior within organizations, and the most basic tribes are those of males and females. Even if men and women share the same values, Neuhauser suggests their thinking is organized differently, which results in different expressions of that thinking" (Robinson-Walker, 1999, p. 29).

> *Women and leadership have always made for an uneasy alliance.* —Nancy Austin

The Feminine Advantage

Such differences in thinking and leadership styles can have significant ramifications, as was pointed out in a brief piece related to military force (*Sexes differ on military force,* 1985). This piece asserted that having more women in the House and Senate could significantly alter decision making in the American political arena. It reported on the work of two Canadian researchers, who concluded that women were less likely than men to support funding for nuclear weapons and missile testing and more likely to favor deterrence through disarmament rather than a cold war. Men, these researchers noted, not only tended to be more "pro-force" than women but also tended to see military defense issues in more "simplistic terms." Women tended to view the same issues from a more complex, "holistic" perspective that included the "human dimension." These researchers concluded that men and women organized their thoughts differently: "If nothing else, males had a much simpler perspective on things and tended to see issues in black and white terms . . . but women saw shades of gray" (*Sexes differ on military force,* 1985, p. 7). Although cold war issues are not the major concern in our society that they were in 1985 when this report was issued, conflict, crisis, change, and war remain significant factors in our lives. Therefore, the findings of this study regarding women's perspectives, their tendency to be more nurturing and "other-oriented," the factors that enter into their decision making, and the ways in which their thinking and potential leadership differ from men are worth noting.

Rosener (1990) described four major areas of difference in style exhibited by the women leaders she studied: (1) they tended to encourage participation; (2) they shared power and information quite readily; (3) they were concerned about enhancing the self-worth of others; and (4) they worked to energize others. This is consistent with other descriptions of women leaders as nurturing, caring, intimate, "more sensitive to the needs of other people, less competitive and more collaborative" (Keohane, 2010, p. 129); it also is consistent in its contrast to descriptions of male leaders as valuing autonomy, objectivity, and fairness. Rosener's work also supports men's tendency to use the power of their position in transactional exchanges (e.g., exchanging rewards for services rendered or punishment for poor performance).

These differences are supported by Helgesen (1990a), whose research revealed several dimensions in which women offer perspectives and reflect values that are a source of their uniqueness and their strength. Women, she says, value "an attention to process instead of a focus on the bottom line; a willingness to look at how an action will affect other people instead of simply asking, 'What's in it for me?'; a concern for the wider needs of the community; a disposition to draw on personal, private sphere experience when dealing in the public realm; an appreciation of diversity; [and] an outsider's impatience with rituals and symbols of status that divide people who work together and so reinforce hierarchies" (pp. xx–xxi).

Such attributes of women leaders also were supported in a study of several hundred women in the Houston area (May, 2001). These researchers found that the following six factors emerged as the most important skills and attributes of leaders, as identified by the women who participated in the study:

- **Personal integrity:** being guided by ethical standards and a moral compass; being trustworthy and credible
- **Strategic vision/action orientation:** finding the path; seeing possibilities and the big picture; crafting and communicating a vision, a preferred future
- **Team building/communication skills:** building coalitions, teams, and consensus; communicating clearly and directly; promoting debate and encouraging discussion; acknowledging the contributions of everyone
- **Management and technical competencies:** making decisions; thinking critically; solving problems; being technically proficient
- **People skills:** demonstrating respect, cultural sensitivity, and an ability to inspire others; allowing followers to make mistakes; sharing information; advocating for others
- **Personal survival skills:** being politically sensitive; possessing an entrepreneurial spirit, being comfortable with competitiveness, self-direction, and self-reliance; demonstrating candor and courage

This study concluded that women need to view themselves as leaders with something to offer the community, for "when women 'sit at the table,' the manner of discussion changes and different priorities are frequently set [which] enable the discussion to become more inclusive" (p. 122). Similar conclusions have been offered by Kunin (as cited in Keohane, 2010, p. 132), who pointed out that "gender differences affect policy because women bring different life experiences into the debate. They change conversations."

The women in Sylvia and colleagues' study (2010) saw themselves as leaders in their rural communities, though few exercised that leadership through elected or political positions. In this study of women in rural Kansas, the researchers set out to identify factors that influenced these women to take on a leadership role. They acknowledged that there are many opportunities for leadership in rural areas because leadership "relies on influence—made possible by repeated interactions and development of trust—to get things done" (p. 23) and wanted to learn what helped certain women "step up to the plate" to provide such leadership. The 133 participants in this qualitative study that used interviews reported that they enabled members of the community to act together to pursue shared objectives, built coalitions, and developed social capital in their communities. The researchers concluded that the following themes described these women and helped determine their success as leaders in their rural communities:

- They were lifelong learners who continued to grow and gain skills as they aged.
- They were flexible with their leadership skills, able to multitask, and not limited by the biases or discrimination they faced.
- They felt a strong sense of responsibility to the community as a whole and worked to ensure that everyone was involved.
- They saw themselves as being able to determine their future by their own efforts and were confident in their ability to succeed, yet they were humble about these strengths.
- Their mentors were likely to be their parents, grandparents, and teachers who instilled in them a strong sense of value and integrity.

Although Sylvia and colleagues' study (2010) did not attempt to compare women and men leaders, it does point out characteristics of women leaders in rural areas and factors that influenced their development and success as leaders.

In the continuation of his seminal work on megatrends, Naisbitt (1982) partnered with a female forecaster to address 10 "new directions" for the 1990s (Naisbitt & Aburdene, 1990). One of the trends they predicted for the last decade of the 20th century was that it would be the "decade of women in leadership" (p. 216). These authors asserted that as individuals and organizations continue to evolve, they demand true leadership—leadership that respects people, encourages individuals to grow and contribute significantly, inspires commitment, and "empower[s] people by sharing authority" (p. 219). The individual who will provide this kind of leadership is a "self-developer" (a term initially proposed by Maccoby, 1981), "an individual who values independence, dislikes bureaucracies, and seeks to balance work with other priorities like family and recreation" (Naisbitt & Aburdene, 1990, p. 221), as well as a "teacher, facilitator, and coach" (p. 227). Women, these authors say, are extremely well positioned to function in such roles. The last decade of the 20th century is far behind us, but the ideas expressed by Naisbitt and Aburdene (about qualities needed in leaders and the fact that women often possess such qualities) are still valid points for reflection.

> *A true leader has the confidence to stand alone, the courage to make tough decisions, and the compassion to listen to the needs of others. He does not set out to be a leader, but becomes one by the quality of his actions and the integrity of his intent. In the end, leaders are much like eagles ... they don't flock, you find them one at a time.* —Anonymous

Book (2000) agreed. In her study of 14 of the most powerful women in American business, she found that these organizational leaders fostered a more collegial environment, played down their own egos, led "from the ground up" (p. 235), and displayed empathy, all of which engendered loyalty from and the respect of those with whom they worked. This researcher concluded that while women were better at communicating, empowering others and being positive, they also were "more decisive [and] better at planning and . . . facilitating change than men" (p. xv). Overall, Book (2000) concluded, "Evidence is mounting that the style of leadership women offer is beneficial not only to employees but also to the bottom line" (p. xv).

The perspectives and evidence cited here contribute to what has been referred to in the leadership literature as the "feminine advantage" theory, proponents of which contend that "women are more concerned with consensus building, inclusiveness, and interpersonal relations; they are more willing to develop and nurture subordinates and share power with them" (Yukl, 2010, p. 450). Caution must be taken, however, to examine the assumptions underlying this theory, whether or not gender stereotypes are exaggerated, and what the findings of empirical research show.

Web and Hierarchical Structures

Without question, women have made important contributions to how we think about the way organizations can and should work. For example, women-run organizations often reflect a "web" structure (Helgesen, 1990a, 1990b), rather than a pyramid or typical hierarchical one.

Helgesen (1990a) reported that the women in business whom she had studied tended to disdain the hierarchical ladder and preferred to create webs rather than pyramids. In these webs, the leader is in the center of things, rather than at the top, which these women perceived as "a lonely and disconnected position" (p. 13). Webs allow everyone in the organization to be connected by invisible strands that emanate from the central goal or mission, and they value affiliation and win/win situations instead of intense competition and win/lose situations. In such a structure, "talent is nurtured and encouraged rather than commanded, . . . a variety of interconnections exist, influence and persuasion take the place of giving orders, . . . the lines of authority are less defined, [there is more dependence] upon a moral center, [and] compassion, empathy, inspiration, and direction"

(p. 225) all play significant roles. Finally, webs allow the group to take full advantage of every person's talents and skills, permit a more effective exchange of information, and minimize conflicts that arise from misunderstanding or lack of communication.

This type of "connective leadership" (Lipman-Blumen, 1992) is endorsed as a style that fits with today's organizations. It incorporates networking, relationship building, empowerment, and mutual responsibilities between the leader and followers.

Leadership in this kind of organization encourages interdependence, increased involvement of all members of the group, communication, and consensus, all of which are needed in the chaotic world of today and tomorrow. Helgesen (1990a, 1992) asserted that women possess the skills, perspectives, and values needed to engage in this type of leadership. Indeed, in contrast to the Great Man Theory of leadership, which claims that some men are born leaders, Weddington (1991) asserted, "some leaders are born women." One would expect, therefore, that women will continue to assume stronger positions of leadership as we progress in the 21st century.

COMBINING THE BEST OF FEMALENESS AND MALENESS

Research on gender and leadership yields conflicting findings about whether or not one gender or the other is more effective in leadership roles. As summarized by Yukl (2010), some reviewers conclude that there is no evidence of important gender differences in leadership behaviors or skills; and others conclude that there are gender-related differences for *some* behaviors or *some* skills in *some* situations. Indeed, the issue is complex, and there are no easy answers to the question of who is more effective as a leader.

Work and Family Interface

Schein (1989) cautioned us to be careful when talking about "feminine leadership" and said that the assumption that women lead differently than men is dangerous and perpetuates sex role stereotyping. She reported that research shows more differences within each sex than between the sexes, noting, "as individuals, executive women and men seem to be virtually identical psychologically, intellectually and emotionally" (Morrison, White, & Velsor, as cited in Schein, 1989, p. 156). This author did suggest, however, that women might lead differently if our organizational systems were changed, and she urged America's corporate executives to restructure the work setting so that work and family are no longer separate but interface, a model similar to the one that exists in Norway and is quite successful. For example, if either parent needs to pick children up at school in the afternoon, the workday is structured to accommodate this "out of the office" responsibility.

In a work setting that values both career and family and that is more understanding of and willing to struggle with accommodating this interface, women would be likely to be more successful (Schein, 1989). In light of women's tendency to prefer "webs" to "pyramids" in the work setting and in other arenas (Helgesen, 1990a, 1990b) and the growing number of women-run businesses that reflect this organizational approach, we may, indeed, see the emergence of women as major players in making significant changes in our society, as Naisbitt and Aburdene (1990) suggested more than 20 years ago.

Androgynous Leadership

The new leadership paradigm that is emerging (and will continue to be needed in the complex, chaotic future) calls for individuals who facilitate interaction among leaders and followers, who empower followers, and who can successfully combine "maleness" and "femaleness" as an androgynous leader (Cann & Siegfried, 1990; Lipman-Blumen, 1992; Park, 1997; Schein, 1989). The androgynous leader blends dominance, assertiveness, and competitiveness—all of which are needed in a world where resources are increasingly limited—with concern for relationships, cooperativeness, and humanitarian values, which also are needed in a world characterized by chaos, uncertainty, and ambiguity. Box 6–1 suggests what women and men both need to do in order to be androgynous, and the case study illustrates the different styles of a male and a female unit manager, as well as how each adopted characteristics of the other to enhance her or his effectiveness as a leader in the institution.

BOX 6-1 **Becoming Androgynous**

For women to be androgynous, they need to:
- Be powerful, forthright, and have a direct, visible impact on others.
- Be entrepreneurial.
- State their needs and refuse to back down.
- Recognize the equal importance of accomplishing the task and being concerned about the relationship.
- Build support systems with other women and take collective action.
- Be able to intellectualize and generalize.
- Deal directly with anger and blame, thereby rejecting feelings of suffering and victimization. Be invulnerable to destructive feedback.
- Talk and cry at the same time.
- Respond directly with "I" statements rather than "you" statements.
- Be analytical and systematic and share abstract models.
- Take more risks with power.
- See themselves as agents of change.
- Continue to be supportive and passionate, and become more autonomous and independent.

For men to be androgynous, they need to:
- Understand how men value women—as validators of masculinity, as a haven from the competitive male world, as the expressive partner in the relationship.
- Be aware of how physical and political power determine behavior.
- Openly express feelings of love, fear, anger, pain, joy, loneliness, and dependency.
- Personalize experience as opposed to relying on objectivity and rationality.
- Build support systems with other men, sharing competencies without competition and sharing feelings and needs.
- Learn how to fail at a task without feeling one has failed as a man.
- Value an identity that is not totally defined by work.
- Assert the right to work for self-fulfillment rather than to play the role of provider.
- Listen empathetically and actively without feeling responsible for problem solving.
- Enjoy friendships with both men and women.

Case Study

Natalie and Sean were nurse managers on different units of the local medical center. Both had qualified staff who respected their managers, and the patient care delivered on both units was considered by many in the institution to be exceptional. Natalie and Sean both participated regularly in the institution's management council, though Sean often was more assertive in offering solutions to problems being discussed and contributed more often to the critical conversations underway.

Natalie admired Sean's assertiveness, his willingness to offer an idea despite knowing it was not likely to be received very well, and his ability to remain objective even in highly charged situations. Sean, on the other hand, was impressed with Natalie's consistent concern for how proposed changes would affect and be received by staff, the network and support system she seemed to have created for herself and on which she called in difficult times, and her ability to energize her staff and the management council.

One day after a particularly difficult meeting, Sean and Natalie went to the coffee shop before returning to their respective units. They talked about the meeting, how the conversation evolved, the decisions that were made, and the contributions made by various participants, including each other. Each shared what they admired about the other's leadership skills and expressed a desire to "be more like the other" in some ways.

These colleagues, who were two of the most influential members of the management council, talked about how they could help each other. Sean agreed to use his comfort with being assertive to "open the door" for Natalie to speak more freely and perhaps disagree with or offer an alternative to what has been proposed, saying something like, "It looks like Natalie has some ideas swirling around in her head about this issue. Natalie, is there something you can share to help us think this through more effectively?" And Natalie agreed to "push" Sean to always consider how his ideas—though they may lead to an acceptable and quick solution—might be more effective if staff were involved in making decisions, saying something like, "Sean, your idea sounds quite reasonable, but what if we all asked our staffs to brainstorm about it before we go ahead and implement it? They may have an even better approach."

As a result of this dialogue and the willingness and concerted efforts of Sean (to take on more "female" leadership qualities) and Natalie (to incorporate more "male" leadership qualities), each grew as a more effective manager and leader. Their contributions to the management council were consistently valuable, and all members of that group looked to them to outline a vision for future directions, suggest ways to empower staff, and lead organizational change. The staff on each of their units grew professionally, and many of them were soon providing leadership, not only on their unit, but also in the institution and in their specialty organizations and communities.

Interestingly, work related to creativity (Csikszentmihalyi, 1996) concludes that "creative individuals to a certain extent escape the rigid gender role stereotyping . . . creative and talented girls are more dominant and tough than other girls, and creative boys are more sensitive and less aggressive than their male peers" (p. 70). It would seem that blending "maleness" and "femaleness," along with focusing on the strengths and similarities of both men and women, could have a positive influence on the development of leaders and the effectiveness of both male and female leaders.

In her analysis of women leaders, Keohane (2010)—former president of both Wellesley College and Duke University, where she was the first women to hold that position—noted that individuals like Golda Meir, Indira Gandhi, and Margaret Thatcher often "behaved in ways usually associated with masculinity, partly in order to be accepted as 'real leaders'" (p. 133). This illustrates that not all women lead in a nurturing or empathetic fashion. Individuals like Jane Addams led by focusing on problems to be solved and needs to be met, thereby engendering a sense of "community" among those wishing to improve living and learning conditions in the industrial districts of Chicago. And Eleanor Roosevelt helped reform the role that women would assume in helping the United States come out of the Great Depression by asserting and living the creed that women must be ready to "stand up and be shot at," thereby emphasizing the risk-taking involved and courage needed of all leaders. Likewise, men like Martin Luther, Thomas Jefferson, Winston Churchill, Steve Jobs, and Martin Luther King, Jr. have demonstrated the effectiveness of "male leadership."

Women do think and act differently than men, and nurses have a perspective that is different from that of physicians. Instead of this being something about which we should apologize, however, or something women and nurses should try to change, it is something we should celebrate. The differences are something both men and women should exploit and use to benefit the increasingly diverse patients, families, and communities to whom we provide care. By combining the best of "female leadership" and "male leadership," our visions can be more clearly articulated and better communicated. We can be more effective in guiding change and enhancing the abilities of followers. We can strengthen our organizations and improve patient care, and the nursing profession can become more powerful.

The humanitarian qualities that women leaders tend to possess need to be guarded carefully against erosion; however, the pragmatic orientations that male leaders tend to possess cannot be ignored. In an age when resources are increasingly scarce and competition reigns, organizations and professions must be focused, firm, bottom line–oriented, and realistic. In an age when any means may be used to reach the desired end (e.g., reducing standards to fill positions, failing to encourage self-care in patients so that they remain dependent, and cutting professional staff to make the bottom line look healthier), it is increasingly important that humanistic leadership be exercised!

STRATEGIES FOR WOMEN AND MEN TO BE SUCCESSFUL LEADERS IN THE FUTURE

In his initial examination of the trends that seemed to be shaping our lives, Naisbitt (1982) did not address the female/male phenomenon, suggesting, perhaps, that in 1982, women were not thought to be a significant force in shaping the future of our society. In subsequent writings (Naisbitt & Aburdene, 1990), however, the role of women became more prominent and even became the subject of a trends book in and of itself (Aburdene & Naisbitt, 1992).

Thus, we are increasingly aware of the significance women have in shaping the future of our world. We also are increasingly sensitive to the different perspectives women and men "bring to the table." What we also need to be fully aware of, however, are the strides being made by both genders to maintain their uniqueness while at the same time incorporating characteristics of the other.

Don't accept the dictates and little boxes that say, "This is how the world operates." You really have to push outside the hierarchy. —Vera Martinez

According to Gordon (1991), "Women do not change the world by becoming more like men" (p. 15) and giving up the "female perspective" totally. Instead, they must work to "create a much needed sense of collaboration and community within the workplace" (p. 285) and other settings so that feminine values can be practiced alongside masculine values.

To become influential leaders and effective agents of social change, women—and men—will need to engage in individual and collective action. The following strategies may be helpful as women and men pursue leadership goals, particularly because many women—as they do approach leadership roles differently from men—lack self-confidence in that role (Farley, 1999):

- Participate fully in the mainstream of broad social and political activity, as well as in arenas of power and influence. Do not allow yourself to be isolated.
- Abandon your self-image and the public image of powerlessness and helplessness. Do not be naive about the realities of power and its uses.
- Refuse to align yourself with the culturally stereotypical female or male expectations. Do not let your need to achieve be sublimated to your need to nurture and serve, or vice versa.
- Continue to advance your education. The nurse influentials in Vance's (1977) study—individuals who had shaped the profession's thinking about education, practice, scholarship, and its potential for power—listed scholarship and intelligence as the most important attributes needed by nurse leaders of the future, qualities that are still seen as critically important (May, 2001).
- Do not allow yourself to be affected by the "impostor syndrome" (Harvey, 1985; *The impostor syndrome*, 1986), a phenomenon common to women (Goleman, 1985; Jacobs, 1985). Those with the syndrome are convinced that they are frauds and do not deserve the success they have achieved, despite evidence of their accomplishments. Such accomplishments are dismissed as resulting not from competence but from luck, timing, or "fooling" others. To avoid this syndrome, both women and men must believe that they have achieved success because of their skills and talents, not because of some "fluke" or sheer luck.
- Develop collective strategies for action. Engage in teamwork and be willing to help others rather than distrusting them and seeing them as competitors, disaffiliating from each other, devaluing alliances, and seemingly wanting to "go it alone."
- Be politically and intellectually astute.
- Get involved with decision-making and policy-making boards.
- Be goal directed, and include "providing leadership to achieve a vision" among those goals.
- Take advantage of the positive leadership traits you possess. Acknowledge those strengths.
- Assure others of your competence by earning the right credentials and receiving competitive job offers and outside acclaim.

- Learn how to give and receive help from men or women without having those interactions become sexual encounters.
- Dress powerfully, not like someone of no importance.
- Take a visible seat at meetings and participate actively.
- Seek assignments to ensure that "the woman's/man's point of view" is represented.
- Seek mentor relationships or apprenticeships with others who have been successful in exercising leadership (May, 2001). Women may particularly want to seek other women as mentors.
- Be sure that others know of your accomplishments and achievements.
- Develop a positive sense of yourself and your abilities.
- Be supportive of others, but be careful not to take on their responsibilities.
- Develop your own support systems.
- Take a stand rather than "play it safe."
- Shape your world rather than just fit into it.
- Make your presence felt.
- Be proactive. Position and prepare yourself to take advantage of opportunities that present themselves or that you might create.
- Act based on power and choice, not fear.
- Learn confrontation skills and how to manage conflict effectively.
- Know yourself—your strengths, your vulnerabilities, your goals, and so on.
- Develop teamwork experiences for others (e.g., students, staff nurses).
- Take charge of your own destiny.

> *The best way to predict the future is to create it.* —*Yogi Berra*

CONCLUSION

In her examination of "The 100 Most Influential Women of All Time," Felder (1996) noted that these women—who were more likely to be writers and social reformers than scientists—have had a great and long-lasting "historical and cultural impact, have inspired us, and . . . have much to teach us about past and present culture, society, and selfhood" (pp. ix–x). She asserted the "indisputable significance of women's past, present, and future contributions to the world" (p. x).

Likewise, Schiff's (2005) analysis of nine women who changed modern America showed that they "influenced the political agenda [regarding segregation, child labor, reproductive rights, and other significant social issues] in creative, innovative ways" (p. xii). Thus, women need to take pride in the unique role they can play in providing leadership.

More recently, we have seen the influence of three women in leadership roles in the city of San Francisco (Breslau, 2005). In 2004, Mayor Gavin Newsom appointed Joanne Hayes-White as Fire Chief, Heather Fong as Police Chief, and Kamala Harris as District Attorney; Fong's tenure ended in 2009, but Hayes-White and Harris continue to serve in these positions. In making these appointments in 2004, Mayor Newsom acknowledged the strength of these women to be compassionate; collaborative; practical; and able to communicate effectively, multitask, put egos aside, and solve problems. They have successfully combined the positive qualities of male and female leadership in providing for the public's safety.

Women and men both need to hold onto the strength of their uniqueness but also to incorporate talents typically exhibited by the other. In other words, a movement toward more androgynous leadership and organizations that combine the benefits of hierarchies with those of "webs" may be most effective for the individuals in those groups or organizations, the individuals and communities they serve, and the professions they represent.

CRITICAL THINKING EXERCISES

Observe a female nurse and a male nurse in interaction with patients, physicians, and each other. What are the similarities between their communication and interpersonal styles? What particular differences do you notice regarding what seems to be important to each, what values each conveys in his or her communications and actions, how each approaches a problem or conflict, and so on? How do your observations compare with the similarities and differences discussed here?

_____

_____

Think about your own childhood and current situation. What were some of the "rules" by which you were expected to behave? Were those rules made explicit to you, or were they merely implied or suggested? What differences, if any, do you recall about how boys and girls behaved in grammar school and high school and what each group seemed to value? Do you think your experiences were fairly typical? If so, what can you conclude about how parents, schools, and the larger society socialize boys and girls into stereotypical roles? Also, discuss this with your colleagues, who may be 10 to 20 years older or younger than you! Have we "come a long way, baby" in terms of a more androgynous approach to grammar school education, for example?

_____

_____

Select one of the women listed in Felder's (1996) book (e.g., Eleanor Roosevelt, Margaret Sanger, Harriet Tubman, Rosa Parks) and read a more extensive biography about her. To what extent did she reflect the characteristics of women leaders discussed in this chapter? To what extent did she also incorporate "masculine leadership" behaviors to be more androgynous? What strategies can you identify from this analysis that might help you be more effective as a leader?

_____

_____

CRITICAL THINKING EXERCISES—cont'd

Write a poem of 20 lines or less that conveys the essence of the strength of "feminine leadership" and that of "masculine leadership." Now read that poem out loud. Given all that you have read and thought about this topic and all the many things you could have said, what points were most significant to you that you absolutely had to include them in your 20 lines? Why do you think these points are so significant to you?

_____

_____

References

Aburdene, P., & Naisbitt, J. (1992). *Megatrends for women*. New York, NY: Villard Books.

American Association of University Women. (1992). *How schools shortchange girls. Executive summary*. Washington, DC: American Association of University Women.

Austin, N. K. (2002). The buzz about women leaders. *Leader to Leader, 26*(Fall), 56–60.

Babcock, L., & Laschever, S. (2003). *Women don't ask: Negotiation and the gender divide*. Princeton, NJ: Princeton University Press.

Book, E. W. (2000). *Why the best man for the job is a woman*. New York, NY: Harper Business.

Breslau, K. (2005). A new team in town. *Newsweek*, October 24, 64–66.

Brooks, A. (1983). For the woman: Strides and snags. *The New York Times*, October 16, 1983, p. 31.

Cann, A., & Siegfried, W. D. (1990). Gender stereotypes and dimensions of effective leader behavior. *Sex Roles, 23*(7/8), 413–419.

Csikszentmihalyi, M. (1996). *Creativity: Flow and the psychology of discovery and invention*. New York, NY: Harper Perennial.

Farley, S. (1999). Leadership. In R. C. Swansburg & R. J. Swansburg (Eds.), *Introductory management and leadership for nurses: An interactive text* (2nd ed., pp. 456–478). Boston: Jones & Bartlett.

Felder, D. G. (1996). *The 100 most influential women of all time: A ranking past and present*. New York, NY: Citadel Press.

Goleman, D. (1985). Feeling like a fake. *The Executive Female, 8*(5), 34–37.

Gordon, S. (1991). *Prisoners of men's dreams: Striking out for a new feminine future*. Boston, MA: Little, Brown.

Grunwald, L. (1992). If women ran America. *Life, 15*(6), 36–46.

Harvey, J. C. (1985). *If I'm so successful, why do I feel like a fake? The impostor syndrome*. New York, NY: Pocket Books.

Helgesen, S. (1990a). *The female advantage: Women's ways of leadership.* New York, NY: Doubleday Currency.

Helgesen, S. (1990b). The pyramid and the web. *The New York Times Forum,* May 27, 1990, p. 13.

Helgesen, S. (1992). Feminism and nursing—"Feminine principles" of leadership: The perfect fit for nursing. *Revolution: The Journal of Nurse Empowerment, 2*(2), 50–57, 135.

The impostor syndrome. (1986). *Management Solutions, 31*(8), 18–19.

Jacobs, S. (1985). How businesswomen overcome a malady—"Impostor syndrome." *New England Business, 7*(E), 66–67.

Kaufman, E. K., & Grace, P. E. (2011). Women in grassroots leadership: Barriers and biases experienced in a membership organization dominated by men. *Journal of Leadership Studies, 4*(4), 6–16.

Kellerman, B., & Rhode, D. L. (2006). Viable options: Rethinking women and leadership. In W. E. Rosenbach & R. L. Taylor (Eds.), *Contemporary issues in leadership* (6th ed., pp. 257–267). Boulder, CO: Westview Press.

Keohane, N. O. (2010). *Thinking about leadership.* Princeton, NJ: Princeton University Press.

Klenke, K. (1996). *Women and leadership: A contextual perspective.* New York, NY: Springer.

Kram, K. E., & Hampton, M. M. (1998). When women lead. The visibility-vulnerability spiral. In E. B. Klein, F. Gabelnick, & P. Herr (Eds.), *The psychodynamics of leadership* (pp. 193–218). Madison, CT: Psychosocial Press.

Lambert, L., & Gardner, M.E. (2009). *Women's ways of leading.* Indianapolis, IN: Dog Ear Publishing.

Levenstein, A. (1981). Leadership and sex. *Supervisor Nurse, 12*(1), 15–16.

Lipman-Blumen, J. (1992). Connective leadership: Female leadership styles in the 21st century workplace. *Sociological Perspectives, 35*(1), 183–203.

Long, S. (1998). Discourse and corporate leadership. Transformation by or of the feminine? In E. B. Klein, F. Gabelnick, & P. Herr (Eds.), *The psychodynamics of leadership* (pp. 219–245). Madison, CT: Psychological Press.

Maccoby, M. (1981). *The leader: A new face for American management.* New York, NY: Simon and Schuster.

May, L. K. (2001). *Leadership skills and attributes for Houston women in the 21st century.* Bellaire, TX: Greater Houston Women's Foundation.

Melia, J., & Lyttle, P. (1986). *Why Jenny can't lead: Understanding the male dominant system.* Saguache, CO: Communication Creativity.

Naisbitt, J. (1982). *Megatrends: Ten new directions transforming our lives.* New York, NY: Warner Books.

Naisbitt, J., & Aburdene, P. (1990). *Megatrends 2000: Ten new directions for the 1990's.* New York, NY: William Morrow.

Paludi, M. A., & Coates, B. E. (Eds.). (2011). *Women as transformational leaders: From grassroots to global interests* [Volumes I and II]. Santa Barbara, CA: ABC-CLIO Greenwood.

Park, D. (1997). Androgynous leadership style: An integration rather than a polarization. *Leadership and Organization Development Journal, 18*(3), 166–171.

Robinson-Walker, C. (1999). *Women and leadership in health care: The journey to authenticity and power.* San Francisco, CA: Jossey-Bass.

Rosener, J. (1990). Ways women lead. *Harvard Business Review, 68*(6), 19–24.

Salas-Lopez, D., Deitrick, L.M., Mahady, E.T., Gertner, E.J., & Sabino, J.N. (2011). Women leaders – Challenges, successes, and other insights from the top. *Journal of Leadership Studies, 5*(2), 34–42.

Schein, V. E. (1989). Would women lead differently? In W. E. Rosenbach & R. L. Taylor (Eds.), *Contemporary issues in leadership* (2nd ed., pp. 154–160). Boulder, CO: Westview Press.

Schiff, K. G. (2005). *Lighting the way: Nine women who changed modern America.* New York, NY: Hyperion.

Sexes differ on military force. (1985). *Higher Education and National Affairs, 34*(23), 7.

Staines, G., Travis, C., & Jayerante, T. E. (1973). The queen bee syndrome. *Psychology Today, 7*(8), 55–60.

Stivers, C. (1991). Why can't a woman be less like a man? Women's leadership dilemma. *Journal of Nursing Administration, 21*(5), 47–51.

Sylvia, E., Grund, C., Kimminau, K. S., Shmed, A., Marr, J. M., & Cooper, T. (2010). Rural women leaders. *Journal of Leadership Studies, 4*(3), 23–31.

Vance, C. N. (1977). *A group profile of contemporary influentials in American nursing.* Unpublished doctoral dissertation, Teachers College, Columbia University, New York, NY.

Vance, C. N. (1979). Women leaders: Modern day heroines or social deviants? *Image, 11*(2), 37–41.

Weddington, S. (1991). Some leaders are born women (the Novello Lecture). Paper presented at the National League for Nursing Convention, Nashville, TN, June 11, 1991.

Yukl, G. (2010). *Leadership in organizations* (7th ed.). Upper Saddle River, NJ: Prentice Hall.

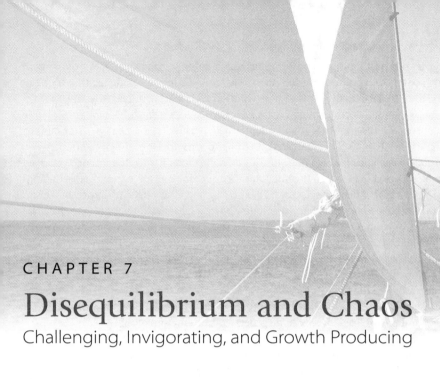

CHAPTER 7

Disequilibrium and Chaos
Challenging, Invigorating, and Growth Producing

LEARNING OBJECTIVES
- Describe the process by which leaders and followers can thrive and grow despite the chaos of today's health-care system.
- Describe how chaos and complexity science can propel individuals and organizations to accomplish goals.
- Analyze how nurse leaders can use the change process effectively in the realization of a vision.
- Formulate strategies that decrease resistance to change.
- Describe how purposeful introduction of conflict can generate change.

INTRODUCTION

Surviving the tumultuous "white water" of the current health-care system—with its redesign and increased emphasis on cost containment—is a tremendous challenge for nurses and other health-care providers, as well as for patients, families, communities, and organizations. Providers must continue to create new and effective delivery systems, partner more effectively with one another and with patients, and work cohesively to provide cost-effective quality care and achieve desired patient outcomes (Ford, 2011). Care delivery must evolve to include the patient and family/significant others as important stakeholders in their own health.

As we move from the Scientific (or Newtonian) Age to the Relationship (or New Leadership) Age, nurses must incorporate a new perspective—that chaos is a good thing because it is what makes us evolve and grow. Nursing leaders need to be willing to make educated guesses, use their intuition, and be comfortable with uncertainty and ambiguity, rather than expecting to rely on formulas that a computer may generate from patient acuity codes. Nurses must take the time to develop leadership ability so that they can be the force that drives the profession's evolution and creates our preferred future.

Nurses can no longer remain as they were. Instead, they must become comfortable with chaos and disequilibrium and adopt a new perspective on change. For example, Wheatley (2006, p.137) remembered listening to a geologist during a radio interview regarding his perspective on a huge hurricane in the Outer Banks. The interviewer asked what he expected to find after the hurricane. Instead of saying all of the negative findings one would expect, the geologist said: "I expect to find a new beach." In organizations, nurses also have to be willing to "find a new beach." They need to appreciate "how life is capable of so much change, so much newness," and "embrace this newness instead of trying to control it" (Wheatley, 2006, p. 139). They need to find time to use their intuition to solve problems, rather than focusing all of their energy on finding the parts that are not working and trying to fix them, as they so often do. By taking a new view of problems, nurses can identify "images, words or patterns that surface" (Wheatley, 2005; Wheatley, 2006, p. 141) that will help them focus on the whole and anticipate how growth and positive outcomes can be generated from the situation.

Nurses must develop adaptive skills to manage conflict, the ability to delegate effectively to other health-care workers, creativity to develop new caring strategies, maturity to recognize their lifelong learning needs, and the astuteness to position themselves in arenas where significant decisions are being made. In other words, it is time to begin "walking the walk," rather than merely "talking the talk," and this requires leadership.

ADJUSTING TO THE LEADER ROLE AND THE PRACTICE OF LEADERSHIP

Nurses must acclimate themselves to feelings of uneasiness, ambiguity, and the unknown. By applying quantum theory principles (Malloch & Porter-O'Grady, 2009), we can realize that all systems work from the inside out, not from the top down or bottom up, and appreciate that relationship is as significant as control in maintaining effectiveness. Although systems cannot be predicted with certainty, we know that tension between stability and chaos creates change. The new leader, therefore, must do the following:

- Create new models and paradigms for care delivery.
- Collaborate with and obtain information from all members of the interdisciplinary team (*never, never work in a silo by oneself or just with other nurses*).
- Be aware of new methods, listen to ideas that may not make sense today, and embrace a degree of uncertainty.
- Engage in continuous quality improvement.

Leadership has changed from a more individualized, unit-focused perspective to a more participative, collaborative focus. In fact, the Center for Creative Leadership (CCL) (2011) strongly recommends that groups of individuals from the same organization participate in their leadership development workshops if possible. The CCL offers multiple workshops and programs on leadership at their various sites, which can be accessed at their Web site at http://www.ccl.org/leadership/programs/DSLAgenda.aspx?pageId=793.

One of the workshops offered is *Developing the Strategic Leader(s)* (CCL, 2011). Developing the Strategic Leader(s) is a 5-day workshop that includes simulated learning scenarios in which the attendees participate in building strategic leadership skills as individuals and as a team to create change and a more effective work culture. The familiar 360-degree assessment strategy or 365-day assessment (Scott, 2009) is also available as a tool for individuals to obtain data on their own regarding their performance in a specific area, such as, for example, adaptation to change. It allows an individual to view data privately from people with whom they come in contact but do not necessarily work for as well as to avoid sharing of data with specific people in their work organization. It is very important, however, to engage in face-to-face discussions with people giving feedback. Otherwise, the individual receiving the feedback might not give much importance to following the feedback. Assessment tools are available on the Internet.

> *Use the constant change around you as your opportunity to change people's perceptions of you, and to prove your skills and ability to contribute.*
> —Susan Rehwaldt and Mary Lou Higgerson

DEFINING CHAOS

Chaos, or extreme, unpredictable disorganization and surprise, is most apparent in the world today. Lorenz (1993, p.4) defined chaos as "processes [systems] that appear to proceed according to chance, even though their behaviour is in fact determined by precise laws." Wheatley and Kellner-Rogers (1996) remind us that a "system maintains itself only if change is occurring somewhere in it all the time" (p. 33). So, one must view chaos or disorder as a means to survival. In other words, if there were no arguments or differences of opinion, the status quo would be maintained, and there would be no individual growth. In addition, organizational survival would be threatened. The following questions were posed by Wheatley (2006, p. 73) to those who tend to believe that everything has to have a place and be labeled and filed away:

- Why would we stay locked in our belief that "truth" exists in objective form?
- Why would we stay locked in our belief that there is one way to do something, or one correct interpretation to a situation, when the universe welcomes diversity and seems to thrive on a plurality of meaning?
- Why would we avoid participation and worry only about its risks?
- Why would we resist the powerful visions and futures that emerge when we come together to co-create the world?
- Why would we ever choose rigidity or predictability when we have been invited to be part of the generative dance of life?

Questions such as these invite one to discard old ways and embrace new ideas like chaos theory. Many creative, motivated, and enthusiastic individuals thrive on chaos and are most successful in their personal and professional lives, despite the incredibly confusing climate in which they function. Hawking (1987) views this uncertainty as opening the way to randomness and unpredictability that are perceived by many as refreshing. Others may become depressed and wallow in the disorder. For example, some nurses who are temporarily assigned to a different unit see that situation as an opportunity to expand their knowledge, skills, and networks. However, other nurses get angry with having to work on a different unit and may become so absorbed with that anger that they cannot rise to the assignment; barely maintain safety; and complain to anyone who will listen, including patients, their families, and nursing students. Is it this latter group of nurses' insecurities, fear of the unknown, or inability to deal with change that prevents them from turning what is seen as a bad situation into something positive? If situations such as these were to be seen as opportunities for learning new things, fear of the unknown could be minimized, and individuals would learn new skills and decision-making abilities. As a result, one would expect such individuals to grow more confident and increase their ability to survive the "chaos" associated with having to work on different units.

The way we perceive our situations in life, at work, and in our personal lives will greatly affect the outcome. Leaders need to see the whole picture, realize the old adage "see the glass half full rather than half empty," and know to keep "shuffling the cards" until visions are realized (Hader, 2005, p. 6). For example, conducting patient rounds during which nurses share their approaches to caring for a patient allows new and experienced nurses to dialogue, learn a great deal from one another, and refocus the negative energy that may accompany new experiences. When everyone and everything can link together, systems form that create more possibilities for all. "This is why life organizes, why life seeks systems . . . so that more may flourish" (Wheatley & Kellner-Rogers, 1996, p. 19).

This perspective helps explain why nurses need to start leading as soon as they graduate and why they need to develop their leadership skills as they grow and evolve throughout their professional careers. The Institute of Medicine (IOM) and Robert Wood Johnson Foundation echo this point in *The Future of Nursing: Leading Change, Advancing Health* (IOM, 2010), in which they recognize that nurses will be well positioned to lead and make positive changes in health-care and offer the following recommendations:

1. Nurses need to use their education and experience to the fullest.
2. Nurses need to obtain higher levels of education, and the educational system needs to provide seamless progression.
3. Nurses need to collaborate and be full partners with other health-care workers in changing care delivery in the United States.
4. Improved health policy and planning of health-care delivery will need a better information infrastructure.

This is an excellent start, but each nurse must make a commitment to continue to develop his or her leadership ability in both professional and private life. This should assist nurses to lead in the changes regarding care delivery. An effective leader generates increased patient satisfaction and is a necessary part of quality care delivery (Chen, Beck, & Amos, 2005).

The introduction to Michael Crichton's book, *Prey*, (2002), is entitled, "Artificial Evolution in the 21st Century." In this piece, this physician author notes, "If we were to grasp the true nature—if we could comprehend the real meaning of evolution—then we would envision a world in which every living plant, insect, and animal species is changing at every instant, in response to every other living plant, insect, and animal. Whole populations of organisms are rising and falling, shifting and changing. This restless and perpetual change, as inexorable and unstoppable as the waves and tides, implies a world in which all human actions necessarily have uncertain effects. The total system we call the biosphere is so complicated that we cannot know in advance the consequences of anything that we do" (p. ix). Health care is similar, in that one cannot know in advance what is going to happen to each individual patient. In attempting to attain the most positive outcome for each patient, nurses need to manage multiple variables and be alert to the possible influence of variables we do not even know about.

Crichton further explained, "The fact that the biosphere responds unpredictably to our actions is not an argument for inaction. It is, however, a powerful argument for caution, and for adopting a tentative attitude toward all we believe, and all we do" (p. x). It is this tentative attitude that nurses need to assume so that when change occurs, they can be flexible and still succeed in attaining optimal patient outcomes. Last, Crichton said, "We are one of only three species on our planet that can claim to be self-aware [human beings, chimpanzees, and orangutans], yet self-delusion may be a more significant characteristic of our kind" (p. x). Nurses who are leaders do not decide themselves. Instead, they attend to the realities and possibilities of chaos inherent in time and learn and grow as a result of the unanticipated occurrences in our lives every day.

CHAOS IN NURSING

From a Newtonian perspective, a leader is expected to help organizations adapt to change by establishing goals, obtaining commitment to the goals from employees at all levels in the bureaucracy, and decreasing uncertainty (Malloch & Porter-O'Grady, 2010). Such behaviors reflect the following assumptions:

- If something works once, keep trying it.
- If employees' needs are identified, managers can manipulate the employee to improve the organization but not necessarily the employee.
- Large effects have large causes.
- Each employee should confine himself or herself to his or her specific job description.
- Given the organizational structure, one should know that lines of authority and information flow are similar.

One can see that this view emphasizes management, planning, and controlling, rather than leadership and empowering a group. The new leadership paradigm helps us realize that individuals are more effective leaders when they can keep their organization on the edge of confusion because it is only then that the whole organization can grow in a creative and productive fashion.

The uncertainty of health care flows from the quantum and chaotic nature of the world over time. Nurses should, therefore, stop trying to plan every step and predict each happening. They must realize that they can never come close to knowing all there is to know about a topic, nor is it possible to plan every step. Hence, they have to accept that no matter how much they know about the world, there are far more questions than answers, and uncertainty is a natural part of their lives.

It is paramount that nurses interconnect with members of the other disciplines for making innovative changes. By using diverse skill sets, incorporating multiple perspectives for improving care for various needs of patients, and seeing the patient/family as the focus of care, nurses will be more successful in accomplishing the profession's goals. Each and every nurse needs to think innovatively and not accept the status quo when planning quality and efficient care for patients.

Nurses also have to realize that the lengthy "to-do" task lists they routinely develop at the beginning of a workday can be nothing more than skeletal frameworks because such lists cannot possibly encompass all that nurses will need to do that day. Being extremely task oriented and using a minute-to-minute structure to organize one's work must give way to critically thinking and constantly adapting as new problems and challenges arise. Because of the exceptional complexity of the nursing role today, organizational charts, time management lists, and critical pathways have served almost as survival techniques by giving some structure in a highly chaotic environment. Unfortunately, to-do lists and predictive pathways inhibit our ability to see things globally. Instead of trying to block out the chaos and unpredictability inherent in health care, nurses need to learn how to embrace it. One must embrace relationships with others and be aware that the order of life is based more on principles of emergence than on predetermined order. Variables such as communication and cooperative relationships among individuals energize a system and help it be effective.

Nurses, however, also cannot simply "wait and see" how things evolve. Haigh (2008) reported on a strategy to use chaos theory to help an acute Pain Practice (with an overwhelming 20% patient growth each year) plan more effectively for providing nursing services. Although it is impossible (and perhaps contrary to chaos theory) to predict for the details of each desired outcome, one can plan to reach specific levels of effectiveness in fulfilling the various components of planned outcomes. This is made possible by creating various ranges of what constitutes effectiveness. The next step involves developing numerous possibilities (i.e., not just the number of professionals needed for safe and quality care delivery in the growing Pain Practice) that can be used to achieve each outcome. This is accomplished using a population equation that can help with service forecasting regarding appropriate provider-to-patient care delivery. Chaos theory assisted this organization to obtain insight into the number and types of patients that would most likely present at the Pain Service; as a result, reasonable staffing could be positioned with the right resources to potentially succeed. Nurses could accomplish this by hiring more diverse staff to work with the more diverse patient population, focusing on retaining current staff instead of recruiting new staff in order to regenerate their energy and passion, trying methods that do not require the same expensive resources that have been used in the past, and assisting staff in experimenting with new ideas that will help develop new practice models.

COMPLEXITY OF THE REGISTERED NURSE'S ROLE IN THE CURRENT HEALTH-CARE SYSTEM

What seems to be a key to success in these ever-changing times is having the ability to appreciate the interrelationships among multiple variables. For example, when a practice or clinic is bought out or acquired by a different care system, several chronically ill patients may be forced to transfer to a new primary care provider. When that happens, no patient–provider relationship exists, and all involved parties must begin again. In addition, it probably will take more time for the new provider to care for these complex patients, compared with the original provider, because he or she does not know the patient. The payer will have to pay for more visits, the patient has to worry about getting to the new office and building trust with the new provider, and the patient and provider will have to invest energy into starting a new relationship. The RN can be the consistent piece and assume the role of coordinating patients and providers so as to provide some type of consistency with the patient and family and the health-care system. This type of case management is needed more than ever before to advocate for the maximal quality of patient care. Fortunately, most health-care delivery practices currently have or are instituting electronic records so that patients' health history can easily be transferred.

Complexity and collaboration are two sides of the same coin. —Kathleen Dracup

Many health-care agencies and institutions have experienced change through merging or acquisition or from an internal governance model shift. Nurse leaders can help avoid some of the problems that have accompanied such change and be more successful with the ultimate change if they (Ponte, Gross, Winer, Connaughton, & Hassinger, 2007):

- Obtain representation from every health-care group that is involved, especially those who are directly engaged in patient care.
- Be sure to keep each representative accountable—by assuring that the representative go back to his or her constituents to gather their ideas and share what is happening in the planning meetings for a redesign of governance model.
- Define each leader's role (including oneself) involved in the change initiative and be sure each of these leaders are part of defining their responsibilities and that these duties are transparent to the entire staff.
- Be very cognizant of developing a governance model that promotes safe, high-quality patient/family-centered care.
- Build in metrics that measure the model's effectiveness regarding quality, patient and staff satisfaction, cost-effectiveness, productivity, and safety.

They also gained some "lessons learned" from this governance model redesign: go slow; have a defined purpose, accountability, and membership; have clear executive leadership; use data to drive decision making; and be patient (Ponte et al, 2007).

FACILITATING LEADERSHIP IN CHAOS

Tonges (1997) suggests the following principles for leaders to succeed where chaos reigns:

- Stay informed about the players in your work setting.
- Know and be guided by your values.
- Learn and use new technology.
- Accept and work with change.
- Renew yourself.

Neubauer (1998) agrees with these principles and recommends that people concentrate on renewing themselves, a process she defines as continuous self-assessment, being aware of one's own reactions, obtaining feedback, caring for oneself, and setting goals. Leaders also should call on the diverse perspective of followers to brainstorm solutions and create the vision, focus on ongoing learning and the continued development of critical thinking skills, and communicate effectively. Further suggestions for providing strategic leadership in uncertain times are enumerated by McDaniel (1998, pp. 358–361):

- Stop planning and being preoccupied with order so that you can learn to cope with the unknowable.
- Move to the edge of chaos to find creative and new directions.
- Expect many people to be leaders because this will make for a vibrant organization.
- Allow for nurse autonomy so that people can learn to adapt and adjust to change in their own way.
- Improve the connections between colleagues because "the quality of connections between workers is more important than the quality of each individual" (p. 359).
- Do not allow people to say, "That's not my job." Instead, teach them what other people are doing and help them appreciate that everyone is important if the vision is to become a reality.
- Assist peers to become "skilled at handling ambiguous issues, revealing differences, and generating new perspectives" (p. 360).
- Assist organizations and people to discover goals themselves.
- Work smarter, not necessarily harder.
- Provide for the emergence of new visions.

It is wise to realize that no matter how much energy is spent trying to lead through chaos, the stability one might long for is not really the solution because stability will only dampen the growth that occurs when some degree of chaos remains. Thus, each of us must become comfortable with constant change.

Nothing endures but change. —*Heraclitus*

CHANGE

It has been said that the only permanent thing in society is change. As humans, one of the most pervasive and significant concepts affecting our lives is that of change—change that comes about through our own development and maturation, change that takes place as a result of our education and our interactions with others, change that is imposed on us from outside sources, and change that we impose on ourselves and others. If we are to cope effectively with change and use it to our advantage, we must be able to recognize when it occurs, when it needs to occur, how to facilitate it, how it can be blocked, and the impact various changes and change strategies have on individuals and groups.

Change is the making of something that is different from the way it was. It is an alteration; it results from differences and conflicts in a system, from information, or sometimes from unfulfilled needs. Change potentiates or allows the possibility of accomplishment of goals. It can be planned, or it may be an unexpected result of a decision or other event. Change can evolve over time, or it can be a spontaneous, revolutionary occurrence. Change in one's personal and professional life can involve a transition period, during which adjustment may be successful or not. No matter what the change, a true change does not affect only a single person; instead, it permeates the ambiance of a setting and triggers some type of change in anyone who comes in contact with the individual or setting that changed.

An example of a change that has profoundly affected most health-care workers and patients is social networking sites, such as Facebook (Shih, 2011). This site is used by one in three of all American adults and can be an avenue to achieve the following:

- Communicate as a health-care team.
- Gain more personal information about coworkers.
- Share ideas about learning to use social Web sites.
- Learn from others who may be engaged in a similar change initiative or subject.

Belasco (1990) says organizations are similar to elephants in that they both learn through conditioning. He describes this phenomenon with the following illustration (p. 2): "Trainers shackle young elephants with heavy chains to deeply embedded stakes. In that way the elephant learns to stay in its place. Older elephants never try to leave even though they have the strength to pull the stake and move beyond. Their conditioning limits their movements with only a small metal bracelet around their foot—attached to nothing." Like powerful elephants, many individuals are bound by conditioned constraints. "We've always done it this way" is as limiting to an individual's progress as the chain around the elephant's foot.

It is time to move the nursing profession forward by listening to new ideas and trying new ways of doing things. Nurses have to start "dancing" rather than feel chained to an invisible stake in the ground and need to start paving their own road to their dreams. Many people often remark that they would change their lives dramatically if they could, and they say the change would focus more on gaining self-respect and increasing quality time with family and friends, rather than on gaining power and affluence.

The secret to leadership is . . . to think of your position as an opportunity to serve, not as a trumpet call to self-importance. —J. Donald Walters

Denhardt and Denhardt (2006) also speak to the dance of leadership. They assert that leadership can be perceived as being "drawn directly from the arts" (p. 6) and of being an "intense textured interplay of space, time, and energy" (p. 6). These authors also differentiate leadership from management by saying leadership is all about "what energizes people," and to energize others, a leader must try one thing and then another until a path reveals itself (p. 10). Additionally, "leadership is a way of working within a world of openness and change," whereas, "management is a way of working within a world of order and regulation" (p. 10).

It seems that many people are dissatisfied with their lives but do not know how to change. They have, in a sense, been conditioned to accept their lot in life and do not know how to move away from their routine—no matter how uncomfortable or dissatisfying that life has become. Perhaps by better understanding some principles of change (Box 7–1), we can be more willing to engage in it and change our lives.

THE LEADER AS A CHANGE AGENT

As nurses acquire new abilities and transform into leaders, they will demonstrate courage by involving others in clarifying the vision and making decisions about how to realize it. Decisions about quality of clinical outcomes, work content, and performance effectiveness of workers will be more readily incorporated if they are influenced by nurses and not just the manager. Nurses are responsible for their own practice; thus, they should exercise leadership and direct that practice. The days of "my nurses are such good workers" and "I need one more RN for the Saturday eleven-to-seven shift, can't you do me a favor and work a double?" must come to an end. It is not the nurse manager's unit but the staff's. In fact, the "power" of the nurse manager will not be diminished—and may actually increase—when he or she empowers others to make change.

BOX 7-1 **Principles of Change**

- A change in one part affects other parts and other systems.
- People affected by the change should participate in making the change.
- People should be informed of the reasons for the change.
- Concrete and specific feedback about the process of change will enhance its acceptance.
- People need assistance in dealing with the effects of the change.
- People's suggestions and contributions about the implementation of change should be sought and incorporated.
- A change must be reinforced, or the system will revert to its old practices.
- Conflict may occur at any step during the change process.
- The more compatible the new ideas are with one's values and needs, the more easily a change will be adopted.
- The more trust one has in the initiator of change, the more likely one is to support the change.
- One's past experience with change can profoundly affect one's willingness to support a new idea.

Kouzes and Posner (2007) believe that leaders do not always seek the challenges and consequential ramifications of change that occur, but that these challenges seek the leaders. They also believe that challenge is the motivating milieu for excellence. They have found through their research that "ordinary" men and women are able to accomplish extraordinary feats, and those who function as leaders in the group realize they have skills they never knew they had, including the ability to manage change.

An important skill for a leader to exercise when involved in change is that of coaching. This is the ability to facilitate others' understanding of themselves and their own abilities. It is the process by which one person (the coach—the leader) helps followers understand that answers to questions or solutions to problems lie within themselves. Being able to role-model behaviors that assist individuals' adaptation to change is also helpful. Leaders who can help facilitate connections among followers should be successful in orchestrating change. Dolci (2005) emphasizes this idea with his statement that "leadership focuses on flexibility, collaboration, crossing boundaries and collective leadership" (p. 4). This validates the importance of mentoring and coaching and confirms that the emergence of leaders is quite likely to result from such processes (Grossman, 2007). What nurses do in their lives every day produces a certain type of wisdom, and this wisdom will assist nurses to lead others. By following what Kilburg (2006) calls "executive wisdom," the leader can help staff rise to their highest level of competency.

The new leadership is about forming relationships and connecting with others to challenge old, bureaucratic organizational structures and old ways of doing things. The delay in committing to a decision allows followers or all those affected by the decision to discuss all issues fully and explore all possible options. Change requires giving up old behaviors so that new ones may be taken on, and it undoubtedly will cause conflict; however, if this conflict is addressed effectively, the new behaviors will be adopted, and the ultimate outcome will be better. It is likely that as followers explore various options and points of view, turmoil in the group or organization will occur. Rather than being distressed by this turmoil, however, leaders are excited by it because it is exactly what the organization needs if change is to be successful. Teams of followers should be expected to cause continuous change in the group's or organization's strategy as they generate ideas for action and identify new directions. Reducing the existing hierarchy and challenging the group's or organization's belief system are necessary components to prevent an organization from maintaining the status quo. When an individual, group, community, or team is able to empower itself, effective leadership has occurred, positive change is likely, and the organization can grow tremendously. With this new perspective, the importance of developing self-directed teams of effective followers in any organization is made abundantly clear (Fig. 7–1).

FACILITATING THE CHANGE PROCESS

Leaders are necessary to facilitate change. The environment must be ripe or made ripe. There must be a reason for the change to occur, and the players must be willing to try to change. The change must also yield growth—positive or negative. Such actions require that the leader be willing to think in new ways and try new approaches despite the barriers to change that they confront.

Implications for Nurses To Be Successful Change Agents

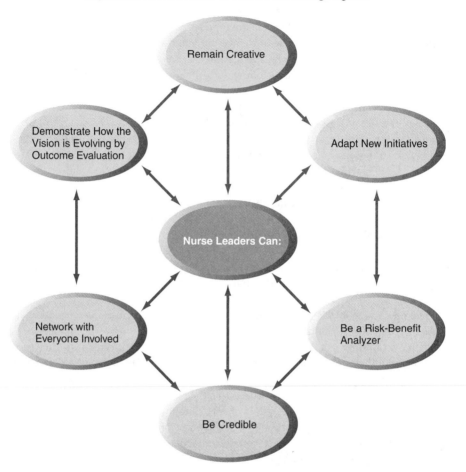

FIGURE 7-1 • Implications for nurses to be successful change agents.

Many times patients do not comply with taking their medications, following a diet, stopping smoking, and the list goes on. What about nurses facilitating change in the patient arena? Change revolves around patient behavior, and essentially much of the discouragement that nurses, staff, and advanced practice nurses experience is due to their patients not listening or complying with their treatment protocol, both pharmacological and nonpharmacological. A method for assisting patients in changing their behavior is the Change Framework by Prochaska, DiClemente, and Norcross (1992). This Model for Health Behavior Change is often used in setting up a contract between a patient and a health provider regarding the steps the patient will follow to make a change that will positively affect his or her health. An important aspect of this Model is that the goals of the contract are mutually decided by the patient and provider. For example, when working with a patient who overeats and needs to change his or her eating habits, the nurse and the patient mutually develop a contract with goals and target dates for measuring changes and outcome results of the change. Communication methods are set up according to what is appropriate to share between the nurse and the patient and includes a list of the consequences the patient will have to deal with if the change in eating habits does not occur. There has been much success with this framework with all health-care providers and their patients. Some suggestions regarding communicating with patients who are in need of changing a health behavior include the following (Van Servellen, 2009):

- Change can occur in very small steps.
- An individual must be motivated to change for the change to be permanent.
- Outside reinforcement of changed behavior can be negative or positive but still be productive for the person making the changes.
- The patient must see the importance of making the change for overall health.
- The patient needs a social network for support in making the change.
- Patients must feel they have the ability to make the change.
- Nurses need to show confidence in the patient making the change.

Effective communication, recognition of staff welfare as well as patient safety during a transition, and empowerment of staff to accomplish the processes necessary for the change to evolve are necessary components for a successful change similar to the above principles of change with patients. Currie (2006) studied how nurse managers contribute greatly to strategic change in health-care organizations and found that part of the success they garnered was a result of their partnerships with agencies outside their own organization. Again, it is the relationships established between nurses and others that assist in making a difference and leading change (Nagelkerk, 2006).

There is no doubt that effective change requires leadership; however, both leaders and followers must be motivated and energized to implement positive changes and thrive in the chaos that will ensue. Having informal discussions face to face or on a unit or department's blog regarding new ideas for changing care is one way to stimulate nurses' thinking about how they can shape future changes in health care and how open they and their organization are to change. Continuous dialogue can offer insight into nurses' and organizations' readiness for the changes confronted by health care today and can help leaders who want to implement a change. Readiness to Change Assessment Tools are available on the Internet to formally assess a unit or department's ideas about change. It is important to create a work culture supportive of change so that individuals develop an appreciation for change, adapt values that motivate them to seek change when needed, and realize that successful change yields positive incentives for both patients and staff.

PROCESS OF CHANGE

The current and predicted rate of change in society in general and in health care in particular is phenomenal. Such change requires professions, groups, and institutions to reassess their goals, structure, culture, and planning processes. Leaders are faced, therefore, with enormous challenges that are energy consuming but are also revitalizing and rewarding. Leaders must help others see the need for change, work with others to implement change, evaluate the effect of change, and participate in each stage of the change process. They also must understand what people experience as they go through change.

Perhaps one of the most useful theories to help us understand this phenomenon is that espoused by Lewin in 1951. He identified three stages of change:

1. *Unfreezing,* in which people are preparing for change
2. *Moving,* in which people have accepted the need for a change and actually engage in implementing the change
3. *Refreezing,* in which the new change is integrated into the system and becomes part of the new norm or culture

For example, a unit practicing primary nursing is experiencing turmoil related to staffing and reporting, as a result of the increased acuity of patients and decreased number of registered nurses (RNs). It becomes obvious that old assignment methods are no longer working, and some unfreezing must occur. The staff and nurse manager engage in brainstorming activities and decide, after exploring many options, to institute a charge position for each shift. Once the new charge position is started, the unit enters Lewin's moving stage and works to refine the position and its duties to make it most effective. As the unit adjusts to and incorporates the new position, refreezing, or the integration of the position into daily work, occurs. This approach to change is congruent with the new leadership style because it is a dynamic process planned or facilitated by the leader and followers, but then allowed to evolve spontaneously and mesh into the system.

Whenever applying Lewin's change theory, it is important to realize that the stages of change are merely categories to help our thinking, not discreet steps that begin and end abruptly. In other words, change typically is not a clearcut process that can be achieved by following a formula. In fact, it is often the case that a change process may advance to stage 2 and then move back to stage 1 when using Lewin's Change Model. Transformational change, as noted earlier, is an evolving process that tends to be the product of a group's vision over time, and revolutionary change follows no clearcut formula. Perhaps nursing is in the process of a revolution. It appears the profession has moved through the unfreezing stage and is now moving toward a more autonomous role in the health-care arena. Advanced practice nursing is taking hold in every setting of health-care delivery, and patient outcomes are beginning to validate the significance of nurses' contributions. RNs and hiring institutions are realizing the need for continuing education as the staff nurse position becomes more integrated into the health-care team structure. RNs and physicians are collaborating more than ever before, and patient outcomes are being tracked to identify both the nursing and medical interventions responsible for outcomes. As outcomes become publicized, our profession must move toward the refreezing or integration of change stage. Buonocore (2004) used Kurt Lewin's Theory of Change to describe the change her institution experienced. She identified some common barriers her organization faced as including self, the target environment, and the external environment. Each individual must be aware of the need for change, and it is up to the change agent to seek agreement from the majority of people the change will affect. Buonocore highlights the concept that nurses, the target group, are generally resistant to change and that multiple variables in the health-care setting can influence a successful change.

Perhaps the following "rules" for achieving change in an organization will be helpful to nurse leaders during the unfreezing, moving, and refreezing phases of change (Porter-O'Grady & Malloch, 2011):

- Participants need to be oriented to the specific concern of their own environment.
- The purpose of learning new ideas is to foster improvement.
- Participants need to be empowered to learn and gain the maximum they can.
- There must be room for risk taking in the organization.
- Participants need to be allowed the time to learn new knowledge and ideas.
- Learning needs to be part of everyday thinking in order to promote innovation and new knowledge on a continual basis.
- Participants need to receive praise for their work.

Kotter (1996) developed a more specific Model of Change built on Lewin's framework. He offers his first four steps as Lewin's first stage of unfreezing; steps 5 through 7 are stage 2, or moving; and the step 8 is Lewin's stage 3, or unfreezing. The following is Kotter's Eight Step Plan for Integrating Change:

1. Identify a need and communicate the necessity for implementing a change.
2. Gather the stakeholders and create power in numbers to lead the change.
3. Develop a vision and strategies to enforce change to lead the initiative.
4. Communicate the new vision for the change to everyone in the organization.
5. Encourage risk taking and creative troubleshooting to move the change along.
6. Move the change and offer incentives for success.
7. Evaluate the implications of the change as it takes hold and offer suggestions to improve it as it progresses.
8. Evaluate the change and offer reinforcement of the successful outcomes of the change.

There is a certain relief in change, even though it is from bad to worse; as I have found in traveling in a stage-coach, that it is often a comfort to shift one's position and be bruised in a new place. —Washington Irving

BARRIERS TO CHANGE

The captain of a ship steers the vessel from one port to another using carefully plotted coordinates. Why then does the ship veer off its course, sometimes miles off track of the destination? Why does the ship end up beached on a shoal not marked on the charts? Why does an iceberg cut up the ship? The answer to all these questions is that life is unpredictable, and captains must consider many other factors besides coordinates when navigating their ships. Nurse leaders must also consider multiple factors and anticipate potential problems when instituting changes.

Many factors can serve as barriers to change, including decreased resources, lack of support, resistance, poor communication mechanisms, or pressures to get the day-to-day work done. The more barriers there are to the change, the more effort will be needed to deal with those barriers and, consequently, the less energy will be available to institute the actual change.

DEALING WITH CONFLICT GENERATED BY CHANGE

Leaders work to implement changes that will have positive outcomes, but they also need to realize that there may be negative outcomes as well. Those seemingly negative outcomes, however, may actually be positive ones. One of the most common outcomes of change is *conflict*, something that historically has been viewed as negative but can be quite positive. The positive results of conflict are growth, an ability to accept that what was can no longer be, and collaboration, which builds healthy relationships.

In the new science of leadership, conflict can be an outcome of change or serve as an instigator of change and ultimately growth. To deal with the conflict generated, some goals may need to be abandoned, the vision may need to be altered, and an extraordinary amount of energy may need to be invested to help the group move through the change. The evolution of individuals, groups, and organizations experiencing the change, however, far surpasses the time and effort involved. Dreher (1996) reminds us that the Tao says one can develop better harmony by looking for it within—by decreasing one's anxiety and defensiveness in conflict. Using both the yin (patience, process, and empathy) and yang (courage and positive action), Taoism suggests the leader must balance opposites within herself or himself and be able to manage and grow from conflict.

Tentative efforts lead to tentative outcomes. Therefore give yourself fully to your endeavors. Decide to construct your character through excellent actions and determine to pay the price of a worthy goal. The trials you encounter will introduce you to your strengths. Remain steadfast . . . and one day you will build something that endures, something worthy of your potential. —Epictetus (Roman teacher/philosopher)

Leaders must be confident, focused, and able to balance personal and professional goals to successfully orchestrate a change. This gives them the energy needed to take on the challenge of change. People must have a "clear perspective and life balance." To lead in the midst of change and chaos, it is necessary to have a clear vision and support from one's followers. Ultimately, it is better to choose to change and design one's own approach to change than to have a change imposed by some external force.

It appears that many nurses use avoidance to manage conflict. Although this may seem like a good approach initially, avoiding a conflict ultimately causes tension among team members and negatively influences the care environment (Kelly, 2006). An example that portrays the conflict of many nurses follows.

Case Study

Susan, an RN, and her colleagues on a high-acuity medical unit have extremely challenging patient assignments. Additionally, they are usually assigned new unlicensed assistive personnel (UAPs) to assist them. Susan and the other RNs usually feel that it would be easier to do the work themselves because they have to spell out every detail to the UAPs, and they hardly ever have any consistency with the UAPs. Generally, there are different UAP assignments each day. Often, like today, the RNs have to orient a float RN who has his own separate patient assignment and who has been told by the supervisor to ask the staff RN for assistance with anything about which he feels uncomfortable. The staff RN has a new UAP to orient, another staff RN not familiar with the unit's policies and staff who is asking questions, and responsibility for an extremely challenging patient assignment. The staff RNs are likely to expend only so much energy and accept this type of working condition only so many times before becoming angry and unwilling to follow this patient assignment model any longer. Whether the nurses stay in this job or not depends greatly on how effectively the leader can help them manage the anger or conflict; create a new model of orienting float nurses; and, even more importantly, assist in retaining nurses so that there is less need for floating. Leaders must know how to deal with change and the conflict typically associated with it. It is important for the leader to assist the staff in developing champions for a new model of orientating and cross-training RNs. Being confident that a change can be made and that the staff RNs can be responsible for creating a new way of thinking about floating will be paramount for success (Vivar, 2006). Some ideas to manage this case include the following:

- Create a champion among the staff who believes in the need for a change and who will guide the creation of a new orientation and cross-training policy.
- Brainstorm so that all staff RNs (those assigned to the unit and those who float to it on occasions) can participate in developing the new cross-training model.
- Obtain feedback regarding the change from other units, an objective party, and administration.
- Facilitate collaboration between representatives of the staff RN group and nursing administration to find a solution that incorporates both parties' perspectives and allows for a win-win outcome for all.
- Evaluate the effect of the change after piloting it.
- Incorporate findings from the pilot to revise the new practice policy.
- Periodically evaluate the effects of the new cross-training policy.
- Implement the new policy on a broader scale.

It is important to teach nurses how to be assertive and communicate their feelings and ideas. Because nurses are responsible for their patients' care, it stands to reason they should be part of planning how to best make patient assignments and how to most effectively orient new staff—both permanent staff and temporary floats. By using the above-mentioned strategies, nurses can better manage conflict and facilitate change on their units.

CONCLUSION

There is no doubt that nurses are experiencing enormous change in their practice and the environments in which they practice. Although nurses may bemoan the fact that leaders cannot control or predict what will happen in these uncertain times, they need to think of this situation as a good thing because the chaos that exists can be used to promote extraordinary growth for the profession, the organization, and all individuals involved in it.

Leaders must have the ability to know when the strategies selected to realize a vision need to be altered, and they must surround themselves with a team of effective followers who bring diverse and innovative perspectives to the situation. Networking, partnering, and collaborating are skills with which nurses have been successful, and they need to draw on those skills to coach followers and help them identify their strengths and build their self-esteem so that they can more effectively manage the many changes the profession faces.

Leaders should strive to make changes in educational programs to focus on learning more than on knowing, changes in incentives for bedside nurses that recognize their significant contributions and allow them to continue to develop their expertise in that role, and changes that create more opportunities for nurses to engage in collaborative efforts with their nurse colleagues and other health-care workers. As we experience the chaos of the 21st century, it is even more important for nurses to lead and participate in change projects that reshape health-care practices and policy. Groups, organizations, and professions that survive will be ones that encourage all members to think beyond what is currently possible and continuously participate in change.

CRITICAL THINKING EXERCISES

Several authors assert that resistance to change grows out of fear. Talk to your nurse colleagues about why they have resisted change. Is the bottom-line reason that of fear? If so, what seems to be feared? If not, what is the bottom-line reason given?

_____

_____

What strategies have you used or experienced being used that have resulted in reduced resistance to and a successful outcome of change?

_____

_____

Given the "state of the art" of nursing, do we need a revolution? Do your nurse colleagues agree with your position?

_____

_____

CRITICAL THINKING
EXERCISES—cont'd

Listen to the song "The Times They Are a-Changing" by Bob Dylan (1967). How is it that new expectations seem to emerge slowly yet still demand change? See Web site: http://www.lyricsfreak.com/b/bob+dylan/the+times+they+are+a+changin_20021240.html.

_____

_____

Listen to the song "Revolution" by the Beatles (Lennon & McCarthy, 1968). Why would some people prefer a quicker, revolutionary approach to change? See Web site: http://www.beatleswiki.com/wiki/index.php/Revolution.

_____

_____

Read an article about chaos in nursing in the journal *Complexity and Chaos in Nursing*. Describe how the new science of leadership correlates with how nurses practice leadership in a state of chaos.

_____

_____

View one of the Harry Potter movies. These movies portray how a group of people work effectively together to solve challenges. What strategies can you take from one of these films to apply in your job to improve group work?

_____

_____

Use a personality inventory such as the Myers-Brigg to identify your individual personality style. Discuss how the results affect your ability to communicate and to resolve and grow from conflict. Use the following Web site to choose which personality assessment tool you think would be best for you: http://www.discoveryourpersonality.com/testlist.html.

_____

_____

References

Belasco, J. (1990). *Teaching the elephant to dance: Empowering change in your organization.* New York, NY: Crown.

Buonocore, D. (2004). Leadership in action. Creating a change in practice. *AACN Clinical Issues 15*(2), 170–181.

Center for Creative Leadership (2011). *Developing the strategic leader.* Retrieved from http://www.ccl.org/leadership/programs/DSLAgenda.aspx?pageId=793

Chen, H., Beck, S. L., & Amos, L. D. (2005). Leadership styles and nursing faculty job satisfaction in Taewan. *Journal of Nursing Scholarship, 37*(4), 374–380.

Crichton, M. (2002). *Prey.* New York, NY: Harper Collins.

Currie, G. (2006). Reluctant but resourceful middle managers: The case of nurses in the NHS. *Journal of Nursing Management, 14,* 5–12.

Denhardt, R., & Denhardt, J. (2006). *The dance of leadership: The art of leading in business, government, and society.* Armonk, NY: M. E. Sharpe.

Dolci, J. (2005). The changing world of leadership. *Association Executive,* November/December, 4.

Dreher, D. (1996). *The Tao of personal leadership.* New York, NY: Harper Business.

Dylan, B. (1967). The times they are a-changing. *Bob's Dylan's Greatest Hits,* CBS Records Inc.

Ford, E. (2011). Chaos and organization in health care. *Journal of Legal Medicine, 32*(2), 245–248.

Grossman, S. (2007). *Mentoring in nursing: A dynamic and collaborative process.* New York, NY: Springer.

Hader, R. (2005). Success is one leadership strategy away. *Nursing Management, 9,* 6.

Haigh, C. A. (2008). Using simplified chaos theory to manage nursing services. *Journal of Nursing Management, 16,* 298–304.

Hawking, S. (1987). *A brief history of time.* London, UK: Bantam Press.

Institute of Medicine and Robert Wood Johnson Foundation. (2010). *The future of nursing: Leading change, advancing health.* Retrieved from http://www.iom.edu/nursing.

Kelly, J. (2006). An overview of conflict. *Dimensions of Critical Care Nursing, 25*(2), 22–28.

Kilburg, R. (2006). *Executive wisdom: Coaching and the emergence of virtuous leaders.* Washington, DC: American Psychological Association.

Kotter, J. P. (1996). *Leading change.* Boston, MA: Harvard Business School Press.

Kouzes, J., & Posner, B. (2007). *The leadership challenge: How to keep getting extraordinary things done in organizations* (4th ed.). San Francisco, CA: Jossey-Bass.

Lennon, J., & McCartney, P. (1968). Revolution. *The Beatles, Past Masters,* EMI Records Ltd.

Lewin, K. (1951). *Field theory in social science: Selected theoretical papers.* New York, NY: Harper & Row.

Lorenz, E. (1993). *The essence of chaos.* London, UK: UCL Press.

Malloch, K., & Porter-O'Grady, T. (2009). *The quantum leader: Applications for the new world of work* (2nd ed.). Sudbury, MA: Jones & Bartlett.

McDaniel, R. (1998). Strategic leadership: A view from quantum and chaos theories. In W. J. Duncan, P. Ginter, & L. Swayne (Eds.), *Handbook of healthcare management* (pp. 339–367). Malden, MA: Blackwell.

Nagelkerk, J. (2006). The process of change in healthcare organizations. *Clinical Nurse Specialist: The Journal for Advanced Nursing Practice, 20*(2), 93–94.

Neubauer, J. (1998). Thriving in chaos: Personal and career development. In E. C. Hein (Ed.), *Contemporary leadership behavior: Selected readings* (5th ed., pp. 247–258). Philadelphia, PA: Lippincott.

Ponte, P. R., Gross, A. H., Winer, E., Connaughton, M. J., & Hassinger, J. (2007). Implementing an interdisciplinary governance model in a comprehensive cancer center. *Oncology Nursing Forum, 34*(3), 611–616.

Porter-O'Grady, T., & Malloch, K. (2011). *Quantum leadership: Advancing innovation, transforming health care* (3rd ed.). Sudbury, MA: Jones & Bartlett Learning.

Prochaska, J., DiClemente, C., & Norcross, J. (1992). In search of how people change: Applications to addictive behavior. *American Psychologist, 47*, 1102–1114.

Scott, S. (2009). *Fierce leadership: A bold alternative to the worst "best" practices of business today*. New York, NY: Broadway Business.

Shih, C. (2011). *The Facebook era: Tapping online social networks to market, sell, and innovate*. Upper Saddles River, NJ: Prentice Hall.

Tonges, M. (1997). The white water of change. *Nursing Management, 28*(10), 64–69, 70, 72.

Van Servellen, G.(2009). *Communication skills for the health professional*. Sudbury, MA: Jones & Bartlett.

Vivar, C. (2006). Putting conflict management into practice: A nursing case study. *Journal of Nursing Management, 14*, 201–206.

Wheatley, M. (2005). *Finding our way: Leadership for an uncertain time*. San Francisco, CA: Berrett-Koehler.

Wheatley, M. (2006). *Leadership and the new science: Discovering order in a chaotic world* (3rd ed.). San Francisco, CA: Berrett-Koehler.

Wheatley, M., & Kellner-Rogers, M. (1996). *A simpler way*. San Francisco, CA: Berrett-Koehler.

CHAPTER 8

Shaping a Preferred Future for Nursing

- Analyze how current societal health-care trends can affect the future of nursing.
- Examine projections for the future that are likely to have an impact on the nursing profession and health care.
- Describe characteristics of leaders needed to shape a preferred future for nursing.
- Propose partnerships and collaborative relationships that can help nurse leaders shape a preferred future.
- Suggest strategies whereby nurses can create their own preferred future.

INTRODUCTION

Leaders in nursing have the responsibility to prepare today for tomorrow's challenges. Although nurses must be fully aware of the past so that they can learn from it, and fully aware of their present so that they can survive in it, it is perhaps most critical that they have some sense of the future, so that they can try to plan for it and shape it to their benefit. Leaders are responsible, through their vision, creativity, ability to facilitate change, and ability to manage and survive chaos, for articulating a preferred future for the profession and its practitioners, whether they are in clinical, administrative, educational, research, health policy, or other roles.

Leaders can articulate a preferred future for the nursing profession by creating bridges, or interconnections, between people that empower them and that change their focus from merely doing their jobs to having a larger purpose. They can do this by taking on a number of different roles:

- **Leaders as integrators:** leaders must see beyond the differences of various group or team members and use divergent talents and perspectives to benefit the group.
- **Leaders as diplomats:** leaders must help people get past their conflicts with one another and facilitate their working together.
- **Leaders as cross-fertilizers:** leaders must bring the best attributes out of each group or individual and allow those attributes to be shared with the entire team.
- **Leaders as emotionally intelligent thinkers:** leaders must be creative and open to new possibilities that have not been thought of before.

In essence, leaders foster collaboration among individuals and keep lines of communication open among all group members to best secure goals with the available resources. In the corporate world, there is a growing trend for "shared power models" in the work environment, and certainly the future will display increased numbers of mergers and acquisitions of industry conglomerates as well as health-care groups (Bennis, 2007). Smith (2006) and Nedd (2006) both reinforce the importance of an efficiently led care environment to generate strong individual and organizational performance by leaders. It is important to realize that the organizational system needs to be more dynamic and allow for flexibility between various care environments and not necessarily be focused on the individual employee who works at the different settings. There are multiple similarities just in the care environments that would benefit a collaboration. Employees can be re-tooled to work in various care environments.

An orientation toward the future involves having an idea of societal trends and awareness of the social, political, economic, and organizational forces that create, influence, or are influenced by those trends. Certainly, anyone would agree at the time of this writing that it is very difficult to predict how these forces will transpire. With the chaotic governance structures of the emerging countries in the world, the ever-changing nature of health-care reform in the United States, and the volatile global and national economic markets, it seems that much of the future is really difficult to imagine, let alone attempt to predict. It is, however, imperative that the nursing profession be a participating member of the group charged with making predictions and decisions about health care.

The profession needs to be a leader in providing ideas and creative solutions so that health-care reform will evolve successfully. Leaders, however, cannot shape the future alone; they must engage others to achieve this goal. In the future, it will be even more important to have an emphasis on cultivating followers. As Bennis (2007) says, ". . . leaders do not exist in a vacuum . . . leadership in its simplest form is a tripod [consisting of] a leader or leaders, followers, and the common goal they want to achieve" (p. 3). Nursing leaders and followers must analyze scientific, technological, and health-care trends and identify innovative strategies to maximize the nurse's role in leading change in health-care delivery.

Hillburn, McNulty, Jewett, and Wainwright (2006) and Matter (2006) urged nurses to use evidence-based practice protocols to participate in developing more reflective practice. They suggest that one of the ways to create the future is through using advances in science and technology. It is time for each individual nurse to get involved and make a difference in his or her practice area and in the profession as a whole, engaging in more reflective practice, which will (hopefully) improve morale and increase quality of care, as well as increase measurements such as patient satisfaction scores to reflect positively on nurses. This, in turn, will assist nurses to have the confidence and voice necessary to lead change initiatives in health-care reform. For example, the patient satisfaction survey assessment scores are a meaningful benchmark for institutions to use to market their successes. These outcome measurements are also significant for a successful Magnet application, which recognizes nursing's contributions and gives a reason for senior leadership to reflect on nursing and how nurses make such a significant difference. Nurses must use their emotional intelligence, critical thinking, negotiating skills, and vision to create their preferred future.

An example of leading excellence with evidence-based research in health care is the Magnet Model developed by the American Nurses Credentialing Center (American Association of Nurse Credentialing, 2011), which includes five components:

1. **Transformational leadership,** which is how nurses need to lead in order to make a difference and consistently provide the highest quality of care
2. **Structural empowerment,** so that nurses will be supported for innovative change that improves morale and ultimately practice
3. **Exemplary professional practice,** which demonstrates the highest competency possible of nurses in all types of practice
4. **New knowledge, innovations, and improvements** that indicate that evidence-based practice is transforming care and achieving high-quality patient outcomes
5. **Empirical quality results,** which are the ultimate goal of the first four components

Ingersoll, Witzel, Berry, and Qualls (2010) share how they created a hospital-based research center as the infrastructure to support this Magnet Model of evidence-based practice and research at their institution, and were able to transform their care. Abad-Corpa, Meseguer-Liza, Martinez-Corbalan, and their colleagues (2010) give an example of how they implemented an evidence-based model of practice on their oncohematology unit using participatory action research. The authors discuss how this new model assisted them in improving the nurse-sensitive outcomes, increasing nursing knowledge, and changing the nurses' attitudes and behavior. It is mandatory for nurses working in an evidence-based clinical setting to be knowledgeable of the new therapies and treatment and also to be aware of their contribution to sustaining this care model. The nurse, in many situations, will be the most knowledgeable about specific new evidence-based care and will need to lead the interdisciplinary team. Ideally, nurses who work in this type of health care setting will:

- Not feel overwhelmed and paralyzed in their thinking
- Be able to do something new or learn about a new topic even though they may be thinking in very task-oriented manners about their patient assignments shift after shift
- Think that change may be the solution to why they are feeling so overwhelmed and paralyzed

PREDICTING THE FUTURE

When listening to someone talk about things they expect to see in the future, it is often difficult not to laugh or roll one's eyes. Ideas that sounded like science fiction only a few years ago—Wikipedia (an online encyclopedia to which anyone can contribute), cars that drive themselves with GPS guidance, gene therapy, battery-powered city cars used for short or long distances and then parked to recharge, cars that are programmed to self-park, iPhones, Androids, Skype for one-on-one and group interactions, recycling waste centers, using oysters or other natural organisms to purge the garbage from what can be reused—are very real in today's world. Kaku (2011) shares some of the information he obtained by interviewing multiple scientists regarding their ideas on predictions in their fields of medicine, nanotechnology, computer science, and energy production over the next 100 years in his book, *Physics of the future: How science will shape human destiny and our daily lives by the year 2100*. The predictions he shares revolve around potential possibilities of all types of technology that will emerge over the next 100 years. In health care, multiple trends are shaping a new future: the change to palliative care instead of hospice, addressing nursing staff and faculty shortages, and managing health care better financially. Publications such as *Futurescan: Health Trends and Implications 2011–2016* (American College of Healthcare Executives, 2011) cite multiple predictions that imply some big changes for health care, including some that are already in process:

- The use of social networks in the hospital environment—maintaining top security of the hospital's organizational files
- Electronic documentation for every aspect of record keeping
- Use of globalization to engage health-care professionals in other countries to interpret images and laboratory findings and to collaborate on differential diagnoses
- Reimbursement (or not) focused on government or private insurance–driven outcomes—health-care reform
- Nurse practitioners and physician assistants as the main workforce for primary health-care delivery
- Robotic surgical technology such as the da Vinci microsurgery technology
- Institution credentialing for nonprofessional health-care workers

Nursing leaders need to be aware of these trends so that the profession will be influenced positively and be a leading force in creating the future of health care, not merely reacting and adapting to those changes. Nurses need to adapt new leadership skills that include a forward-thinking perspective in order to accomplish the following (Canton, 2006):

- Recruit talent
- Create innovative work environments to retain staff
- Set the highest possible expectations and vision for the unit, department, or practice
- Execute the new leadership profitably

There is only one direction for a leader: FORWARD.
—*Advertisement*

Kouzes and Posner (2007) recommend that nurses think of the future as a time for great things and that, in most instances, things will improve. These authors surveyed leaders about the future and found that terms such as "foresight," "focus," "forecasts," "future scenarios," "perspectives," and "points of view" are common in discussions of visions of the future. It is important, however, that leaders be able to translate these global terms into detailed descriptors as much as possible when sharing the vision so that followers can better understand what the vision represents and more fully participate in making it a reality.

There are methods that futurists use to try to determine future happenings. Leaders must know a particular area well, understand how certain occurrences in this area started and evolved, and be knowledgeable about how patterns of related happenings might affect the area currently and in the future. This kind of information will assist the leader in knowing how and where to notice trends and determine whether they are indicators of future patterns. Aburdene (2011) reminds nurses to use past occurrences as they attempt to predict future ones. By examining these past trends and how they affected the world, nurses will be more prepared to anticipate consequences of the new trends and not be surprised.

Futurists recommend that leaders read what is new and predicted for the future, review the histories of significant developments, maintain a global perspective on new issues and economic growth, and review information from sources like the Census Bureau and the Bureau of Labor Statistics. Every individual and every profession or group need some context within which successful plans for the future can be made, and resources such as these help a leader create that context.

Four kinds of futures are addressed in the literature (Valiga, 1994):

1. The *probable future* is what is likely to occur if things continue as they are and no changes are made.
2. The *possible future* is what can occur if some changes are made in the current state of affairs.
3. The *plausible future* is what is likely to occur when specific efforts are made to accomplish goals.
4. The *preferred future* is what one would like to see happen.

Using this framework is a good way to brainstorm about the future. Small groups of nurses can create various scenarios to increase their ability to visualize different futures and to strategize how they can create the future they want for nursing. This might occur in a retreat setting where nurses engage in strategic vision planning, or it can begin at staff meetings or during discussions over coffee.

By analyzing changes in societal values, public policies, and individual behaviours that are significant to the future of health, rather than dwelling merely on medical breakthroughs, nurses can significantly influence the general welfare of humanity. For example, if society does not deal with poverty and illiteracy, both of which are related to illness, more people will use hospital emergency departments for their basic health care, thereby increasing costs; less emphasis will be placed on health promotion and disease prevention; and the poor will be likely to have more illness complications. If nurses become involved in developing health policy that mandates health promotion for the uninsured, impoverished, and illiterate, people will likely have a greatly improved future.

> *Leadership is a process rather than an event. We don't always know how, when, or what we will lead. Each of us wants our life to stand for something. Being able to have an impact—to make a difference—is perhaps the biggest benefit of being a leader. —Sarah Weddington*

Nurses can make strong contributions to improving health care in multiple areas and can significantly change the quality of life for many, as well as enhance cost savings and health-care quality, by accomplishing the following:

- Educating the public
- Providing testimony for changes in health-care policy
- Providing wellness care to the poor and underserved
- Creating nurse-driven initiatives to maximize quality outcomes for a more patient-centered health-care reform
- Speaking out about issues or injustices in one's workplace

Most nurses would probably agree that the preferred future depicts a healthier, more educated population. Health promotion will reign, and wellness-focused health centers will populate the country and outnumber disease management clinics. Nurses, as leaders of health, must propel their visions forward and begin thinking in a future-forward frame of mind so that they can have more input into how the future will transpire. Nurses in every aspect of care have the power, for example, to spearhead a massive antiobesity campaign by educating all people about obesity's negative impact on health. Who better than nurses to teach the population how to manage health, prevent illness, reduce complications of illness, and choose health resources?

Molitor (1998) reminds us to be aware of possible "wild cards," such as meteor strikes, volcanic eruptions, and other disastrous events that could disrupt the best laid plans. Since Molitor provided us with this warning, we have seen the effects of many natural disasters, including devastating earthquakes, tsunamis, typhoons, tornados, and hurricanes. We have also witnessed the events of September 11, 2001, during which terrorists flew two hijacked airliners into the Twin Towers of New York City's World Trade Center, toppling them and killing thousands. We also need to realize that things no one had dreamed or thought to be so significant, such as individuals wanting to learn how to fly jumbo jets but not how to take off or land them, can have a significant influence on future developments. This is an example of what no one could have possibly conceived of coming true. Nurses, being in the grassroots of health care, are confronted with multiple events every day that no one would have predicted could occur. When new graduate nurses or nurses who have not worked in the "trenches" are faced with patients with complex injuries resulting from trauma, many "freeze" and cannot process the situation. Perhaps these nurses need to practice in a simulated health-care laboratory so that they can gain experience and knowledge for when they are confronted with real-life patients with extreme injuries. Uncertainty and unpredictability can result in positive change if they cause nurses to think and change.

Today's new science of leadership makes us more open to the unknown becoming a reality and to accepting that the future holds endless possibilities for us. Despite this unpredictability, however, nurses must attempt to shape the future because "foresight enhances abilities to capitalize upon opportunities, decrease adversities, gain lead time for responding, and assert leadership in trying to manage change" (Molitor, 1998, p. 59).

A preferred future does not just happen. We dream about it and shape it to some extent every day. Whenever a change is proposed, no matter how small, that change influences the future and can contribute to the growth of the organization or profession. Change of any type ultimately will have ramifications for any number of people.

> *There are three kinds of people: those who make things happen; those who watch things happen; and those who wonder what happened.* —Anonymous

An example from clinical practice may help illustrate this notion of interdependence and how a change can have a "ripple effect." A nurse in the cardiothoracic intensive care unit draws on research data to suggest that every nurse use the forced warm air blanket instead of the fluid-filled blanket to rewarm postoperative patients. The nurse implements this change for her patients and monitors their rewarming times, frequency of cardiac dysrhythmias, cost, and electrolyte balance. Consistent with reported research findings, this nurse finds that rewarming times are shorter, dysrhythmias are less frequent, electrolyte imbalances are reduced, and the cost of care is less. As a result of this change, this nurse's idea becomes a hospital-wide protocol. This nurse then disseminates her findings in a publication and is invited to address critical care nurses at a regional conference. The nurse's findings are validated at other institutions, and eventually a state-of-the-art postoperative rewarming standard of care is accepted (Grossman, Bautista, & Sullivan, 2002). This is an example of how one idea, tested by one nurse, then acted on and followed through by other nurses, can generate a significant difference for patients and have a positive impact economically.

Perhaps more nurses need to advocate for "killing sacred cows" by not always sticking to a plan and encouraging an "if-it-ain't-broke, break-it" philosophy. Such thinking allows more participation in developing a vision that is exciting, creating a future that is challenging and with new opportunities.

Nurses continue to be the largest health-care occupation; 2.6 million full-time registered nurses (RNs) are employed in the United States, with about 60% of the RNs employed by hospitals (Bureau of Labor Statistics, 2011). In March 2011 alone, 37,000 new jobs were added to hospitals, long-term care facilities, and other ambulatory care centers, and the highest percentage of health-care workers hired were RNs (Bureau of Labor Statistics, 2011).

Despite this, Buerhaus, Auerbach, and Staiger (2009) predict there will be a new RN shortage in 2018. The current nurse shortage is masked; health-care facilities have few openings in many geographical areas of the United States because many older nurses are working longer than they expected owing to the sluggish economy and financial uncertainty. Once the economy turns, many of these older nurses will retire and create new positions. Buerhaus and colleagues (2009) project that the 2018 shortage of RNs will continue to expand. Only 50% of the RNs in the United States are prepared at the baccalaureate or graduate level, whereas the other 50% are prepared with an associates degree (American Association of Colleges of Nursing [AACN], 2011). The nursing profession needs to be sure RNs are educated to lead and make the necessary changes in health-care reform.

The Institute of Medicine (IOM) and the Robert Wood Johnson Foundation created *The Future of Nursing: Leading Change and Advancing Health* Report in 2010, which provided several recommendations for the profession that have a direct bearing on leadership ability of RNs:

- Nurses should practice to the full extent of their education and training.
- Nurses should achieve higher levels of education and training through an improved education system that promotes seamless academic progression.
- Nurses should be full partners with physicians and other health-care professionals when redesigning health care in the United States.
- Effective workforce planning and policy making require better data collection and an improved information infrastructure.

The IOM is advising nurses to continue their education and wants nursing schools to offer more flexible programs. Nurses, with all other health-care professionals, need to bring their ideas to the table and make strong contributions toward guiding health-care reform. If nurses are well educated, they most likely will have the ability to lead more successfully and also be knowledgeable about informatics. This message from the IOM is imperative for nurses to follow so that nurses will have a preferred future in health care. Nurses are in an opportune position currently, and each nurse needs to propel himself or herself further so that the profession will be a strong contributor in reforming the health-care system. Additionally, making international partnerships between universities is essential, and to be successful must be established as a priority during resource allocation. The nursing profession needs to network with nurses and health-care workers globally. Nurses need to gain more creative and innovative ways of delivering care and educating nurses, as well as anything else that can help make the largest health-care profession the strongest. Wildavsky (2010) offers exemplars and advice on how globalization is changing higher education around the world in his book, *The Great Race: How Global Universities Are Reshaping the World*. Not only can the profession gain an exponential amount of ideas for improving nursing education, but also it can garnerinnovative ways to "reshape" the world by using culture- and country-specific health-care delivery with the opportunity to connect electronically for global access to patients' medical records.

It is important to be aware of the work being done by the 34 current nursing workforce centers and the new initiatives in education, policy, service, and health services research they support (National State Nursing Workforce Centers, 2011). Just about each state has a Web site operated by their State Nursing Workforce Center that can be helpful to nurses interested in furthering their education and gaining entry into the state's health policy arenas. The growing diversity of our population, aging baby boomers, technological advances, the genome model, and palliative care movement are trends that have had an impact on health care and will continue to influence the role of the nurse.

GENERAL PREDICTIONS ABOUT THE FUTURE

It is difficult not to be slightly pessimistic when considering some of the current issues and predictions about the future: climate change and the possibility of ecological deterioration, nuclear or biological warfare, terrorism, increased violence, economic demise, and infectious diseases that are resistant to antibiotic therapy. Such challenges and predictions, however, also can serve to challenge us to plan proactively to minimize these possibilities and their negative effects. Challenges can promote enthusiasm for countering negative trends, for example, by developing super antibiotics, connecting to possible alien civilizations in space, increasing the quality of life and life span, benefiting from the ability to map all 80,000 genes in human DNA, strengthening the total world infrastructure, and using solar power and other renewable energy sources.

If there is no struggle, there is no progress.
—*Frederick Douglass*

Advancements in consumer electronics will assist in greater communication, easier access to services, at-home jobs, less traveling time, increased leisure time, and new education avenues. Just for a moment, think about this possibility: all roads and cars are removed from the earth; the old roads are made into moving sidewalks where one steps on and, with a handheld apparatus, controls the direction and speed of one's trip. Just think of the decrease in trauma that would result if there were no automobile crashes. The reality is that most people still have cars, and traffic jams and crashes still exist. We can still envision, however, a preferred future in which energy is clean and conserved, and more travelers use super-fast rail systems, mini battery-charged city cars, and suborbital space travel. Changes such as these will affect global trade, influence how people interact with one another and how they spend their time, and possibly assist people in living a more productive life.

In addition to infrastructure changes, dramatic changes in family structures and population demographics will continue to occur. The family unit is undergoing great change. There are more single-parent families, grandparent families, and blended families than ever before. The U.S. population is approximately 313,232,044. About 20.1% of the people in the United States are younger than 14 years, 66.8% are between the ages of 15 and 64 years, and 14% are older than 65 years (CIA World Factbook, 2011).

The U.S. population currently makes up less than 5% of the world population, but it will make up only 4% of the world population in 25 years. Thus, America is not growing in population the way many other countries are growing. There will be fewer young people in America, and the United States will have less of a voice regarding national and global issues. Currently, the median age in the United States is 36.9 years, and the life expectancy is 75.92 for men and 80.93 for women. Of today's U.S. population, 14% is at least 65 years old, and 20% of the population is expected to be at least 65 years by 2030; thus it is accurate to say a large portion of the health-care business is and will continue to be caring for older adults (CIA World Factbook, 2011).

Because of the increase in the elderly population (currently one in eight people in the United States is older than 65 years) and the decrease in the percentage of the younger population, the United States may give more priority to issues affecting the old compared with those issues influencing the young. The result of this improvement in life span is a vast increase in the number of older adults within the population and a definite change in focus for health care. Nurses can do the following:

- Lead initiatives to help older adults stay in their homes
- Advocate for reimbursement for self-care and for elders' taking responsibility for their own health issues
- Set up volunteering, mentoring, role modeling, and pay-for-time jobs for older adults to participate in their communities
- Create specific health-care policies to protect older adults' rights regarding health

With the increased number of retirees and decreased number of workers, there is great uncertainty regarding solvency of the Social Security system in 30 years. Ethical considerations for caring for the elderly, critically ill individuals with multiple-organ disease, the disabled, and those found to have genetic defects will be more prevalent, which will force the health-care system to explore new alternatives to providing care for the very ill and dying. There will continue to be a paradigm change of providing palliative care to people with advanced chronic illnesses, as well as to the terminally ill.

PREDICTIONS ABOUT THE FUTURE OF HEALTH CARE

Between 2009 and 2010, the cost of health care increased at a rate of 3.9%, similar to the gross domestic product (GDP), which increased at 3.8% (Davis, 2011). This slower than usual increase in health-care cost, however, was due to the high unemployment rate in the United States. Unemployment has prevented about 5 million health-care visits in the past 2 years because many unemployed people have lost their private insurance coverage and choose to go without preventive care (Davis, 2011). Health-care costs in the United States are predicted to consume about 21% of the GDP in 2020 (Davis, 2011). In 2009, 50.7 million Americans were uninsured (Davis, 2011). It is no wonder, then, that cost is a major issue in health care today. Some governmental and corporate organizations have started to import their members' drug prescriptions and imaging interpretation from other countries to attempt to decrease costs. Some individuals even have elective surgeries in countries other than the United States to save costs.

"Health-care quality" seems to be the buzz phrase today and a factor that individuals use to choose a health-care agency. Likewise, health-care organizations are focusing more of their attention and resources on measuring and marketing their patient outcomes. The American Nurses Association (2011) has responded by developing nursing-sensitive quality indicators to implement in acute care settings and home care, and these can help nursing claim a significant leadership role in health care. The emphasis on the quality of services provided at a reasonable cost has many benefits, including the following:

- More educated consumers
- Certification for health-care providers
- Choice of health-care provider (e.g., nurse practitioner, nurse anes-thetist, nurse midwife, physician)
- More health partnerships
- More independence for nurses and other nonphysician providers
- Telehealth
- An outcomes-driven system
- Improved care for patients, families, and communities

The emphasis on quality and the measurement of outcomes require that all health-care professionals be accountable and responsible for providing competent interventions that generate positive patient outcomes. Robert and Sebastian (2006) provide an example regarding implementation of a Tele-Intensivist Program that improved patient safety, and quality was demonstrated when computer physician-order entry, evidence-based hospital referrals, and intensive care unit physician staffing were implemented. Another good example of how nurses were able to improve care significantly is the integration of a nurse-driven electronic system for communicating reliable outcome information (Johnson, Hallsey, Meredith, & Warden, 2006). Improvements included cost-effectiveness, less time with nurse-to-nurse reporting and documentation by nurses of care rendered, and improved nurse satisfaction with communication change.

In the future, health care will focus increasingly on the prevention of illness and the promotion of health. More care will be provided in short-stay units, urgent-care centers, subacute facilities, and homes. Except for some very rural providers, most health-care agencies are now affiliated with a large corporation. Health care has moved from independent, freestanding agencies to integrated networks that focus not only on primary or tertiary care but also on the entire continuum of health-care delivery. It is expected that all health-care agencies will continue to develop affiliations with other hospitals, home-care agencies, rehabilitation centers, subacute care facilities, community centers, long-term care facilities, and laboratories, as well as satellite centers in the community to provide primary and secondary care to neighborhoods. Hospitals no longer will deal merely with health restoration but also with health promotion and maintenance. In fact, some policies in place today allow individuals with a normal body mass index (BMI) to get reductions on their health-care insurance premiums (About.com, 2009). Multiple possibilities will be beneficial in the future, such as anti-aging antidotes, medications that decrease insulin resistance before the patient is diagnosed with diabetes mellitus, antiobesity remedies, and drugs that can decrease lipid accumulation that are already being used. New techniques in diagnostic technology and genetic research are expected to move us from a "diagnose-and-treat" scenario (once symptoms are manifested) to a "predict-and-manage-in-a-proactive-fashion" scenario (even before symptoms are evident) that would include measures like gene therapy to create new peripheral vessels for extremities.

Computerization will continue to allow all providers to access the patient's record, regardless of location, and patients/consumers will be able to access their records freely. Multidisciplinary teams involving physicians, nurses, social workers, physical therapists, psychologists, occupational therapists, and other providers one cannot even envision today will follow evidence-based protocols to deliver quality care to patients. They will be delivering that care in the patient's home or community, including schools, malls, workplaces, satellite health centers, and other access points.

PREDICTIONS ABOUT THE FUTURE OF NURSING

Nursing shortages and patient safety are two of the most significant issues facing nursing in the future. Employment of RNs is expected to grow by 22% in the next decade to 2018. RNs needed for physician offices will increase by 48%, in home health care by 33%, in nursing homes by 25%, in employment services by 24%, and in hospitals by 17% (U.S. Department of Labor, 2008). It seems there must be different ways to deliver nursing care so that the next predicted shortage will not mitigate the ability to provide safe and high-quality patient care. Some care delivery methods that may be considered are making group patient appointments for routine diabetes, hypertension, and asthma evaluations; having all electronic prescriptions; and assigning a member of a patient's family (after appropriate teaching by the professional physical therapist) to conduct physical therapy exercises or ambulation therapy, rather than a nonlicensed paid individual.

Many elements of the chaos in health care, such as downsizing of health-care institutions, changing from an illness to a wellness perspective, moving from private physician–dominated providers to multidisciplinary systems, and using capitated payment systems, all have had an impact on nursing. In addition, many demographic changes, such as the increasing elderly population, single-parent families, ethnic diversity, homelessness, and underprivileged people needing health care in their communities, provide increased opportunities for delivering care outside the hospital.

The nursing workforce needs more nurses who practice autonomously, use evidence-based nursing interventions that generate positive patient outcomes, are respected as experts in certain areas of patient care, provide input to the development of health policy, and participate fully on multidisciplinary health-care teams. Both RNs and advanced practice registered nurses (APRNs) *must* be accountable for patient outcomes and eliminate old ways of thinking. In the past, "A nurse reports to the physician and merely needs to notify the physician about a change, or document a finding about a patient in the patient record." To create a preferred future for nurses, they must be responsible for identifying problems and seeing them through to a positive patient outcome. The future of the profession depends on nurses following through, taking responsibility, and documenting the outcomes of their research-based interventions. Only then will nurses truly be able to negotiate with colleagues from other health-care disciplines and be recognized for contributing significantly to quality and cost-effective care. As stated earlier, nurses must become involved not only in predicting the future but also in creating the future they prefer.

High technology, including patient monitoring systems, computerized medication administration, interactive computer communication, and computerized patient data storage, is a good example of how nursing can benefit from change. Technological advances such as those just mentioned maximize the potential for nurses to spend more time with patients, allow more independent clinical judgments, provide immediate communication with other members of the health-care team, and help nurses manage patient data for quick retrieval when analyzing patient outcomes. Another way that technology benefits health care is through distance education. Several models of educating health-care providers through course management modalities have been successfully instituted around the world and demonstrate how attitudinal, technical, and structural barriers were overcome so that more nurses could become educated on a variety of topics (Lewis & Farrell, 2005).

To shape a preferred future for nursing, all nurses should be involved with developing health policy, networking with legislators and political groups, and spearheading changes in the delivery of health care to consumers by participating on boards and taking on leadership positions in policy-making organizations. To accomplish these actions, however, nurses need to be taught how to advocate for a change in health policy or how to initiate a new health policy. They also need to learn the politics of health care and the value of being a member of their state nurses' association. Gaining some experience during undergraduate and graduate nursing programs in sitting on a board, developing health policy, stepping up to the leadership position on a taskforce or committee in their work setting, or volunteering in a community health project by writing a grant for funding of an aspect of the project would assist nurses in shaping a preferred future for nursing. Such actions will enable nurses to influence necessary changes in health care that will improve the profession's image as a competent and powerful contributor to the health of the American people.

No longer can nurses focus solely on their particular unit or specialty area because nurses need to be specialty trained so that they are cross-trained to work on multiple units. Today's nurses cannot expect to work for the same employer throughout their careers because the technology and care of patients is changing exponentially. Many nurses who work in acute care institutions will need to be educated to work in outpatient delivery units. Nurses will need to constantly engage in learning new techniques, knowledge, and methods to communicate and document. They must be aware of the larger arena of health care, continue their education, and remain flexible. Nurses also will do well to focus on measuring nursing care outcomes, being attuned to cost-effectiveness, ensuring high-quality nursing interventions, participating in ethical debates, providing access to health care for all, working collaboratively with one another and with other health-care professionals, increasing educational preparation standards, and being a vital voice in health-care policy making. A good example of integrating nurse-sensitive outcomes with the assistance of performance and workload indicators to justify nurse staffing ratios is explained by Griffin and Swan (2006). They were able to identify specific actions that were performed by nurses (nurse-sensitive outcomes), and given this number of nurse-needed interventions, they could justify an allocation of a specific number of nurses to perform the necessary work needed on a unit.

> *Quality is never an accident; it is always the result of intelligent effort.* —*John Ruskin*

By studying patterns of change, being aware of important trends in one's specific area of nursing, keeping abreast of general health-care literature, and talking to others involved in health care, nurses will be able to deal more effectively with the unexpected that the future is bound to bring.

All nurses need to be knowledgeable about multiple views of issues facing health care, nursing education, and the nursing profession, as well as to be flexible and capable of making a decision when the need arises. For example, a staff nurse directs the care of patients and reviews, and in many instances, determines or coordinates what transpires between the health-care team and each patient. In addition, he or she plays a negotiator role regarding what the patient should receive, what type of services, and when. The nurse also oversees ancillary workers, builds consensus to successfully implement patients' plans of care, takes risks in demanding that patient safety and high-quality care be given, and empowers patients and other staff to speak up and be counted among those who will make a difference. Nurses need to be knowledgeable about the health-care delivery system in which they work, as well as about the newest knowledge on which their practice is based.

It is important to realize that no single individual can determine what the future will be, but nurses can shape their own future by being cognizant of multiple possibilities and open to trying new, and even radical, changes. Nurses cannot sit back passively and accept everything the future hands them; instead, they must create a preferred future of nursing. How can they do that? The following discussion is intended to help nurses become more effective in increasing their own ability to shape a preferred future for the profession and for health care.

Approaches to Shaping a Preferred Future for Nursing

Nursing education must prepare graduates who have the ability to participate as full partners in health-care delivery and shape health policy. Nursing curricula should emphasize patient safety, patient education, health promotion, rehabilitation, self-care, alternative methods of healing, and palliative care while maintaining the concern for acute and tertiary care. Both accreditation bodies in nursing, the National League for Nursing Accrediting Commission (NLNAC) and the Commission on Collegiate Nursing Education (CCNE), recommend that nursing educators, along with nurse executives and clinicians in practice settings, shape practice. All curricula should include, at appropriate levels, case management, health-care policy, research, quality indicators, outcome measures, financial management, legislative advocacy, and management of data. The notion of lifelong learning for all nurses to maintain competency must also be continually addressed, perhaps through mandatory continuing education or certification.

> *You don't have to be brilliant to be a good leader. But you do have to understand other people—how they feel, what makes them tick, and the best way to influence them.* —John Luther

Nursing Image

Nurses also must clearly define what they do and communicate it to the public so that consumers will be able to understand the role of the RN and APRN. Malloch and Porter-O'Grady (2010) recommend that nurses expand their roles to work as consultants to the public, patient or professional specialty groups, health-care equipment or pharmaceutical corporations, day-care centers, or any group interested in health. These exemplary entrepreneurs in nursing say that the skills of the staff nurse, grounded in practice and framed by the discipline of nursing, more than adequately prepare the nurse to take on the expanding demand of the consultant's role. In the future, more nurses who are competent in their specific area will be expected to serve as consultants, thereby increasing the public's knowledge of what nurses do.

Influencing Change

The nurse leader must go further than identifying that there is a need for change and assisting others to be a part of the evolution of this change. Rather, nurse leaders need to promote alternative practice models (e.g., health teaching on the Internet by assigned nurses, mobile satellite stations that provide care scattered in a community housing project, and telehealth technology to follow-up with discharge instructions) in order to maximize the use of expensive resources and conserve costs. Another idea that could greatly assist with making the future of health care brighter is to develop programs that allow older adults to stay in their own homes for a longer period of time before going to a long-term care facility. These changes in care delivery would positively affect health care even in the midst of a nursing shortage, high patient acuity, and escalating health-care costs. Also, nurses can help each other visualize that many traditional nursing activities could become a part of the patient's own care process. For example, nurses could have monthly group meetings to check blood pressure, weight, and blood work and offer a 15-minute interaction time between patients with similar problems regarding their best hints for managing their health problem. Families and patients can be instrumental in decreasing costs and increasing quality of health care. This new paradigm drastically changes what nurses will be doing in the future. The uncertainty that exists at present regarding this paradigm change provides nurses with an opportunity to create and "test" new care models that increase accountability of patients and families for their own health. At the same time, nurse leaders must be sure nurses are involved in hospital initiatives regarding work flow, physical plant changes, and communication-related issues because these areas are closely related to patient safety issues (Thompson, Navarra, & Antonson, 2005). An example of how collaborating nurses and physicians decrease medication errors using safe practices is described by Rogers, Alper, Brunelle, Federico, Fenn, and Leape (2006). This project involved 50 hospitals. The most significant factors identified as positive predictors for increasing safe practice regarding medications (both prescription orders and delivery of medications) included active physician and RN involvement at point of care, administrator participation, collaborative team engagement, and small-step procedure changes regarding the changes in medication prescription and delivery.

Nurses also need to receive ongoing education regarding knowledge and technical expertise to assist them to be prepared to care for their patients. Once again, there is the question of resources. Are there enough nurses to have a few nurses not assigned to patients and teaching other nurses, or should all nurses, similar to physicians, have a patient care responsibility during some portion of their work day? One would think there will continue to be a need for centralized staff development by staff nurse educators; however, there is a trend for more of the nursing support functions, such as orientation, training nurses on new equipment, and annual competency-based learning evaluation, to be conducted by unit-specific staff or by podcasting or video streaming. This is a controversial issue, and some acute care institutions do maintain a small centralized staff of nurse educators.

All nurses have a professional responsibility to maintain their competency by attending continuing education programs and in-house health-care symposiums. Advanced practice nurses need to spend direct clinical hours with patients and participate in continuing education to maintain their certification and thus their license. It would be excellent for the profession of nursing if each nurse were also involved in a nursing organization that was actively working to create a preferred future for the profession. Sigma Theta Tau International (STTI) and other organizations (e.g., American Association of Critical Care Nurses, American Nurses Association, American College of Nurse Practitioners, and Emergency Nurses Association) are committed to creating a positive future by offering leadership institutes, helping members expand their networks through the Internet or newsletters, and offering recognition through awards and citations as a way to motivate nurses to work at their highest level. Whether working at the local or chapter level as a committee member or officer, serving on a board of directors, working on an international committee, or reviewing manuscripts for an organization's journal, nurses are working to advance the future of nursing and are shaping that future by leading a health policy change, volunteering in the community to provide pro bono health care or knowledge, or keeping the image of nursing visible to the public. Senge, Scharmer, Jaworski, and Flowers (2004) remind us that the ultimate focus for the future is to lead in a just and human way and advocate for all.

Research

Research must be conducted to determine the extent to which research-based protocols are implemented and the cost-effectiveness of the patient outcomes. Nursing science must continue to be developed, so that nurses can provide care that will increase positive health-care outcomes (Bae, Mark, & Fried, 2010). For example, Bae, Mark, and Fried (2010) found that the turnover of RN staff was significantly linked to poor patient outcomes, which included patient falls, medication errors, patient satisfaction scores, and length of stay on the unit. Nurses can create a work milieu that is conducive to having a productive but friendly atmosphere, which should prevent RN turnover. This will foster more of a team approach and collaborative "think tank," where nurses work together for the greater good of the unit and, ultimately, the patients. Krapohl, Manojlovich, Redman, and Zhang (2010) also found that a positive workplace environment allowed for empowerment of each nurse by each other. They show how a strong and supportive workplace environment is associated with a higher number of certified nurses. Although more research needs to be conducted between the number of certified nurses and improved patient outcomes, it is still implied that there is a significant relationship. Similar findings linking a positive work environment and successful patient outcomes were found by Trinkoff, Johantgen, Storr, Gurses, Liang, and Han (2011a). In another study by this same group of nurse researchers, adverse patient outcomes were associated with poor work schedules and demands on nurses (Trinkoff, Johantgen, Storr, Gurses, Liang, & Han, 2011b). Nurse leaders can propose multiple interventions for staff in order to retain them, maintain a good work culture and attitude, and foster passion, excitement, and success.

Hesselbein and Goldsmith (2009) share multiple examples of how organizations that provide work environments that foster commitment and pride can be pivotal in creating long-lasting and positive organizational change for the future. Their book gives suggestions on what they believe are imperative steps for organizations to follow in order to secure a preferred future:

1. **Strategy and vision:** one must be able to identify and be able to follow a vision that is not stagnant but continuously evolving and relates to positive patient outcomes
2. **Organizational culture, values, emotions, hope, ethics, spirit, and behavior:** each organization needs to incorporate their values, emotions, hopes, spirit, and behavior and ethically create an organizational culture that transforms their employees and collaborative communities
3. **Designing the organization of the future:** a discussion of the "perfect storm" merging five socioeconomic shifts and how they affect organizations, from nonprofits to large corporations
4. **Working together:** to have successful organizations, it is paramount that there is a team spirit and that leaders and followers are working together
5. **Leaders:** a display of how the leaders of the future will lead, including examples of dynamic duos and corporate mavericks

Nurses must study the effectiveness of what they do and provide leadership, perhaps using Hesselbein and Goldsmith's (2009) suggestions, regarding the nursing aspect of multidisciplinary research. They must continue to study the health-care practices of various groups, as well as patient responses to specific interventions. Such patient responses might include pain management, understanding of one's health status, stress level, and ability to perform self-care to maintain or enhance function. In other words, nurses must measure the specific effect of nursing care and not merely describe problems that exist in health-care or nurses' perceptions of what the problems may be.

Dissemination of results should be done in publications and presentations, including those that are multidisciplinary in nature and those accessed by the public.

There must be a commitment to using research results as a basis for practice, and being involved in the conduct of research must be integral to every nurse's ongoing practice.

Today's chaotic world needs more than just a few leaders at the top. Leadership is not a position but a process and a role that everyone can and must assume at some point in time. Staub (1996) suggests that nurses look for leaders at all levels of society in all types of organizations, and that such people are the ones who are comfortable with "fuzzy logic" and "approximations" (p. xv). Consider the light switch, which turns a light on or off, and a dimmer switch, which allows a light to vary in degrees of brightness. According to Staub (1996, p. xv), the dimmer switch, which can be compared to fuzzy logic or approximations, "allows for a greater range of response and therefore flexibility to the requirements of the environment. . . . So too, in real life, [where] the range of options can be extended to many more iterations between the two fixed positions of off or on, right or wrong, black or white. In approaching the challenge of our complex world, it is important to remember that while white matters and black matters, where it really counts is in gray matter(s)." Thus, leaders who will help shape a preferred future for nursing will benefit from the use of "fuzzy logic."

In essence, everyone has something to offer; there is a place on the team where each person can make important contributions. Perhaps if the strengths of all individuals were appreciated, and they were empowered, members of a team would develop the self-confidence to do their very best and make significant contributions to shaping a preferred future. This attitude of people working hard, feeling good about themselves, and having their contributions acknowledged can significantly affect the accomplishment of a once seemingly distant vision.

> *The reward of a thing well done, is to have done it.*
> —Ralph Waldo Emerson

Partnering implies teamwork, with every member being equal and all connecting horizontally, or through a web structure (Helgesen, 1990), rather than vertically or through a hierarchical structure. Using principles of partnership such as equity, accountability, and ownership, each member contributes a unique set of talents to achieve the common goal (e.g., quality patient care), each partner is patient centered, and no one tells another partner what to do or when to do it. Indeed, the health-care system of tomorrow will not support the old type of authoritative behavior; instead, it will expect each person do her or his job with excellence. Such a paradigm supports collaboration, dialogue, patient participation, freedom of expression, and empowerment, all of which are crucial to success. Nurses must take pride in the responsibility they have to monitor patients and provide health surveillance in all health-care settings. Nurse must take pride in the leadership they provide as case coordinators and the role they play in "holding the system together." This is what nurses do, and it is their unique contribution to health care. With the increase in equal partnering, nursing has a new frontier to pursue and new roles to assume.

CHARACTERISTICS OF NURSE LEADERS NEEDED TO CREATE A PREFERRED FUTURE FOR NURSING

Leaders of tomorrow must be transformational ones. Transformation leaders are those who can propel a vision, recruit the new generation of nurses, empower followers to work enthusiastically to realize a vision, meet change "head on" and grow from it, harness conflict to ensure people are thinking in different ways, and keep harmful stress at a minimum for themselves and the organization. They must be designers, teachers, and stewards (Senge, 2006): *designers* assist in developing the vision; *teachers* help followers develop the skills and gain the knowledge to work toward making the vision a reality; and *stewards* act as spokespersons for the group, keep the group focused on the vision, and facilitate the long-term growth of all followers.

Leaders have ideas about what the future can bring and what it could be like, but they do not just sit around and wait for things to happen. In fact, Bennis (2007), who has interviewed multiple leaders and identified common talents they possess, concludes that exemplary leaders have six skill competencies that define them as leaders:

1. Create a sense of mission
2. Motivate followers to work with them on the mission
3. Develop a social ambience for their followers
4. Create trust and optimism
5. Develop others to lead
6. Obtain results

Leaders for the future take action, engage in self-evaluation, seek feedback from colleagues, set goals and periodically evaluate progress in meeting them, advance their own knowledge, and try new things (Valiga, 1994). Being able to envision the future and create a sense of vision separates leaders from others. To accept the challenge of leading is a decision each of us must make. When nurses accept that challenge, they also accept responsibility for shaping a preferred future for nursing. Nurses may be more successful in shaping a preferred future if they incorporate the following guidelines (Kouzes & Posner, 2007):

- Be ready to embark on the vision.
- Maintain your credibility, integrity, and competence and think of the future.
- Stay grounded but think *big*—try something new but be realistic!
- Be aware you cannot do it by yourself—you need a team.
- Every individual needs to use her or his leadership abilities.

As long as a person has a vision, articulates it clearly, enlists others to help make it a reality, is aware of factors that influence it, and is able to keep the vision on course, that individual really is a leader and is shaping a preferred future. Johansen (2009) suggests the following characteristics for leaders to acquire in order to be well prepared to lead in the future:

- **Maker instinct:** try to create your own and connect with all that you possibly can.
- **Clarity:** think logically and present a plan to manage the complications and hard times that may present . . . keep motivated and on track.

- **Dilemma flipping:** turn dilemmas, which are problems that cannot be solved and just have to be accepted, into challenges and opportunities.
- **Immersive learning ability:** immerse yourself into the digital environment and gain new skills.
- **Bio-empathy:** if you try to see issues and problems through nature's patterns, you will gain new and successful solutions.
- **Constructive depolarizing:** assist all from diverse backgrounds to connect with each other.
- **Quiet transparency:** be open and authentic with everyone and do not brag about yourself.
- **Rapid prototyping:** try out your new ideas spontaneously and see if any catch on . . . if not, try another one.
- **Smart mob organizing:** always network, even when you think there is no use.
- **Commons creating:** be sure to have a common asset that is respected and generates competition between the group members to work a little harder.

It is much more exciting to help determine what the future will be than to merely react to it as it happens around us. True wisdom and true leadership come from learning from the past, enjoying and growing in the present, preparing for the future, and creating the future.

Never give up your credibility by saying, "This may be a dumb question, but . . ." —Elizabeth Tegues

Phenomenon of Leadership: What Is New? Should You Change Your Practice?

Everyone knows there are as many definitions of leadership as there are books on the topic. Nurses must continue to review the literature on leadership and integrate new ideas and findings into their practice in order to grow personally and strengthen the profession. Because there is no procedure book on the leadership skills necessary for nurses to acquire (contrary to the clinical skill procedures that are described specifically), nurses must be prepared to help each other lead in the dynamic health-care arena of the future. They lead based on what has been successful in the past and what they learn from others (e.g., through reading, listening to presentations, observing or studying others). The following case study illustrates how nurse practitioners made significant differences in their practice by collaborating daily on a communication board.

This example of a common situation illustrates how nurses in any practice setting can choose to exercise leadership. Assimilating similar assessment data, detecting patterns, and finding commonalities among the data helped these nurse practitioners make a difference in the care they provided. These nurses were empowered to take the time and make a difference because they cared enough to discuss their intuitive thoughts. Nurses have much

Case Study

At a college health clinic, the nurse practitioners are seeing several patients complaining of pruritus from a rash randomly scattered on their legs. The lesions are isolated to the lower extremities, and the nurses soon determine that it appears to be poison ivy. Upon discussion with one another, they realize that the patients include many athletes from the track team that participated in a tournament presently going on in a nearby state. When more details are shared among the nurse practitioners, it is determined that the method of transmission is by droplets from running through puddles on the dirt road leading to the competition field. None of the students remember having direct exposure to poison ivy or any plants. One of the nurse practitioners calls the university where the tournament took place and shares the findings collected regarding the multiple cases of contact dermatitis resembling poison ivy. Representatives from the hosting university recall that the grounds had recently had some pruning in preparation for the tournament and determine that clippings of poison ivy could very well have had blown into the puddles. It is most reasonable to conclude, therefore, that as students run through these puddles, they are infected by the droplets.

The nurse practitioners identified a pattern, realizing there was a correlation with being at the tournament university and contracting poison ivy, communicated their findings with each other and the host university, and recommended that action be taken to prevent other athletes and bystanders from further exposure during the ongoing tournament. After seeing the positive outcomes of this experience, the nurse practitioners decided to institute the daily use of a whiteboard inside their office to document high-frequency or unusual diagnoses they see in the clinic.

This collaborative communication whiteboard has come to be a most helpful method of assisting with diagnosing. Because these nurse practitioners cared enough to get to the bottom of the poison ivy epidemic, they were able to make a difference. Likewise, the practitioners have been very successful in recognizing community-acquired methicillin-resistant *Staphylococcus aureus* in wounds, identifying a scabies-infected group of students, educating the wrestling team regarding impetigo, and finding other problems sooner than had occurred when they saw patients in isolation of each other and did not communicate as effectively.

to share and can lead others in providing improved care to patients if they use their leadership competencies. Some nurses would greatly benefit by expanding their knowledge and using new leadership skills to assist them in changing the way they practice.

CONCLUSION

The world around us is changing dramatically, and the role of the nurse will continue to expand and evolve. In light of this, nurses must decide how they want the role to develop and then plan to make that happen. It would seem that all nurses can embrace the vision of providing quality health care to anyone in need. What they need to do now is work collaboratively to make this vision a reality. They must think critically, not on a linear trajectory but with a multidimensional perspective, and communicate effectively with their equal partners on the health-care team to determine the evidence-based interventions that will result in the highest quality of patient care.

Leadership must be everybody's business. That means each nurse has to believe that every nurse does have the power to make a difference with maximizing the health outcomes of patients. Just like nurses work with experienced nurses to gain clinical expertise, nurses need to shadow expert leaders and be mentored by someone who can help an individual nurse grow. Every nurse must stand up for a cause, bridge a gap, network with others, and do what needs to be done to move the profession forward toward *the future she or he wants.*

CRITICAL THINKING EXERCISES

Imagine that it is the year 2020 and you will be interviewed by an international nursing journal about the significant difference you have made to the nursing profession. What will you talk about? What significant differences have you made? How will you respond when the interviewer asks what you plan to do in the next 5 years to continue to make a difference?

_____

_____

Draw a picture of your vision of the future role of the nurse. What could you do to make this vision a reality? Share your ideas with your professor, nurse manager, or colleagues.

_____

_____

Identify three positive events related to your nursing career or your education as a nursing student that you experienced in the past. Describe why each may have happened. Review these positive events and determine a pattern. What can you learn from this analysis that could help you shape your own professional future?

_____

_____

Identify three negative events related to your nursing career or your education as a nursing student that you experienced in the past. Describe why each may have happened. Review these negative events to see if a pattern emerges. What can you learn from this analysis that could help you shape your own professional future?

_____

_____

Given the predictions about the future in general, the future of health care, and the future of nursing, what kinds of nurse leaders will the profession need to shape a preferred future? Are these same qualities needed today? Why or why not? How will globalization affect these predictions?

_____

_____

Informally interview a variety of people (e.g., child, older adult, health-care provider, nurse colleagues, new college graduate) about the future of the health-care system. Ask them what they think things will be like in the year 2025 and beyond. Also, ask them what they think we need to do now to achieve the positive things they envision and avoid the negative things they think could happen. Are the views of nurses different from those of other groups? Are there differences in the views of nurses from different cultures?

_____

_____

References

Abad-Corpa, E., Meseguer-Liza, C., Martinez-Corbalan, J. T., & Zarate-Riscal, L., Caravaca-Hernandez, A., Paredes-Sidrach de Cardona, A., Carrillo-Alcaraz, A., Delgado-Hito, P., & Cabrero-Garcia, J. (2010). Effectiveness of the implementation of an evidence based nursing model using participatory action research in oncohematology: Research protocol. *Journal of Advanced Nursing, 66*(8), 1845–1851.

About.com (2009). *Business insurance.* Retrieved from http://businessinsure.about.com/b/2009/01/09/obesity-wellness-programs-and-health-insurance-savings.htm.

Aburdene, P. (2007). *Megatrends, 2010: The rise of conscious capitalism.* Charlottesville, VA: Hampton Roads Publishing.

American Association of Colleges of Nursing. (2011). *Nurse Shortage.* Retrieved from http://www.aacn.nche.edu/media/factsheets/nursingshortage.htm.

American Association of Nurse Credentialing (2011). *Magnet Model.* Retrieved from http://www.nursecredentialing.org/Magnet/ProgramOverview/New-Magnet-Model.aspx.

American College of Healthcare Executives. (2011). *Future scan: Health trends and implications 2011–2016.* New York, NY: Health Administration Press.

American Nurses Association (2011). *Nursing sensitive indicators.* Retrieved from http://www.nursingworld.org/MainMenuCategories/ThePracticeofProfessionalNursing/PatientSafetyQuality/Research-Measurement/The-National-Database/Nursing-Sensitive-Indicators_1.aspx.

Bae, S., Mark, B., Fried, B. (2010). Impact of nursing unit turnover on patient outcomes in hospitals. *Journal of Nursing Scholarship, 42*(1), 40–49.

Bennis, W. (2007). The challenges of leadership in the modern world. *American Psychologist, 62*(1), 2–5.

Buerhaus, P., Auerbach, D. I., & Staiger, D. O. (2009). The recent surge in nurse employment: Causes and implications. *Health Affairs, 28*: 4w657–w668.

Bureau of Labor Statistics. (2011). U.S. Department of Labor, *Occupational outlook handbook for RNs, 2011.* Retrieved from http://www.bls.gov/oco/pdf/ocos083.pdf.

Canton, J. (2006). *The extreme future: The top trends that will reshape the world for the next 5, 10, and 20 years.* New York, NY: Penguin Group.

CIA World Factbook. (2011). *Population.* Retrieved from https://www.cia.gov/library/publications/the-world-factbook/geos/us.html.

Davis, K. (2011). *Health spending continues to moderate: Cost of reform over estimated.* Commonwealth Fund, Retrieved from http://www.commonwealthfund.org/Blog/2011/Jul/Health-Spending-Continues-to-Moderate.aspx

Griffin, K., & Swan, B. (2006). Linking nursing workload and performance indicators in ambulatory care. *Nursing Economic$, 24*(1), 41–44.

Grossman, S. Bautista, C., & Sullivan, L. (2002). Using evidence based practice to develop a re-warming protocol for postoperative SICU patients. *Dimensions of Critical Care Nursing Journal, 21*(9), 206–214.

Helgesen, S. (1990). *The female advantage: Women's ways of leadership.* New York, NY: Doubleday Currency.

Hesselbein, F., & Goldsmith, M. (Eds.) (2009). *The organization of the future: Visions, strategies, and insights on managing in a new era.* San Francisco, CA: Jossey-Bass.

Hillburn, K., McNulty, J., Jewett, L., & Wainwright, K. (2006). Build upon strengths and leadership practices using EBP. *Nursing Management, 37*(11), 15–16.

Ingersoll, G. L., Witzel, P. A., Berry, C., & Qualls, B. (2010). CNE Series: Meeting Magnet research and evidence based practice expectations through hospital based research centers. *Nursing Economics, 28*(4), 226–236.

Institute of Medicine (2010). *The future of nursing: Leading change and advancing health.* Retrieved from http://www.iom.edu/Reports/2010/The-Future-of-Nursing-Leading-Change-Advancing-Health.aspx

Johansen, R. (2009). *Leaders make the future: Ten new leadership skills for an uncertain world.* San Francisco, CA: Barrett–Koehler Publishing.

Johnson, K., Hallsey, D., Meredith, R., & Warden, E. (2006). A nurse-driven system for improving patient quality outcomes. *Journal of Nursing Care Quality, 21*(2), 168–175.

Kaku, M. (2011). *Physics of the future: How science will shape human destiny and our daily lives by the year 2100.* New York, NY: Doubleday.

Kouzes, J., & Posner, B. (2007). *The leadership challenge: How to keep getting extraordinary things done in organizations* (4th ed.). San Francisco, CA: Jossey-Bass.

Krapohl, G., Manojlovich, M., Redman, B., & Zhang, L. (2010). Nursing specialty certification and nursing-sensitive patient outcomes in the ICU. *American Journal of Critical Care Nursing, 19*(6), 490–499.

Lewis, J., & Farrell, M. (2005). Distance education: A strategy for leadership development. *Nursing Education Perspectives, 26*(6), 362–367.

Malloch, K., & Porter-O'Grady, T. (2010). *The quantum leader: Applications for the new world of work* (2nd ed.). Sudbury, MA: Jones & Bartlett Publishers.

Matter, S. (2006). Empower nurses with evidence-based knowledge. *Nursing Management, 37*(12), 34–37.

Molitor, G. (1998). Trends and forecasts for the new millennium. *The Futurist, 32*(6), 53–59.

Naisbitt, J. (1982). *Megatrends: Ten new directions transforming our lives.* New York, NY: Warner Books.

National State Nursing Workforce Centers (2011). The forum of state nursing workforce centers. Retrieved from http://www.nursingworkforcecenters.org/Resources/files/Forum-response-to-EMSI-study.pdf

Nedd, N. (2006). Perceptions of empowerment and intent to stay. *Nursing Economics, 24*(1), 13–19.

Robert, A., & Sebastian, M. (2006). The future is now: Implementation of a tele-intensivist program. *Journal of Nursing Administration, 36*(1), 49–54.

Rogers, G., Alper, E., Brunelle, D., Federico, F., Fenn, C., Leape, L., et al. (2006). Reconciling medications at admission: Safe practice recommendations and implementation strategies. *Joint Commission Journal on Quality & Patient Safety, 31*(1), 37–50.

Senge, P. (2006). *The fifth discipline: The art and practice of the learning organization* (2nd ed.). New York: Doubleday.

Senge, P., Scharmer, C., Jaworski, J., & Flowers, B. (2004). *Presence.* New York, NY: Doubleday Currency.

Smith, A. (2006). Managing people or places. *Nursing Economic$, 23*(1), 45–46.

Staub, R. (1996). *The heart of leadership: Twelve practices of courageous leaders.* Provo, UT: Executive Excellence.

Thompson, P., Navarra, M. B., & Antonson, N. (2005). Patient safety: The four domains of nursing leadership. *Nursing Economic$, 23*(5), 331–332.

Trinkoff, A. M., Johantgen, M., Storr, C. L., Gurses, A. P., Liang, Y., & Han, K. (2011a). Linking nursing work environment and patient outcomes. *Journal of Nursing Regulation, 2*(1), 10–16.

Trinkoff, A. M., Johantgen, M., Storr, C. L., Gurses, A. P., Liang, Y., & Han, K. (2011b). Work schedule characteristics, staffing, and patient mortality. *Nursing Research, 60*(1), 1–8.

U. S. Department of Labor. (2008). *Health care occupations: Registered nurses.* Retrieved from http://www.bls.gov/oco/pdf/ocos083.pdf

Valiga, T. (1994). Leadership for the future. *Holistic Nursing Practice, 9*(1), 83–90.

Wildavsky, B. (2010). *Great brain race: How global universities are reshaping the world.* Princeton, NJ: Princeton University Press.

CHAPTER 9

Developing as a Leader Throughout One's Career

LEARNING OBJECTIVES

- Describe ways in which individuals can develop as leaders.
- Describe the characteristics of an environment that facilitates the development of leadership skills in oneself and others.
- Relate the concept of empowerment to the development of leaders.
- Analyze the process of mentoring as it relates to the development of leaders.
- Propose a personal plan for leadership development that attends to empowerment, mentoring, role-modeling, networking, self-assessment, and continued renewal.

INTRODUCTION

One of the early leadership theories, the Great Man Theory, espoused that leaders were individuals who had been born into the "right" family at the "right" time. This theory has been challenged over the years as being far from useful in understanding the multifaceted nature of leadership. Indeed, there is now widespread agreement that leaders are made, not born. The question remains as to how an individual can be "made" into a leader.

Individuals who are acknowledged as leaders do not simply declare that they will be leaders and expect that others will accept such a declaration. In addition, success in one role (e.g., faculty member) does not guarantee success in a leadership role (e.g., dean) (Gmelch, 2000). Instead, as demonstrated in our own profession (Houser & Player, 2004, 2007), individuals who are acknowledged as leaders often are nurtured and guided by others, seek and function in environments that encourage leadership behavior, "test" the role, and study others who have been leaders.

177

Thus, the development of oneself as a leader is a purposeful process that is enhanced by guidance and support from others. But what are the ways in which one can develop leadership skills? This chapter explores numerous approaches to leadership development, and several of the strategies that have particular relevance for nurses are examined in depth.

GENERAL APPROACHES TO LEADERSHIP DEVELOPMENT

Emergence as a leader is a developmental learning process in which capacities, insights, and skills gained through one experience or at one level serve as the basis for further growth; thus, leaders go through stages in their development. It also is generally acknowledged that one learns to be a leader by serving as a leader. Merely talking about being a leader or observing others in that role does not make one a leader. One is a leader when he or she exercises leadership.

Based on past performance or promise of future performance, one often is expected to provide leadership to a group. As a person has success in that role, more and more leadership is expected of that individual; thus, one may continually be "promoted" to higher levels of leadership responsibility.

Finally, leadership development is a lifelong process. As nurses progress throughout their careers, they will face new challenges. The need for change will always exist, and groups will need leaders to help them weather the forces of change. Conflict also will always exist, particularly as resources become more scarce and new health-care workers challenge traditional roles; groups will need leaders to help them manage those conflicts. New visions will continually need to be articulated as previous visions are realized or changing societal expectations demand new directions; groups will need leaders to help them see and realize those new visions. As the circumstances of our lives are constantly altered, our leadership skills also need to be refined, renewed, and further developed.

Lecture and Discussion: Formal Course Work

Perhaps one of the most common and easiest ways to develop leadership skills is through participation in lectures, discussions, or formal course work on leadership. Such experiences provide information about the phenomenon, facilitate a "formal" examination of individuals who have demonstrated leadership in the past or in contemporary society, and stimulate thinking about the nature of leadership and followership. Participation in an effective discussion group also provides experience in working with others to reach decisions and helps one develop an awareness of the need for more than single, simple answers to complex problems.

Nursing curricula often include courses related to "leadership and management," though they often focus more on the latter concept than on the former. Sherman and Bishop (2007, p. 295) warn that "the success of nursing as a profession in facing the challenges ahead will hinge on our ability to proactively recruit, develop, and mentor future nurse leaders," and they argue that educational programs need to do more to create a "leadership mindset" (p. 295) in students. To achieve this goal, they advocate that leadership concepts be integrated throughout curricula, rather than being taught as a separate course.

The nursing faculty at Kennesaw State University (Georgia) took this kind of advice to heart when they developed a master's program in Nursing in Advanced Care Management and Leadership, designed to "ensure the development of the next generation of nurse leaders" (Aduddell & Dorman, 2010, p. 1171). This program grew out of evaluation data that showed the community was in need of advanced practice nurses who would possess "the knowledge, skills, and competencies necessary to successfully navigate the ever-increasing complexity of today's health care environment" (p. 168), an environment that clearly requires effective leaders.

In addition to individual or clusters of lectures and discussions about leadership, many universities have instituted programs that focus on leadership. The University of Richmond (Virginia) offered the first baccalaureate program in leadership in 1992, and Chapman University (California) and Fort Hays State University (Kansas) have since added their own majors in this field. Kennesaw State University (Georgia) offers a master's degree in conflict management, and Antioch University (Ohio) offers a master's in conflict analysis and engagement, as well as a doctoral program in leadership and change in the professions. George Mason University (Virginia) offers both a master's and a doctoral program in Conflict Analysis and Resolution, and Gonzaga University (Washington) offers a PhD program in Leadership Studies. Duke University's (North Carolina) advertisements note that strong leadership is the best way to ensure success, and they offer an innovative leadership program to prepare individuals for that role. The University of Denver's (Colorado) Pioneer Leadership Program combines classroom instruction with adventure-based outings as a way to develop leadership abilities, and it leads to a minor in leadership studies. In addition, a growing number of institutions now offer minors in leadership studies.

In 1992, the National Student Nurses Association (NSNA) developed an independent study module that was intended to serve as a model for schools to involve students as active participants in learning about leadership, developing leadership skills, and enhancing professional socialization. Through individualized learning contracts with faculty members, students use their experiences as the chairperson of a local Student Nurses Association (SNA) chapter or committee to study their own leadership style, gain confidence when leading groups, appreciate the many facets of group decision making, and understand the legislative process. This has now evolved to the NSNA Leadership University (www.nsnaleadershipu.org/nsnalu).

Finally, many nursing education programs have credit-bearing courses or noncredit workshops that deal with leadership and its development, and many use creative strategies to help those concepts "come alive" for students (Kirkpatrick, Brown, Atkins, & Vance, 2001; Valiga & Bruderle, 1997). Individuals who want to learn more about this complex concept and the effective exercise of leadership, particularly in nursing and health care, may benefit from enrolling in such courses; however, it would be wise to study the course offering carefully before enrolling to be certain that it does, indeed, focus on leadership rather than on management.

One study (Levine, 2005) examined graduate programs in education to determine their effectiveness in preparing school leaders. Such academic programs have been in existence for many years, and they have produced principals and superintendents who have led our nation's schools and school districts. Despite this success, it was determined that at a time when "the quality of leadership in our schools has seldom mattered more" (p. 5), and in "an era of profound social change" (p. 5), "fundamental rethinking of what [graduate] schools [in education] do and how they do it" (p. 5) was required. Thus, while formal course work in leadership is a viable route to development in this area, one must look carefully at the quality of those learning experiences to ensure they are relevant and effective.

Role-Playing, Games, and Simulation

Although it often makes people uncomfortable, participation in role-playing, games, or simulation exercises is an excellent way to develop leadership skills. By being expected to play the role of leader, one must be articulate, forward-thinking, creative, and able to manage conflict and resolve differences among group members, acknowledge and build on the strengths of followers, and help the group move forward. Role-playing also can serve as a "diagnostic technique," through which one's strengths and areas needing improvement become apparent. For example, it will be evident if the individual playing the role of leader cannot articulate a vision clearly; the individual will then know that this is a particular skill needing more development.

Role-playing and simulation also can serve as a way to "test" various solutions to problems before actually being in the problem situation. For example, a group might construct a scenario in which one of its members plays the passive "sheep" follower role (Kelley, 1992) and the leader must figure out ways to help that follower become more effective. Knowing that reality often presents leaders with many "sheep" followers, being able to address this situation through role-playing gives leaders an opportunity to generate a number of approaches to dealing with such a situation before finding themselves actually faced with it. In addition, this kind of experience provides other participants with an opportunity for vicarious learning in which they have observed which strategies were successful and which were not.

Guthrie, Phelps, and Downey (2011) demonstrated how virtual worlds are a viable venue for leadership education and identified a hierarchy of leadership skill sets that can be developed through virtual worlds. That hierarchy includes technical knowledge (learning more about team functioning, for example), environment knowledge (learning about a particular context), problem solving, organizational skills (learning how to organize and coordinate human and material resources to move toward problem resolution or goal attainment), instruction skills (learning how to coach and mentor others), and facilitation skills (learning how to communicate effectively, share knowledge among team members, and build trust).

Thus, it can be seen that in-person or virtual games, role-playing exercises, and simulations all can be used to help individuals think about and develop their leadership abilities. It is important to keep in mind, however, that such exercises must be carefully designed, implemented with precision, and followed by effective debriefing sessions during which participants are helped to reflect on what has been learned and what personal insights have been attained.

Sensitivity Training

Sensitivity training sessions led by expert facilitators provide participants with an opportunity to focus on openness, how hostilities and defensiveness may be exhibited within a group, and one's personal feelings, perceptions, and biases. Participation also increases one's sensitivity to others' needs and helps one appreciate the significance of shared decision making. Finally, such sessions also assist group members to reflect on the inner workings or processes of the group itself: who assumed what kinds of roles, who emerged as the leader, who was most effective in moving the group forward and why, and so on. Such insights are invaluable for those who will provide leadership in their work settings, professional associations, or communities.

> *There's nothing wrong with a pleasant, good natured approach to people and problems—in fact, there's none better. The strange thing is that we so often forget to use it.* —Dwight Eisenhower

Role-Modeling

Effective leadership skills can be developed by carefully observing individuals who are successful as leaders. By studying what such people do, how they communicate, how they motivate followers to "join in the cause," their level of energy and personal investment, their ability to keep the group focused on the vision despite conflicts and challenges along the way, and how their careers have evolved can be extremely helpful to the novice leader.

Role-modeling occurs whether or not it is planned or purposeful. In other words, many pattern themselves after others, even though they may not be aware of such unconscious "decisions" and may find that they have adapted the negative or nonhelpful behaviors exhibited by others, as well as the positive or helpful ones. Therefore, role-modeling is much more effective when it is done consciously and with deliberation.

Conscious or "formal" role-modeling may be enhanced by attending professional conferences and conventions where one observes how participants conduct themselves, deal with "hot" issues that are open to debate, express opinions, and connect with members of the audience. It also can be achieved by being more observant during meetings. Who is typically able to convince the group that his or her point is the one that should be supported, and what does that person do that makes him or her so convincing? Conscious role-modeling occurs when one reads articles or editorials written by nurse leaders and reflects on their communication style, their willingness to address controversial topics publicly, and the fact that they use print media to convey a strongly held message or to articulate a vision. Finally, leadership can be facilitated by reading biographies about leaders—in nursing (such as the 23 leaders presented by Houser and Player [2004, 2007]) or outside nursing, contemporary or historical—and studying what they did and how they did it.

Institutes and Fellowships

A more formalized approach to leadership development occurs through participation in institutes and fellowships. Such opportunities are announced in professional publications and are open to a wide variety of individuals.

Studying Our Leaders

Although "research on the effectiveness of using cases for leadership training is still limited" (Yukl, 2010, p. 464), the analysis of individuals who have been effective can be a valuable way to help individuals think about leadership and their own skills. Often the subject of the case is someone who has come to be quite well known (e.g., Florence Nightingale or Joan of Arc), but by stepping back into that person's history to appreciate factors that influenced her or him to emerge as a leader or to better understand what "ignited" her or his passion and vision, one can learn about how individuals develop as leaders.

Of course, more contemporary figures—including those in one's own field or organization—also can be used for a case study. Although it may be difficult to identify influencing factors without knowing the outcome of the person's leadership or without the benefit of hindsight, exploring specifics of those providing leadership in the culture and context that are more relevant to a current situation can enhance individuals' understanding of how they might need to develop.

In 1998, for example, the American Academy of Nursing and the American Nurses Foundation formed a partnership to develop an Institute for Nursing Leadership. The aim of this institute was to "build new leadership capacities through self-assessment, skill-building learning modules, and programs designed to connect nurses with mentors, sponsors and other . . . contacts" (Ferguson, 1998, p. 10). It was multifocused and relevant to nurses at all stages of their careers: fostering leadership skill building among undergraduate and graduate nursing students, fostering leadership competencies for nurses at early and emerging career points, facilitating mentoring and networking for nurses in their first managerial position, brokering access to leadership development programs (with executives outside their traditional work settings) for senior executive nurses, and enhancing connections with leaders in the field to maintain leadership capacity in the profession.

Sigma Theta Tau International, the Honor Society of Nursing, has as one of its major goals the development of leadership among its members. The ultimate purpose of focusing on leadership is to promote the discovery, dissemination, and utilization of knowledge to improve the health of individuals and communities worldwide. Through its workshops, programs, conferences, and various leadership institutes, Sigma Theta Tau International serves to address the leadership development needs of nurses who are currently providing leadership at the local, regional, and international level as well as nurses who have the potential to provide such leadership. The goal of these institutes is to help nurses be able to influence others to bring about transforming change.

Florida Atlantic University offers two Nursing Leadership Institutes, one founded in 2002 "to prepare nurse leaders grounded in the essential values of nursing, with the complex knowledge needed to lead competently and compassionately" (http://nursing.fau.edu/index.php?main=6&nav=158), and a Novice Nursing Leadership Institute, founded in 2006, to create a pool of future nursing leaders. In Boston, a consortium of six Harvard Medical School–affiliated hospitals created the Institute for Nursing Health-care Leadership (INHL), a nonprofit organization dedicated to advancing nursing practice through leadership development, research, collaborative activities, and education programs that can be customized for individual nurses and nurse groups from abroad (http://www.phmi.partners.org/News/PHMI-Archive/The-Institute-for-Nursing-Healthcare-Leadership.aspx).

The West Virginia Nursing Leadership Institute is a 12-month program designed to prepare nurses to become effective leaders who can—and will—address and positively affect the critical need for nurse recruitment and retention in their communities and beyond. The Central Virginia Nursing Leadership Institute is an innovative community-wide, year-long experience that builds on management leadership skills in mid-level nurse managers from all sectors of health care, and similar programs exist in Kansas and Kentucky for public health nurses and in North Carolina for school nurses. The University of Illinois at Chicago's International Center for Health Leadership Development conducts leadership development activities that prepare leaders from communities, community health centers, and health professions education to build links and partnerships between communities and institutions. It helps individuals discover their leadership capabilities and helps them see that, in many ways, leadership is a function of the relationship between leaders and followers.

Finally, several prestigious leadership programs are sponsored by nonprofit foundations, including the Kellogg Leadership for Community Change program and the Institute for Sustainable Communities' Leadership for a Changing World program. In addition, the Center for Creative Leadership (North Carolina) is a well-established program that offers workshops, books, and other resources to positively transform the way leaders, their organizations, and their societies confront the most difficult challenges of the 21st century (http://www.ccl.org/leadership/about/index.aspx), and the Center for Courage and Renewal (http://www.couragerenewal.org/) helps participants reflect on "reconnecting who you are with what you do" through programs and retreats that focus on, among other topics, the courage to lead.

All these and many more programs are designed to enhance leadership development. When combined with "on-the-job training" and extensive reflection and self-assessment efforts, individuals can be most effective in developing as leaders in their organizations, communities, and professions.

On-the-Job Training

Perhaps the most effective way to develop as a successful leader is to use such skills "on the job" so that one can learn from experience. On-the-job training may include temporary job rotations to positions that require the use of new skills, assignment as an assistant or apprentice to someone in a leadership role, serving as the chair-elect of a committee, or participation in some leadership internship, such as those described previously or those offered through one's employing agency. On-the-job training also may occur through a mentor relationship, a concept discussed in more depth later in this chapter.

> *Knowing is not enough; we must apply. Willing is not enough; we must do.* —Goethe

Reflection and Self-Assessment

Reflection is generally viewed as having two dimensions: "reflecting on experience after an event occurs and reflection in action—in real time—during an event" (Johns, 2004, p. 24). It involves learning from everyday experiences and gaining insights about oneself and one's actions. By thinking deeply and honestly about your vision, your character, your passion, your ability and willingness to share power, the way you communicate, your persistence, the extent to which you embrace and celebrate differences, and other qualities of effective, transformational leaders, you can identify the strengths you wish to enhance and the limitations you wish to improve as a leader.

Such insights also occur through serious and thoughtful completion of self-assessment tools and careful reflection on what they reveal about you. The *Self Profile* (1987), for example, can help you identify how you relate to others, how you might respond in a given situation, and how you can build more meaningful relationships with others. *Self Profile* statements such as the following offer insights to leadership behaviors and may be particularly revealing: "When in a group, I tend to speak and act as the representative of that group," "When faced with a leadership position, I tend to actively accept that role rather than diffuse it among others," "It's important to me that people follow the advice that I give them," and "Other people usually think of me as being energetic."

Another helpful self-assessment tool is the *StrengthsFinder* (Rath & Conchie, 2008). The extensive research conducted by these authors with 20,000 leaders and 10,000 followers led to three key findings about the most effective leaders (pp. 2–3): (1) they are always investing in strengths, (2) they surround themselves with the right people and then maximize their team, and (3) they understand their followers' needs. The authors concluded that "the path to great leadership starts with a deep understanding of the strengths you bring to the table" (p. 3), and they developed this self-assessment tool to reflect four domains of leadership strength: *executing* (the ability to "catch" an idea and make it a reality), *influencing* (the ability to speak up, take charge, and make things happen), *relationship building* (the ability to serve as the glue that holds a team together), and *strategic thinking* (the ability to keep the group focused on what could be and to continually stretch thinking for the future).

The Center for Leadership Studies (http://www.situational.com/about-us/center-for-leadership-studies/) offers several tools, including LEAD (Leadership Effectiveness & Adaptability Description)—for self and for others—and the Situational Leadership tool, which is based on Hersey's (1985) situational leadership model. These tools help individuals understand their leadership style and their actual or potential effectiveness as a leader.

One other popular self-assessment method is the *Keirsey Temperament Sorter®* (2011), which is based on Keirsey's personality theory of four temperaments: artisan, guardian, rational, or idealist. This test helps you appreciate if you are more of a teacher or promoter, inventor or performer, inspector or mastermind . . . if you are expressive, probing, tough-minded, introspective . . . so that you can better understand who you are and how you relate to others, both of which are critical for effective leaders.

Thus, reflection and self-assessment are important strategies for leadership development and should be integral to the ongoing development of any leader. Seeking feedback from peers and potential followers also is useful in assessing your leadership qualities.

Summary

In essence, nurses who are seeking to develop or enhance their leadership skills and abilities would benefit from attending carefully to those in their work and professional environments (e.g., as potential role models) and considering becoming involved in some type of formal leadership training program. In selecting such a program, one should look for opportunities to examine the complex phenomenon of leadership in depth, be certain one chooses carefully between leadership development and management training programs, and choose a program that provides opportunities to actually experience the role of leader; receive thoughtful, critical feedback on one's performance in that role; and receive guidance in building on areas of strength and developing areas of weakness. Potential and effective nurse leaders also would be best served by practicing in an environment that facilitates their development as leaders. The following case study illustrates how one can purposefully pursue development as a leader, as well as how lack of planning can result in missed opportunities and delayed or limited development in the role.

Case Study

Marty and Josh were classmates during their nursing program, and after graduation, both went to work at the local medical center. Although they both enjoyed successful careers in nursing, each evolved to a very different place in terms of his leadership and the extent of his influence in the field.

Both Marty and Josh identified Dr. Richards as one of the best teachers they had in nursing. She was knowledgeable in the subject she taught but admitted to not knowing things and thought those situations through "out loud" so that students could benefit from her thinking processes. She used innovative strategies to facilitate learning and actively engaged students in designing their own learning experiences. Dr. Richards published extensively in her area of expertise, completed research that influenced patient care, was inducted into the American Academy of Nursing, received numerous awards for her work, consulted with schools of nursing across the country, was invited to speak at national and international conferences, was actively involved in her specialty organization, and most recently was inducted into the National League for Nursing's Academy of Nursing Education. Although she did not brag about these accomplishments, Dr. Richards kept her students informed about her activities and the directions in which her career took her.

Neither Marty nor Josh thought they would pursue an academic position, but they were impressed with Dr. Richards' accomplishments and contributions, and they often talked about their desire to have a career as exciting and productive as hers. Marty took steps to make that happen. Josh did not.

While still a student, *Marty* took advantage of the opportunity to talk with Dr. Richards and other faculty about their careers, how they balanced professional development activities with work responsibilities, and how they got where they are. He asked for advice about jobs, how to get involved in professional organizations, who the "movers and shakers" were in his area of interest (rehabilitation), how to get the most out of conferences one attends, and whether Dr. Richards would mentor him, particularly at the outset of his career. He wrote goals for where he would like to be 5 and 10 years after graduation and began to outline steps to achieve those goals. As an RN, Marty volunteered to serve on several committees at the rehabilitation center where he worked, proposed innovations in patient care that evolved from research reports he read, submitted abstracts for presentation of those patient care innovations at the national convention of the nursing rehabilitation organization, sought feedback from peers and supervisors about his practice, challenged ideas presented by others and offered alternative solutions, and worked with his mentors to advance professionally. Ten years after graduation, Marty was well-known in the field of rehabilitation nursing, was

Continued

Case Study—cont'd

collaborating with experts in that field to design and implement research projects, and was reporting the findings from their research in journal articles and at conferences. Rehabilitation nurses across the country knew of Marty's work and used his research findings and ideas about innovative practices as the basis for their own practice. Without question, Marty was a leader in the field whose own work influenced the work of others and helped shape a preferred future for rehabilitation nursing practice.

Josh, on the other hand, never sought out his teachers while he was a student or afterward. He was dedicated to providing excellent care to the homeless, but he made no effort to actively shape that practice or advocate for the population he served daily. When asked to attend a meeting about care of the homeless, Josh accepted, listened attentively, and prepared a comprehensive report of what took place during that meeting; however, he made no special effort before the meeting to be best prepared for it, did not contribute to the discussion, did not take risks to offer different perspectives (despite the fact that he disagreed with some of what was being proposed), and did not influence the thinking of those at the table. Although he knew of several organizations that worked diligently on behalf of the homeless, Josh did not join or actively participate in any events sponsored by those organizations. He also did not attend professional conferences on the topic, attempt to incorporate research findings into his practice, challenge his colleagues to continually strive for excellence, seek out a mentor, nor expand his professional networks. The care he provided was exceptional, but his sphere of influence was extremely limited, and his plan to advance as a leader was essentially nonexistent.

ENVIRONMENTS THAT FACILITATE LEADERSHIP DEVELOPMENT

Aspiring leaders may not be in a position to create an environment that facilitates leadership development. However, they may be in a position to choose to practice and participate in such environments. What do such environments look like? What should nurses look for in such environments?

Much like those that promote creativity (see Chapter 5) and human development in general, environments that promote the development and enhancement of leadership skills and abilities are open, trusting, and dynamic. In such environments, individuals feel free to raise questions about what is being done, how it is being done, why it is being done in a particular way, and why it is being done at all. Not only is a questioning attitude accepted, it is also encouraged and expected. Bennis (2004) refers to this as a "culture of candor."

Environments that promote the development of leadership do not maintain the status quo and do not put individuals into "boxes," but they do encourage each person to reach his or her maximal potential. A spirit of competitiveness that constantly pushes members to achieve excellence may characterize the environment, but group members are not in competition with each other. Indeed, environments that facilitate the development of leadership recognize the strengths and talents of each member of the group, find ways to build on those strengths, and expect group members to guide, encourage, and support each other as they continue to grow. They are, in essence, environments in which leaders are allowed to emerge and followers are seen as valuable, contributing members of the team.

Individual members of the group are encouraged and expected to take risks and try new roles, even though they may fail. For example, a relatively new nurse may be asked to head up an ad hoc committee that is charged to look at how the working relationships between licensed and unlicensed personnel can be enhanced. With the guidance and support of the nurse manager or more seasoned nurses on the unit, this new nurse would be expected to take the lead in working with group members to formulate the goals for this group, suggesting ways the group could go about achieving those goals, maintaining open communications with other nurses not directly involved in the project about the progress of the committee, and keeping the group focused on preparing a timely report that includes realistic, feasible recommendations for how working relationships can be enhanced. Along the way, this nurse may make some mistakes, but he or she has been provided with an opportunity to develop leadership skills and to think of himself or herself as a leader.

I view mistakes as opportunities to learn. —Zerrie Campbell

An environment that facilitates leadership development does not "recycle" the same people over and again, giving only a limited number of individuals an opportunity to grow. Although there is some merit in "recycling" leaders (Kelly, 1991; Stocker, 1991) (e.g., organizations that do this make the best use of people who have proved themselves to be effective, and they benefit from the experience and history of these individuals), repeated recycling with limited opportunities for involvement of inexperienced nurses does not serve the profession well in the long run because it does little to contribute to the ongoing development of leaders.

Finally, a leadership development environment is characterized by good channels of communication and a sense that all members are free to suggest ideas (e.g., they do not merely wait for the person "in charge" to generate ideas). It "forces" members to address issues of significance to them and the profession, and it encourages the sharing of information, rather than the hoarding of it. The Leadership Environment Assessment Survey (Box 9–1) can be used to help analyze the extent to which one's work settings or professional organizations can facilitate the development of leadership.

EMPOWERMENT

The environment that encourages, supports, and expects leadership development can be thought of as an empowering environment. Empowerment is a process through which individuals feel strengthened, in control, and in possession of some degree of power. It often is "given" by someone in a position of power or authority (e.g., a nurse manager, the home health agency supervisor), but it also can be "taken" by an individual.

"Instead of exercising power over people, transforming leaders champion and inspire them" (Burns, 2003, p. 26). This is empowerment, whereby "leaders encourage followers to rise above narrow interests and work together for transcending goals" (p. 26). In fact, as Burns said, transforming leadership is achieved "not by enslaving followers, but by liberating and empowering them" (p. 27).

When someone in a position of power empowers others, it is through the sharing of that power. People are empowered by others when they are invited to participate in mak-

BOX 9-1 **Leadership Environment Assessment Survey**

Think about your place of employment or a professional organization in which you are involved (e.g., your state nurses' association, your clinical specialty group, your local honor society). With that organization in mind, consider each of the following questions about the nature of the general environment or "culture." **Yes** responses to most questions suggest that the organization supports, encourages, and expects leadership among its members. **No** responses to most questions may suggest that the organization's priorities do not include leadership development.

QUESTION	YES	NO
Is this organization open to new ideas and new ways of doing things?	_____	_____
Do members of the organization feel free to raise questions about what is being done? How things are being done? Why things are being done at all? Why things are done in a particular way?	_____	_____
Is a questioning attitude accepted, encouraged, and expected in the organization?	_____	_____
Does the organization prevent putting individuals into "boxes"?	_____	_____
Does the organization push members to strive for excellence?	_____	_____
Is competition among group members healthy and productive?	_____	_____
Are the strengths and talents of individual members recognized?	_____	_____
Are the strengths and talents of individual members built upon?	_____	_____
Are group members expected to guide, encourage, and support each other as they continue to grow?	_____	_____
Are leaders allowed to emerge in the organization?	_____	_____
Are followers seen as valuable, contributing members of the group?	_____	_____
Are individual group members encouraged to take risks and try new things?	_____	_____
Are mistakes accepted as part of the learning process for group members?	_____	_____
Are different group members given opportunities to develop as leaders?	_____	_____
Are channels of communication clear and open?	_____	_____
Are group members allowed and encouraged to address issues that are of significance to them and the profession?	_____	_____
Is information shared?	_____	_____
Are accomplishments of group members acknowledged and rewarded?	_____	_____

ing decisions that will affect their lives, their work, and their futures. Rather than having "Big Brother" make all the decisions because "he knows best," those people who will have to live with the consequences of decisions are involved in making them. It is clear that this model has relevance for the administrator–staff nurse relationship, but it also has relevance for the nurse–patient relationship, the teacher–student relationship, the parent–child relationship, and any other relationship in which one person typically has more power than others.

Nurses are empowered in their organizations when they are held accountable. Rather than being in a position in which blame can be placed on someone else or "the system" for less than ideal outcomes, empowered nurses know that the quality of care they deliver is their responsibility and that they are accountable for their actions and inactions. By being held accountable, nurses actually have more power in the practice arena.

Nurses are empowered when a shared governance model is in place. In this environment, nurses set their own schedule, formulate goals for their unit or agency, set standards of excellence, participate actively in peer review, and support one another. The structure is more open and interactive than limiting and hierarchical, and the success or failure of the group is the responsibility of all members, not only the nurse manager or supervisor. Such a model requires that nurses are adequately prepared to assume such responsibility and that there is a mix of skills and experiences in the group to implement the model most effectively.

Although we tend to think of empowerment as something someone in power does for those who are have less power, that is far from the only means to empowerment. Nurses who find themselves in work or professional environments that are not designed to be empowering can still feel strengthened and "in control" by their own actions.

Empowerment or strength comes from a number of sources. Among the most significant of those sources is knowledge! Nurses empower themselves when they are knowledgeable and expert in their area of practice: when they know the structure, dynamics, and culture of the organizations in which they work; and when they know how to use resources effectively. They also empower themselves when they know themselves: their strengths and limitations, their values and biases, and what motivates them.

Empowerment also comes from having a sense of control over one's life. This may take the form of choosing where one will work; the level of excellence toward which one will strive, regardless, perhaps, of the standards held by others in the setting; and the degree to which one will accept being spoken down to, taken advantage of, or criticized unjustly. To some extent, it is related to self-esteem, self-worth, personal pride, and one's sense of identity.

> *The secret of joy in work is contained in one word— excellence. To know how to do something well is to enjoy it.* —Pearl Buck

Participating actively in one's work setting, professional association, or community also gives one a sense of having control over one's life and is empowering. By serving on committees, for example, nurses are in a better position to influence decisions that are made, and they are able to ensure that nursing's voice is heard; this is empowering. Holding office in a professional association or engaging actively in the debate of issues presented at a convention of that association is empowering because it gives nurses an opportunity to shape the future of the organization and, perhaps, the profession. Meeting with local legislators and community leaders about ways to enhance the resources available to children and the elderly in one's community is empowering because it reinforces one's ability to advocate for and help improve the lives of those who cannot speak for themselves.

Thus, empowerment need not occur only when someone in a position of power or authority decides to "give" some of that power away. Each nurse can "take" some power by his or her own actions. Perhaps one needs to return to school for an advanced degree, attend a workshop on assertiveness, volunteer to serve on a committee, run for political office, or review and reaffirm his or her values related to excellence and quality patient care. Perhaps one also can feel more empowered by entering into a relationship with a mentor.

MENTORING

Mentor was a figure in Greek mythology who served as the wise and faithful guardian and tutor of Telemachus during the 10-year absence of his father, Odysseus, who fought in and struggled to return home from the Trojan War. The words "mentor" and "mentoring," therefore, typically refer to an experienced individual who befriends and guides a less experienced individual.

Although the word "mentor" is often overused today—with anyone who shows the slightest interest in a person or offers the slightest amount of assistance being referred to as a "mentor"—a true mentor invests a great deal of time and effort in the advancement and growth of a protégé. Such a relationship is conscious, is purposefully designed, and typically extends over a number of years.

What Is a Mentor?

Mentors are close, trusted, experienced counselors or guides. They are accomplished and more experienced individuals, usually, but not always, in the same profession of the neophyte, and they offer neophytes advice, teach them, sponsor them, and guide them through significant points in their careers. As such, they help protégés establish themselves in the profession.

By serving as a mixture of "good parent" and "good friend," mentors provide counsel during times of stress, encouragement during risk-taking endeavors, intellectual challenges, and assistance in the development and enhancement of professional skills. They encourage, cajole, test, teach by example, advise, model, act as a partner, sponsor, and give honest feedback, both positive and negative.

Mentors see some potential in a neophyte, which the neophyte often does not see in herself or himself, and then they do something about that potential. The "something" mentors do is to commit themselves to the neophytes, often for a number of years: helping them develop a clearer professional identity, fostering their growth in personal and professional power, supporting and facilitating the realization of their dreams, and acting as an energizer and a sounding board.

Mentors also inspire neophytes and challenge them to achieve a level of professionalism they may not have known otherwise. By representing a point of development to which neophytes aspire, mentors invite their protégés into a new world, as peers and colleagues, and open doors for them. They help their protégés "learn the ropes" within a broadened community of colleagues so that they can sense the political climate, spot the behind-the-scenes actions, gain insights into the profession, expand their networks, and eventually spread their wings and fly.

Myths About Mentors and Mentoring

Mentoring often is thought of as a panacea for solving the problems of nurses in the health-care arena or women executives aspiring to climb the corporate ladder. Nurses, however, would be wise to be alert to a number of myths surrounding mentors and mentoring (Sandler, 1993):

- *Myth:* The best way to succeed is to have a mentor. *Reality:* Mentoring is important and can make a significant difference in the career development of many individuals, but it is not necessarily essential for success or survival. Similarly, having a mentor does not guarantee success.
- *Myth:* Mentoring is always beneficial. *Reality:* Although there are numerous benefits to a mentoring relationship, there are some limitations as well, such as the difficulty in sustaining the intensity required of both participants over time, the exclusivity of the relationship (e.g., the mentor invests in a very small number of individuals and is not available to work with a larger number of neophytes), the potential for the protégé to rely primarily or exclusively on the mentor for emotional support and guidance rather than interacting with a broader scope of colleagues, and the fact that the mentor, not the protégé, typically "sets the agenda."
- *Myth:* The mentor should be older than the person being mentored. *Reality*: It is quite possible that the more experienced, accomplished individual in the relationship is younger chronologically.
- *Myth:* A person can have only one mentor at a time. *Reality:* Although it may be difficult to maintain close, intense relationships with several mentors simultaneously, it is not impossible. One mentor may be most effective in helping a neophyte write grants, another may be the expert clinician who gives guidance with difficult clinical problems, and a third may be the best resource in gaining entry to a professional association.
- *Myth:* If you are seeking a mentor, you have to wait to be asked. *Reality:* It is perfectly acceptable for a neophyte to approach a potential mentor to discuss the possibility of entering into a relationship.
- *Myth:* Men are better mentors for women. *Reality:* Most mentors throughout history probably have been men largely because women were not socialized (until recently) in the direction of such relationships and many women were not in positions of leadership to serve as

mentors. No evidence supports the claim that men are better mentors. In fact, with women's tendency to attend to personal issues and not merely work or professional ones, a female mentor may be more effective than a male mentor.

- *Myth:* When a man mentors a woman, the chances are great that it will develop into a sexual encounter. *Reality:* This, of course, is a possibility in any relationship, but when the mentoring relationship is focused on the career development and advancement of the protégé, sexuality need not, and, indeed, should not, enter into it.

- *Myth:* The mentor always knows best. *Reality:* Although it is true that the mentor is the wiser, more experienced member of the pair, it also is important to remember that the protégé is a bright, talented individual with ideas and a great deal of potential. Those talents should not be ignored or exploited in the relationship to benefit or stroke the ego of the mentor. The whole point of a mentoring relationship is to promote the career advancement of the protégé, not to make the protégé dependent on the mentor. Thus, the protégé must play a significant role in the relationship and sometimes is the person who "knows best."

What Mentors Look for in Protégés

Mentors and leaders look for novices who have the potential to move the profession ahead. They then invest the time, energy, and caring to create what they believe will be a future leader in the field. With this kind of investment expected of mentors, it is no wonder that they would choose neophytes who show they are worth investing in and are likely to show some measure of reward for the investment made.

Specifically, mentors often seek protégés who possess certain qualities. Box 9–2 presents characteristics that may serve as a guide to determine whether we are the kind of

---

BOX 9-2 What Mentors Look for in Protégés

Mentors often seek protégés who possess certain qualities. The following characteristics may serve as a guide to determine whether you are the kind of individual in whom a mentor might invest:
- Intelligence
- A self-starter: someone who is internally motivated
- Someone who is looking for new challenges
- Good interpersonal and communication skills: someone who is articulate
- A risk-taker
- A hard worker
- Someone who has and understands ideas and is always open to new perspectives and possibilities
- Integrity
- Someone who presents himself or herself professionally: in appearance, through the written word, and so on
- A sense of humor
- Someone who is willing to invest in himself or herself
- A curious mind: someone who asks questions and is not satisfied with the status quo
- Someone who has a vision: for himself or herself and for the profession

individual in whom a mentor might invest. In essence, mentors look for protégés who are beginning leaders or have the potential to be leaders. They then work to help those individuals develop the knowledge, skills, and savvy needed to be effective leaders.

Caveats Regarding a Mentor Relationship

When considering entering a mentoring relationship, both individuals should consider the following caveats or "commandments" (Sandler, 1993):

- Be careful not to confuse a mentor relationship with a personal, emotional one.
- Many people can be mentors—you need not be at the top of your profession to be of assistance to novices.
- The protégé must take personal responsibility for learning.
- The mentor should not be expected to fulfill every need and meet every demand of the protégé.
- The confidences of the mentor must be respected.
- Expectations of both the mentor and protégé (e.g., time, type of assistance) need to be clarified early on in the relationship.
- Protégés should know if they are asking for too much, or too little, of the mentor.
- The feedback from the mentor to the protégé should take the form of praise and constructive criticism, with specific suggestions for improvement.
- The relationship should be used to open doors for future protégés.
- Mentors and protégés need not come from the same educational, ethnic, racial, religious, or any other type of background.
- Recognize that the relationship goes through stages (Loue, 2011)—from dependence, uncertainty, and hesitancy to mutual give-and-take to termination or separation, at which point the protégé is more independent and identifies his or her separateness from the mentor.
- Be careful not to fall into mentoring because "it's the thing to do" or the "in" thing.

Benefits to the Mentor

Although it may sound as if the only person who benefits from a mentor relationship is the protégé, nothing could be further from the truth. Indeed, mentoring is a mutually supportive, mutually beneficial relationship in which the mentor also gains a great deal.

The strength of mentors comes from their own professional experience, self-worth, and autonomy. They must be capable of motivating neophytes to be creative and possess a good sense of their own creative selves. They also must be careful not to direct or control every facet of their protégé's life, and they must be open and willing to learn from the protégé.

As individuals engage in this evolving relationship, the protégé often pursues more sophisticated lines of investigation, develops skills the mentor may not possess, and establishes new networks. The mentor who is open to and willing to learn from a protégé will grow enormously from the relationship.

It is incredibly rewarding for mentors to see novice clinicians, educators, researchers, administrators, and leaders grow and evolve. In many cases, the accomplishments of the neophytes far surpass those of the mentors, and mentors take great pride in seeing their protégés receive awards, make changes in practice, receive offers of significant positions, be elected to office in professional associations, receive competitive grants, and publish articles or books that influence others.

Increasingly, "scholars are recognizing that mentoring is a bidirectional process, with responsibilities falling on both the mentor and mentee and benefits potentially inuring to each" (Loue, 2011, p. 2). The true mentoring relationship is mutually rewarding and results in growth in both the mentor and the protégé. In addition to the personal growth one experiences, both individuals also expand their networks of professional colleagues and "influentials."

Because this relationship is mutually beneficial, those who are more junior in the field may need to take the initiative to seek out those in the field who have the expertise, experience, networks, and scholarly agendas that align with their own career goals. They can call or write to those whose published work they admire or whose research matches their own interests; approach such individuals at conferences; suggest such individuals as consultants at their place of employment or as speakers at conferences they are involved in planning—and then use those opportunities to connect to point out common interests, talk about their career goals, and explore the possibility of a mentor relationship. Likewise, those who are more senior in the field may need to seek out those more junior whose passions are aligned with one's own professional work and who have potential to make significant contributions to the organization or field . . . or to respond positively when more junior colleagues come forward (as noted earlier) and suggest a mentoring relationship. This kind of reaching out and responding to nurse colleagues is a hallmark of mentors and effective protégés.

NETWORKING

As noted, a mentoring relationship can help both participants develop contacts and expand their professional networks, networks they may call on throughout their careers for assistance, support of ideas, and guidance. Although some take offense at the idea of "using" people to one's benefit, the whole concept of networking is built on the assumption that who one knows is important and can be helpful.

Networks form for the purpose of providing access to contacts, referrals, information, support, feedback, understanding, and empathy. They also can serve to help nurses maintain a social and professional identity and provide a means of working toward organizational, professional, or societal reform.

Nurses might "tap into" their networks when they are looking for a guest speaker for a program, a consultant, someone to fill a key position in an organization, someone to nominate for appointment to a community board, or an expert in a clinical area. They might also use their networks to gather data about practices in other institutions that can help advance a proposal for a change in their own settings. Thus, networks serve a number of useful purposes, without the sustained, intense investment of a mentor relationship.

As described, mentoring is a special kind of relationship between two individuals that is intense, personalized, and long-lasting and that has positive outcomes for both participants. Indeed, studies have documented several positive outcomes from engagement in a mentoring relationship.

In a classic study of 1,250 top executives, Roche (1979) found that almost two thirds of those studied had mentors, and most mentoring relationships started when the protégé was in his or her 20s or 30s. Roche found that executives who had mentors moved into successful positions more quickly, earned more money at a younger age, were more likely to follow a personal career plan, were better educated, were more satisfied with their career progress, received greater pleasure from their work, and eventually sponsored protégés themselves.

In a classic study of 71 nurse influentials, Vance (1977) found that 83% of those studied had mentors, and 93% of them were consciously aware of being mentors to others. A follow-up study (Kinsey, 1986) revealed similar findings, namely, that many of those nurses who were thought of as influentials in the profession had, themselves, been mentored by others and had served as mentors to novices.

Does everyone need a mentor to "make it" and "get ahead"? No, but most people do need guides, support systems, sounding boards, and peer "pals" to help during certain times throughout their careers, and this is where one's network can be most effective.

Peer *"pals"* may help each other manage a particularly difficult community health problem or deal with an arrogant physician. *Guides* know easier ways to do something or have experienced a particular situation and share those insights with others. For example, nurses who are enrolled in a master's program may serve as guides to colleagues who are in the process of deciding whether they should pursue graduate education and, if so, what school to attend and what specialty to pursue. Nurses who have particularly good writing skills may review and critique an abstract before it is submitted in response to a "call" for presentation at a conference or a manuscript before it is submitted to a journal for review. *Sponsors* act on behalf of others, promote them, and advance them, much the same way a mentor does, but in more isolated instances, rather than over a lengthy period of time. For example, a faculty member may nominate a graduate for an award or suggest that graduate as a candidate for office in a professional association. All of these are examples of a patron-type system in which nurses "use" their networks but do not necessarily enter into an extended, intense mentoring relationship.

Networks, then, are most effective to enhance one's development as a leader, and nurses should be cautious not to fall into the trap of believing myths such as the following: networking is important only when you are looking for a new job, networking is something you do only outside your own organization and community, networking is an idea that is no longer relevant in the age of social media and the Internet, and networking is relevant to managers and executives, but not to those who are not in such positions (Cardillo, 2001). Instead, we need to broaden our "web" of professional contacts and "use" those contacts to help us face and manage difficult situations, grow professionally, and develop as leaders.

CONCLUSION

The development of leadership knowledge and skills throughout one's career requires (1) purposeful, goal-directed action; (2) honest, extensive self-assessment; (3) a willingness to ask for assistance or guidance; and (4) a willingness to accept help or guidance when it is offered. It is enhanced by the development and effective use of professional networks, as well as by engagement in mentoring relationships.

Regardless of their role, their level of education, or their scope of practice, nurses who are in positions of influence must take on the responsibility of grooming other promising nurses. Those seeking to be more influential and to become leaders must start early to seek experiences and colleagues—and possibly mentors—who will provide the professional and personal nourishment necessary for success. They must identify the people who are in a position to help, let them know they respect their ability, and seek their support. They also must convey to those who are in a position to help that they have something to gain by helping, guiding, and possibly mentoring them.

> *Whatever development process you're comfortable with, do it to the maximum.* —Bonnie Saucier

Each nurse must create a personal plan for leadership development throughout her or his career and then take responsibility for implementing that plan and documenting the results of various actions, perhaps through maintaining a professional portfolio. Such a plan may include advancing formal education or enrolling in courses or workshops that will help develop a better understanding of the phenomenon of leadership or enhance specific skills, such as assertiveness or public speaking. It may include looking for a work setting or professional association that is empowering or one in which strong role models exist. One's personal plan for leadership development may incorporate seeking a mentor, expanding professional networks, becoming more involved in the political process, running for office in one's specialty organization, submitting a manuscript for publication, or responding to a call for paper presentations at a regional or national conference.

Whatever the specific course of action, nurses will develop as leaders through a well-thought-out plan, and not through the waving of some magic wand. Taking responsibility is a large part of what leadership is all about, and such responsibility grows out of honest self-assessment about one's leadership abilities and potentials, as well as positive, focused action. Taking responsibility for one's own development as a leader is an excellent way to achieve professional goals, realize visions, and shape a preferred future for the nursing profession.

Leaders also are responsible for developing other leaders. Leadership in nursing is about "ensuring a well-thought-through succession plan where the future of the profession remains the key focus" (Ang & Fong, 2003, p. 28).

CRITICAL THINKING EXERCISES

Read at least three journal editorials, one by Leah Curtin, one by Chris Tanner, and one by another editor. To what extent do these individuals express controversial ideas and convey a passion about their topic? Do you see any differences in the uniqueness of perspective, challenging nature of the ideas put forth, or passion expressed by the editors? What can you learn from this comparison about the nature of risk taking that is inherent in a leadership role? If you were given the opportunity to write a controversial editorial for a prominent nursing journal, what would you write about? How would you express your ideas? Who would you ask to review your manuscript before you submitted it?

_____

_____

Complete the Leadership Environment Assessment Survey (see Box 9–1). To what extent does "your" organization provide an environment that promotes leadership? What can you do to make "your" environment more conducive to the development of leadership skills?

_____

_____

Review the discussion about what mentors look for in a protégé. How do you "rate" in each of the areas listed? What assets do you think you would bring to a mentoring relationship?

_____

_____

List the qualities you would like to see in your mentor. Whom do you know—in your immediate environment, from your educational program, in your specialty organization, in your local community, through your professional readings—that possesses all or most of those qualities? Consider making a contact with that person to discuss the possibility of establishing a mentoring relationship.

_____

_____

The next time you attend a professional conference or convention, make it a point to meet at least three new colleagues. Talk to each one about his or her interests, areas of expertise, goals, current position, and so on. You also should be prepared to tell them about your goals, interests, and areas of expertise. Exchange e-mail addresses or obtain a business card from each new colleague; note pertinent information about the individual, along with the date and conference where you met the individual, and file it when you return home. This will help you build your professional network.

_____

_____

Continued

CRITICAL THINKING
EXERCISES — cont'd

Reflect on the "results" of the assessments you completed earlier and any other tools you have found. What areas repeatedly emerge as strengths? How can you use those to develop as a leader throughout your career? In what areas do you need to develop? What will you do to overcome those limitations and enhance your leadership potential?

_____

_____

Write your personal career goals: What position would you like to hold 25 years from now? What types of offices would you like to hold? What awards would you like to have won or honors to have been bestowed on you? What types of books or articles would you like to have published? What would you like to be "known for" in the nursing profession? How influential would you like to be on the local, national, and international level? Think big! Now, for each goal, list the types of actions you will need to take to achieve that goal, and plot a timeline for each action. For example, if you would like to publish an article in the _Journal of Nursing Scholarship,_ you may want to take an intensive writing course and carefully read the articles published in that journal during the past 5 years to better understand the nature of what is published and its format. Take a paper you wrote for school or a difficult, challenging patient case study you presented at rounds and rewrite it to fit the guidelines of that journal, then submit it to a former faculty member or a trusted colleague at work for critique and comment. Talk to other nurses who have published in the _Journal of Nursing Scholarship_ or other prestigious journals about their experience "breaking into" the publication arena, and seek a mentor to assist you with writing for publication.

_____

_____

References

Aduddell, K. A., & Dorman, G. E. (2010). The development of the next generation of nurse leaders. _Journal of Nursing Education, 49_(3), 168–171.

Ang, R., & Fong, L. C. (2003). Nursing leadership: The Singapore experience. _Reflections on Nursing, 29_(1), 27–28.

Bennis, W. G. (2004). A leadership discussion with Warren Bennis. Webcast sponsored by the American Society of Association Executives Foundation, April 20, 2004.

Burns, J. M. (2003). _Transforming leadership: A new pursuit of happiness._ New York, NY: Atlantic Monthly Press.

Cardillo, D. (2001). Myths about networking. _Nursing Spectrum (New York/New Jersey edition), 13A_(15), 13.

Ferguson, S. L. (1998). Academy, Foundation launch program to enhance nurses' leadership capacity. *American Nurse, 30*(4), 10.

Gmelch, W. H. (2000). Leadership succession: How new deans take charge and learn the job. *Journal of Leadership Studies, 7*(30), 68–87.

Guthrie, K. L., Phelps, K., & Downey, S. (2011). Virtual worlds: A development tool for leadership education. *Journal of Leadership Studies, 5*(2), 6–13.

Hersey, P. (1985). *The situational leader.* New York, NY: Warner Books.

Houser, B. P., & Player, K. N. (2004). *Pivotal moments in nursing: Leaders who changed the path of a profession.* Indianapolis, IN: Sigma Theta Tau International.

Houser, B. P., & Player, K. N. (2007). *Pivotal moments in nursing: Leaders who changed the path of a profession. Volume II.* Indianapolis, IN: Sigma Theta Tau International.

Johns, C. (2004). Becoming a transformational leader through reflection. *Reflections on Nursing Leadership, 30*(2), 24–26, 38.

Kelley, R. (1992). *The power of followership: How to create leaders people want to follow and followers who lead themselves.* New York, NY: Doubleday Currency.

Kelly, L. S. (1991). The conundrum of recycled leadership (Editorial). *Nursing Outlook, 39*(1), 5.

Keirsey Temperament Sorter® (2011). Retrieved from http://www.keirsey.com/aboutkts2.aspx

Kinsey, D. C. (1986). The new nurse influentials. *Nursing Outlook, 34*(5), 238–240.

Kirkpatrick, M. K., Brown, S. T., Atkins, A., & Vance, A. (2001). Using popular culture to teach leadership. *Journal of Nursing Education, 40*(2), 90–92.

Levine, A. (2005). *Educating school leaders.* Washington, DC: The Education Schools Project.

Loue, S. (2011). *Mentoring health science professionals.* New York, NY: Springer.

Rath, T., & Conchie, B. (2008). *Strengths based leadership: Great leaders, teams, and why people follow.* New York, NY: Gallup Press.

Roche, G. (1979). Much ado about mentors. *Harvard Business Review, 58,* 14ff.

Sandler, B. R. (1993). Women as mentors: Myths and commandments (Opinion). *Chronicle of Higher Education, 39*(27), B3.

Self Profile. (1987). Overland Park, KS: National Press Publications.

Sherman, R. O., & Bishop, M. (2007). The role of nurse educators in grooming future nurse leaders (Guest Editorial). *Journal of Nursing Education, 46*(7), 295–296.

Stocker, S. (1991). Unraveling the leadership conundrum (Sounding Board). *Nursing Outlook, 39*(4), 188–189.

Valiga, T. M., & Bruderle, E. (1997). *Using the arts and humanities to teach nursing: A creative approach.* New York, NY: Springer.

Vance, C. N. (1977). *A group profile of contemporary influentials in American nursing.* Unpublished doctoral dissertation, Teachers College, Columbia University, New York, NY.

Yukl, G. (2010). *Leadership in organizations* (7th ed.). Upper Saddle River, NJ: Prentice Hall.

Bibliography

Bos, S. (1998). Perceived benefits of peer leadership as described by junior baccalaureate nursing students. *Journal of Nursing Education, 37*(4), 189–191.

Breaux, A. L. (2002). *101 Answers for new teachers and their mentors: Effective teaching tips for daily classroom use.* Larchmont, NY: Eye on Education, Inc.

Curtin, L. (1993). Empowerment: On eagles' wings (Editorial). *Nursing Management, 24*(6), 7–8.

Daloz, L. A. (1999). Mentor: Guiding the journey of adult learners. San Francisco, CA: Jossey-Bass.

Fields, W. L. (1991). Mentoring in nursing: A historical approach. *Nursing Outlook, 39,* 257–281.

Gibson, C. H. (1991). A concept analysis of empowerment. *Journal of Advanced Nursing, 16,* 354–361.

Glennon, T. K. (1992). Empowering nurses through enlightened leadership. *Journal of Nurse Empowerment, 2*(1), 41–44.

Gunden, E., & Crissman, S. (1992). Leadership skills for empowerment. *Nursing Administration Quarterly, 16*(3), 6–10.

Hartshorn, J. C., Berbiglia, V. A., & Heye, M. (1997). An honors program: Directing our future leaders. *Journal of Nursing Education, 36*(4), 187–189.

Helmuth, M. (1994). Mock convention: A simulation for teaching leadership. *Journal of Nursing Education, 33*(4), 159–160.

Huang, C. A., & Lynch, J. (1995). *Mentoring: The Tao of giving and receiving wisdom.* New York, NY: HarperCollins.

Johnson, W. B., & Ridley, C. R. (2004). *The elements of mentoring.* Hampshire, UK: Palgrave Macmillan.

Kelly, L. S. (2000). Where leaders are born: Living the mentoring continuum. *Reflections on Nursing Leadership, 26*(3), 8–9, 46.

Kessenich, C. R. (1997). The evolution of a leadership course. *Journal of Nursing Education, 36*(6), 301–303.

Klein, E., & Dickenson-Hazard, N. (2000). The spirit of mentoring. *Reflections on Nursing Leadership, 26*(3), 19–22, 46.

Krichbaum, K. (1997). Preparing students for leadership in practice. *Creative Nursing, 2,* 12–14.

McCall, M. W., Jr. (1998). *High flyers: Developing the next generation of leaders.* Boston, MA: Harvard Business School Press.

Murray, M. (2001). *Beyond the myths and magic of mentoring: How to facilitate an effective mentoring process.* San Francisco, CA: Jossey-Bass.

Olson, R. K., & Vance, C. N. (1993). *Mentorship in nursing: A collection of research abstracts with selected bibliographies—1977–1992.* Houston, TX: University of Texas Printing Services.

Prestholdt, C. O. (1990). Modern mentoring: Strategies for developing contemporary nursing leadership. *Nursing Administration Quarterly, 15*(1), 20–27.

Shea, G. F. (1999). *Making the most of being mentored.* Boston, MA: Course Technology, Inc.

Shea, G. F., & Woodbury, D. (2001). *Mentoring.* Cincinnati, OH: Muska & Lipman Publishing.

Sinetar, M. (1998). *The mentor's spirit: Life lessons on leadership and the art of encouragement.* New York, NY: St. Martin's Press.

Stewart, B. M., & Krueger, L. E. (1996). An evolutionary concept analysis of mentoring in nursing. *Journal of Professional Nursing, 12*(5), 311–321.

Stoddard, D. A., & Tamsay, R. (2003). *The heart of mentoring: Ten proven principles for developing people to their fullest potential.* Colorado Springs, CO: NavPress Publishing Group.

Taylor, D. E., Barrick, C. B., & Harrell, F. H. (1994). Preparing students for health care reform: An innovative approach for teaching leadership/management. *Journal of Nursing Education, 33*(5), 230–232.

Tebbitt, B. V. (1993). Demystifying organizational empowerment. *Journal of Nursing Administration, 23*(1), 18–23.

Tenner, E. (2004). The pitfalls of academic mentorships. *Chronicle of Higher Education, 50*(49), B7–B10.

Tracey, C., & Nicholl, H. (2006). Mentoring and networking. *Nursing Management, 12*(10), 28–32.

Vance, C. (2000). Discovering the riches in mentor connections. *Reflections on Nursing Leadership, 26*(3), 24–25, 46.

Vance, C. (2000). Mentoring at the edge of chaos. *Nursing Spectrum, 12A*(17), 6.

Vance, C. (2001). The value of mentoring. *Imprint, 48*(2), 38–40.

Vance, C., & Olson, R. K. (Eds.). (1998). *The mentor connection in nursing.* New York, NY: Springer.

Wilson, B., & Laschinger, H. K. (1994). Staff nurse perception of job empowerment and organizational commitment. *Journal of Nursing Administration, 24*(4), 39–47.

Yoder, L. (1990). Mentoring: A concept analysis. *Nursing Administration Quarterly, 15*(1), 9–19.

Zachary, L. J., & Daloz, L. A. (2000). *Mentor's guide: Facilitating effective learning relationships.* New York, NY: John Wiley & Sons.

Zachary, L. J., & Koestenbaum, P. (2005). *Creating a mentoring culture: The organization's guide.* San Francisco, CA: Jossey-Bass.

CHAPTER 10

Leadership, Excellence, and Creating the Future of Nursing

LEARNING OBJECTIVES

- Analyze the concept of excellence.
- Discuss the responsibility for promoting excellence that rests with leaders who will create nursing's preferred future.
- Examine the interrelationship among leadership, excellence, and professional involvement.
- Propose strategies for exercising leadership, promoting excellence, and being professionally involved to create nursing's preferred future.

INTRODUCTION

One of the responsibilities of those leaders who will create nursing's preferred future is to promote excellence. Nursing professionals certainly have a responsibility to strive for excellence in their own practice and in the delivery of health care to consumers. As leaders who will create a future for nursing that acknowledges and takes full advantage of the myriad talents nurses bring to the health-care arena, nurses have an even greater responsibility to promote excellence.

This chapter examines the concept of excellence in depth. Excellence is then related to leadership, and the role of leaders in advancing the notion of excellence is explored. Finally, both concepts—excellence and leadership—are blended with the idea of professional involvement throughout one's career as a means to promote nursing and create a preferred future for our profession.

The case studies presented depict two very different approaches to an individual's nursing career—one that accepts mediocrity and makes no attempt to be a leader and the other that is characterized by excellence and leadership. Referring back to these case studies as the concept of excellence is discussed and as it is related to leadership and professional involvement should help those ideas come alive for the reader.

Case Study

Adrienne's Career Track When She Is Willing to Accept Mediocrity and the Status Quo

Adrienne completed a baccalaureate program in nursing 8 years ago. In that time, she has worked in her local community hospital and now holds the position of nurse manager of a 30-bed telemetry unit in the area medical center. She runs her unit very efficiently, patient care is good with few incident reports being filed, and when she attends the mandatory management team meetings of the nursing department, Adrienne reads all material in advance and listens attentively. She occasionally reads a few articles in journals that colleagues bring to the unit, attends all required in-service sessions, and implements new practices as directed by her supervisor. Adrienne does not, however, attend conferences or workshops to advance her learning, is not enrolled in a graduate program, has never sought out a mentor, does not propose new ideas to her staff or at the management team meetings, does not hold membership in her professional association, and is glad to go home at the end of the day, knowing that everything is in order and she does not need to think about her practice until tomorrow.

Adrienne's Career Track When She Strives for Excellence and Is a Leader

Adrienne completed a baccalaureate program in nursing 8 years ago. In that time, she has worked in her local community hospital and now holds the position of nurse manager of a 30-bed telemetry unit in the area medical center. She runs her unit very efficiently, patient care is good with few incident reports being filed, and when she attends the mandatory management team meetings of the nursing department, Adrienne reads all material in advance and listens attentively. She also, however, always goes to those meetings having read about the latest research in her area of nursing practice and having talked with her staff about ways to improve patient care. She shares those ideas, as well as proposals for how change can be implemented in the institution. Adrienne sought out her former nurse manager as a mentor, and she regularly communicates with her mentor about nursing practice issues, career advancement, and other professional matters. In addition, she serves as a mentor to a former colleague who is beginning her career in nursing. Adrienne seeks out opportunities to attend conferences and workshops as a way to learn more and expand her professional networks, and she participates actively in her professional organization at the state level. She aspires to become involved at the national level and is talking with her mentor and others in the organization about how to make that happen. Adrienne is enrolled in a graduate program in nursing administration and has talked with the chief nursing officer about becoming involved in some system-wide change projects that will be implemented at the institution, offering to read and compile background information that will be helpful to the project team. She looks forward to the day when she can be more actively involved in interdisciplinary research studies related to excellence in nursing care delivery to patients with chronic illness and their families.

THE CONCEPT OF EXCELLENCE

"Excellence" is a word we hear tossed about everywhere recently. General Motors says they are in the business of excellence. IBM claims they are all about excellence. The American Nurses Association (ANA) talks about excellence in clinical practice. The National League for Nursing (NLN) promotes excellence in nursing education. Sigma

Theta Tau International advances excellence in scholarship. Our colleges and universities talk about excellence in their program offerings, faculty, students, and facilities. What is excellence? What is meant by this often-used, but little-examined, word?

Excellence means striving to be the very best you can be in everything you do—not because some teacher or parent or other "authority" figure pushes you to do that but because you cannot imagine functioning in any other way. It means setting high standards for yourself and the groups in which you are involved, holding yourself to those standards despite challenges or pressures to reduce or lower them, and not being satisfied with anything less than the very best.

This kind of perspective or approach applies to all spheres of life—writing papers for a course, preparing for a final examination, providing care to elderly patients in a long-term care facility, teaching school-aged children about good nutrition or sexually transmitted diseases, driving a car, or working to secure more resources for the homeless in our community. Individuals who are committed to excellence do not—and will not—settle for second best, mediocre performance, or "getting by."

In all that you do, reflect the excellence that's in you.
—*Martin Luther King Jr.*

When we allow ourselves and the systems in which we function to simply be "OK," "good enough," or minimally adequate, we sell ourselves short and we do little to advance the profession of nursing and ensure quality of care for patients, families, and communities. We fail to be challenged; we fail to grow; we fail to make change; and we fail to help others develop. Excellence means not allowing this state of affairs to exist!

Excellence also means being unwilling to accept the status quo. Wergin (2003, p. xiii) argues, "The most useful way to build and sustain a culture of excellence is to create a culture of critical reflection and continuous improvement." Critical reflection, however, does not mean that all one does is criticize the way things are being done and then walk away in the hopes that someone else will correct what is wrong. Instead, individuals who strive for and expect excellence question and challenge the status quo by asking why things are done the way they are, examining the assumptions that underlie existing practices, and offering thoughtful and realistic alternatives for how things could be done in other ways. They are also willing to invest time and energy to implement those alternatives, evaluate their effectiveness, and orchestrate change so that those new approaches become integral to the system.

Look for the ideal, but put it into the actual.
—*Florence Nightingale*

Excellence means to excel—to surpass—to be the best. It can be equated with accuracy, flawlessness, and even perfection—terms with which many are uncomfortable. Indeed, for many, perfection and the pursuit of excellence represent the "impossible dream." But in a piece about perfection in organizations, Mescon and Mescon (1984) note that "the pursuit of perfection is a challenge and a chase that must be won. . . . We must put to rest the notion that excellence represents fantasy, not fact in organizational life today" (p. 94). Perhaps this statement could be modified to say that "we must put to rest the notion that excellence represents fantasy, not fact in nursing practice today!" According to these authors, "Nothing but perfection is acceptable, [and] nothing but perfection should be rewarded" (p. 94).

> *The real voyage of discovery consists not in seeking new landscapes, but in having new eyes.* —Marcel Proust

Excellence is not an "impossible dream." In fact, if we look at just what excellence is, we see it is not so foreign or so unattainable. Many people have written about excellence, but the description of that concept offered by Diers and Evans (1980) many years ago still is particularly helpful. These authors said that excellence involves several things:

- *Discipline:* drawing on our knowledge and experience to practice in a "systematic" way that is of the highest caliber; in other words, "not settling for second best"
- *Choreography:* successfully balancing competing demands in our pursuit of goals
- *Responsibility:* acknowledging what we have done well or poorly and blaming no one
- *Caring:* consistently demonstrating a concern and a compassion for others (including our colleagues) and for ourselves
- *Skepticism:* keeping a proper distance from what is thought to be the truth and not accepting everything blindly; keeping our minds open to new ideas, new information, and new approaches
- *Perseverance:* continually striving to fulfill a goal or realize a vision
- *Passion:* "the essence of excellence"; being "inflamed" by our work

> *Let me tell you the secret that has led me to my goal. My strength lies solely in my tenacity.* —Louis Pasteur

Diers and Evans (1980) said, "Excellent nurses are inflamed by nursing. . . . To be an excellent nurse is to be suffused with a deep and almost inexpressible passion for humankind" (p. 30).

As made exceptionally clear by W. Edwards Demming more than 25 years ago, quality is never an accident. It is always the result of high intention, sincere effort, intelligent direction, and skillful execution, and it represents the wise choice from among many alternatives. Demming (1986) outlined 14 key principles that, although directed toward managers who wished to transform business effectiveness, have relevance for our discussion of excellence. Among those points are the following:

- Create constancy of purpose toward improvement.
- Awaken to the challenge and take on leadership for change.

- Cease dependence on inspection to achieve quality . . . build quality into the product in the first place.
- Constantly and forever improve the system.
- Institute leadership . . . help people and systems do a better job.
- Remove barriers that rob individuals of their right to pride of workmanship.
- Institute a vigorous program of education and self-improvement.
- Put everyone to work to accomplish the transformation because it is everyone's job.

A commitment to pursuing excellence does not just happen; it does not just randomly occur. Doing whatever it is that must be done requires an ongoing attention that is initiated and maintained by top management in an organization. In fact, Demming (1986) advocated that extensive training was needed to help everyone develop the courage that would be needed to break with tradition and to excel.

Management recruits and may even reward individuals who are committed to excellence and who consistently produce excellent work. Achieving excellence occurs only with individual investment. Top management and "the organization" can do only so much. What each of us needs to remember is that every job is a self-portrait of the person who did it. Each of us, therefore, needs to autograph **our** work with excellence.

> *Excellence is the gradual result of always striving to do better.* —Pat Riley

The pursuit of excellence must be vigorously and relentlessly incorporated into everything we think, say, and do. As Mescon and Mescon (1984) wrote, "It is the little things that count on the road to perfection. But too often it is the little things that we all too often simply forget" (p. 94). The individual who autographs his or her work with excellence does not ignore or forget the little things, just as he or she does not forget the big ones.

Vince Lombardi, former coach of the Green Bay Packers football team, once said, "The quality of a person's life is in direct proportion to his or her commitment to excellence, regardless of the chosen field of endeavor." This is a profound concept when one considers the significant role it suggests excellence plays in our lives.

According to John Gardner (1961), one of the leading experts on leadership, "We must learn to honor excellence (indeed to demand it) in every socially accepted human activity, however humble the activity, and to scorn shoddiness, however exalted the activity. An excellent plumber is infinitely more admirable than an incompetent philosopher. The society which scorns excellence in plumbing because plumbing is a humble activity and tolerates shoddiness in philosophy because it is an exalted activity will have neither good plumbing nor good philosophy. Neither its pipes not its theories will hold water" (p. 102).

> *If a man is called to be a streetsweeper, he should sweep streets even as Michelangelo painted or Beethoven composed music, or Shakespeare wrote poetry. He should sweep streets so well that all the hosts of heaven and earth will pause to say, here lived a great streetsweeper who did his job well.*
> —Martin Luther King Jr.

Each of us who hopes to make a significant contribution to our organization, our profession, our community, or the world needs to make this commitment. The quality of our lives will be enhanced as a result. As Aristotle said, "We are what we repeatedly do." Excellence, then, is not an isolated act, but a habit.

As mentioned earlier, excellence needs to be a way of life, and for those who do make it a habit, it sets up a "vicious cycle." In other words, excellence begets excellence—for ourselves and for those around us.

Striving for excellence is highly contagious because peer pressure and collegial influence have powerful effects and because they can usually do more than management ever could. Evidence exists to support this claim. Curtin (1990) reported on studies that showed that nurses who practice on units where excellent nursing is the norm soon are striving and growing to reach the level of excellence demonstrated by their peers. However, when nurses practice on a unit where the standard of care is poor and everyone is satisfied merely with maintaining the status quo and "getting by," their practice tends to descend to the lowest common denominator on that unit. Thus, the level of excellence found in practice is a function of the collegiality among nurses and the kind of habits they have. It is a reflection of the way they challenge and support each other, and the way they practice, repeatedly.

> *I never had a policy: I have just tried to do my best each and every day.* —Abraham Lincoln

Perhaps each of us needs to take what has been referred to as "the mirror test." Look at ourselves in a mirror and ask if we can honestly tell the person we see there that we have done our very best.

Excellence comes from within, and perfection is impossible without that personal investment. If staff tolerate mediocrity in what they do, practice will be mediocre. Management can create an environment that expects, fosters, and rewards excellence, but it is only when each individual in the organization can "pass the mirror test" and honestly say that he or she has done his or her very best that excellence will occur.

Unless we try to do something beyond what we have already mastered, we will never grow. Excellence, therefore, involves challenging ourselves—accepting challenges that are offered to us (e.g., writing a grant proposal, pursuing advancement through our agency's clinical levels, facilitating a research project on our unit, or accepting an invitation to speak at a professional meeting or to the media). Excellence also involves seeking new experiences (e.g., asking to serve on a committee, agreeing to have our name placed on a ballot for election to a committee or office, assuming new responsibilities with cross-training, submitting an abstract in response to a call for papers). Excellence is not allowing ourselves to get too comfortable or too complacent or so wrapped up in our "little corner of the world" that we lose this broader perspective.

> *The secret to leadership is . . . bearing the larger picture always in mind. Ask yourself, "What are we really trying to accomplish?"* —J. Donald Walters

No one ever attains eminent success by simply doing what is required. It is the amount and excellence of what is done over and above the required that determines the greatness of ultimate distinction.

In our society and in nursing, we have, for too long, accepted the mundane, promoted the average, and rewarded the mediocre. But the organization or the profession that is going to make a difference—to the recipients of its services and to those providing the service—is the one that prizes the absolute best at all levels. It is the organization that never forgets the ideal of excellence and never loses the aspiration to go beyond the merely "acceptable."

This goal of organizational excellence has been advanced in several projects. Between 2002 and 2007, the Robert Wood Johnson Foundation (2005) offered a program entitled, "Pursuing Perfection: Raising the Bar for Health Care Performance," the goal of which was to dramatically improve patient outcomes in a number of health systems in the United States and Europe by pursuing perfection in all major care processes. The evaluation of this project identified five critical elements of a health-care organization's success in moving to sustained, evidence-based improvements that lead to transformation of patient care. Those five elements were as follows: impetus to transform; leadership commitment to quality; improvement initiatives that actively engage staff in meaningful problem-solving; alignment to achieve consistency of organization goals with resource allocation and actions at all levels of the organization; and integration to bridge traditional intraorganizational boundaries among individual components.

In 2003, Wergin published a book focusing on excellence in academic departments in colleges and universities. He offered data from a number of studies to support his recommendations that, in order to "build and sustain cultures of excellence" (the book's subtitle), academic departments must have a clear direction, fully engage students and faculty, discuss explicit and tacit values, engage in "'difficult conversations' about matters of importance" (p. 128, citing Lucas, 2000), encourage experimentation and reflection, engage in peer collaboration and thoughtful peer review, respect and benefit from differences, and make a commitment to excellence.

Finally, a major work about how higher education can and should take greater responsibility for creating social change (Astin & Astin, 2000) offered valuable suggestions on the relevance of transformative leadership in higher education, the role of students in providing leadership, and the significance of a quest for excellence. The authors of this report concluded that "we have the power and the opportunity to transform our institutions" (p. 87), but they acknowledged that "perhaps our most limiting beliefs are concerned with what is *possible*" (p. 88) [emphasis in the original]. Thus, each individual needs to take responsibility for providing leadership that will help us achieve excellence in our lives, our institutions, and our society.

It has been said that only those who dare to fail greatly can ever achieve greatly. In other words, it is only when we strive for excellence, for flawlessness, and for perfection that we will achieve it. In that process, we may fail; therefore, taking risks is a critical component of achieving excellence. Although we may fail along the way, we need to try because excellence also involves action or execution (Bossidy & Charan, 2002). One anonymous writer put this idea into words by saying, "Some people dream of worthy accomplishments while others stay awake and actually do them."

Having a dream is critical, but it is not enough. Each of us needs to be able to articulate that dream clearly, express it to others, and entice others to work with us to make it become reality. This is the essence of leadership.

LEADERSHIP AND EXCELLENCE

Just as excellence is a complex phenomenon, so too is leadership. As noted earlier, Burns (1978, p. 2), in a classic work on the topic, asserted, "Leadership is one of the most observed and least understood phenomena on earth." This assertion was reiterated by Richardson (2000), who noted that "leadership has often escaped precise definition, yet we respect its power to transform and are quickly able to sense its absence" (p. v). Despite a lack of full understanding, however, many elements of leadership are universal, elements that bear reviewing.

First, there is agreement that, unlike management, *leadership is not necessarily tied to a position of authority in an organization*. In other words, there is a need for and opportunities to function as a leader at every level of every organization, society, and institution. One can be a leader as a staff nurse or as a student, just as well as if one is a nurse manager, the vice president for nursing, a faculty member, a dean, or the president of a professional association. In fact, it may be easier to be a leader if one is not in a position of authority because then that individual is not expected to promote any "party line," and it may be easier for him or her to "rock the boat" by raising difficult questions, articulating a vision, and working toward changing the system.

Second, *leadership is a relationship of influence* more than a relationship of authority. People follow leaders by choice, not because they are required to do so.

Perhaps one of the most important characteristics of leaders is that *leaders have a vision;* they see new possibilities, new horizons, and different options. They have some notion of circumstances being able to be better than they are now, regardless of how good they are now. In addition, this vision is their cause or purpose in life, and they are willing to invest enormous amounts of energy to see it realized. Think again about Martin Luther King, Jr., who worked all his life for racial equality and the peaceful resolution of differences. Mother Teresa devoted her life to helping the poor and disenfranchised. Candy Lightner lost her daughter to a drunk driver and established Mothers Against Drunk Driving (MADD). Many other individuals have had a vision of a better world and worked to see it materialize. This is the stuff of which leaders are made. Each of us needs to ask if we are leaders—if we have a vision of a better world.

> *In the quiet hours when we are alone and there is nobody to tell us what fine fellows we are, we come sometimes upon a moment in which we wonder, not how much money we are earning, nor how famous we have become, but what good we are doing.* —A.A. Milne

In accord with this drive toward realizing a vision, *leaders are change agents.* They are innovators who continually challenge the status quo, stick their heads above the crowd, and take the risk of being rejected. They strive to keep people and organizations moving forward. Again, each of us needs to ask ourselves if we are leaders—if we work toward positive change.

If leaders are going to be agents of change, they also must be *comfortable with conflict.* In fact, leaders must be able and willing to seek conflict, introduce it if necessary, and use it to achieve the goals of the group. They do not always want to minimize conflict or "sweep it under the rug" because they know that conflict is healthy and it promotes growth in individuals and organizations. Ask yourself if you are a leader—if you can manage the conflict we face in our daily lives and our professional lives.

Leaders are *willing to use intuition* in making decisions, they are *comfortable with ambiguity and uncertainty,* and they are *creative.* They want to see new forms take shape, and they do not need to rely on predictability or rationality. They *see the "big picture,"* are *"telescopic,"* seem to *have a "get-it-all-together" perspective,* and *want to collaborate* with others to achieve goals, rather than having a narrow, limited, self-centered interest or focus. Each of us needs to ask ourselves if we are leaders, if we are creative, if we can tolerate uncertainty, and if we can look beyond our own needs.

Finally, leaders are *characterized by excellence,* and they work to promote excellence in themselves and others. Driven by their vision, they strive to be the best they can be, and they inspire others to do the same. Dissatisfied with the status quo, they take risks, try innovative approaches, call on their creativity, and work to make change. Energized by a desire to continue to grow and learn, they seek new opportunities, take on challenges, and know how to manage conflict. Appreciative of the diverse and complex world in which we live, they do not allow themselves to become too highly specialized or too narrowly focused. "Social change results only when people take it on themselves to get involved and make a difference" (Richardson, 2000, p. iv).

Leaders promote and create excellence, and since "leadership is an essential ingredient of positive social change" (Richardson, 2000, p. iv), leaders create the future. Ilona Herlinger (1990, p. 4), former president of the interdisciplinary honor society of Phi Kappa Phi, challenged members of that organization to think about what role they would play during the 21st century. The questions she posed are challenges leaders must accept:

- Will you make a significant contribution to or an important difference in the world?
- Will you be a doer or merely an observer?
- Will you be an actor or merely a member of the audience?

In essence, Herlinger challenged us to ponder whether we will strive for excellence or accept mediocrity. She also suggested that we consider whether we will be leaders or apathetic, passive crowd-followers. These ideas are expressed powerfully by Hesselbein (2002, p. 5), who says, "Leadership is a matter of how to *be*, not how to *do* it" [emphasis in original].

PROFESSIONAL INVOLVEMENT

When one thinks about the history of Sigma Theta Tau International, the Honor Society of Nursing, or the interdisciplinary Honor Society of Phi Kappa Phi, one is inspired by what could be characterized as true leadership and true excellence. Sigma Theta Tau was started in 1922 by six nursing students who wanted to create some way to recognize and acknowledge nursing scholarship. Phi Kappa Phi was started in 1897 by one young man who dreamed of scholars from all disciplines being recognized on college campuses to the same extent that athletes were recognized. Those six nursing students and that one young man each had a vision, they banded together or enlisted the support of others, they took action and worked tirelessly, and they formed two of the most prestigious honor societies in our country.

Today, each of these organizations has hundreds of chapters and thousands of members. They are dedicated to scholarship and leadership (in the case of Sigma Theta Tau) and to promoting academic excellence (in the case of Phi Kappa Phi). They are proactive and forward-looking. Sigma Theta Tau is international in scope and purpose. Each organization is clear about its purpose; each is focused in its efforts; and each is highly regarded, well respected, and emulated. All of this from a handful of students who saw a need, had a vision, believed in excellence, and exercised leadership.

Members of Sigma Theta Tau are among the most powerful "movers and shakers" in our field. Dorothy Brooten's research on the effects of nursing care on low-birth-weight infants who have been discharged early from the neonatal intensive care unit to home has received accolades from the nursing and medical professions. Lois Evans and Neville Strumpf's extensive work on restraint-free care of the elderly has humanized that care in countless ways. Imogene King's contributions in theory development have been significant in advancing the science of nursing. Melanie Dreher's commitment to advancing the concept of clinical scholarship has been influential in helping nurses in practice develop more significant insights into their practice and be creative in where and how they deliver quality care. Dan Pesut's writings about the future have opened the minds of many. The late Virginia Henderson helped us crystallize the professional nursing role in a way few others have.

Real leaders are ordinary people with extraordinary determination. —Anonymous

By being involved in organizations like this—or in many other professional organizations—each of us has the opportunity to interact with and learn from outstanding individuals. We have the opportunity to see true leaders "in action," connect with and seek possible mentors, be involved in activities that promote excellence, and learn more about ourselves as potential leaders. Individuals such as these have an intense passion for the profession and their own area of work, and they do not hesitate to reach out to, guide, and help others in the field. They share a commitment to advancing the profession in whatever way they can, and they want to invest in others.

Professional involvement also means participating in organizational, community, and political activities to advance our vision and see it become a reality. Nurses who serve on committees where they work, on the board of the local community health center, on school boards, as local freeholders or mayors, or as U.S. senators, all are in positions of influence and have many opportunities to promote excellence, exercise leadership, and create a preferred future for nursing.

Nurses who publish or give presentations in which controversial ideas are presented or a high standard of practice is put forth are helping to create nursing's preferred future. The same is true for nurses who conduct special projects (funded or not), conduct research and disseminate the findings, mentor others, and engage in collaborative practice with other nurses and with members of other health-care disciplines. The opportunities to promote excellence and function as a leader are limitless, and each time a nurse engages in activities that advance nursing or that demonstrate leadership to realize a vision, he or she is contributing to the creation of a preferred future for the profession.

When we do the best we can, we never know what miracle is wrought in our life, or in the life of another. —Helen Keller

CONCLUSION

As we develop as leaders, each of us should take advantage of the opportunities presented to become involved professionally. We might even create opportunities to become involved. Each of us has a responsibility to participate and to try to make a difference. Through networking, role-modeling, mentoring relationships, and the continued study of leadership and excellence, practice will be enhanced and we will grow enormously. The outcomes will be excellence in our spheres of practice and a preferred future for the nursing profession that we helped create. Indeed, "leadership holds the key to transforming our institutions . . . and our society" (Richardson, 2000, p. v).

Perhaps nursing would do well to systematically study the phenomena of leadership and followership in our field to better understand how we can best prepare, support, and nurture our leaders and effective followers. A few research questions are offered to stimulate our thinking about these concepts:

- What is the relationship between learning experiences designed to help prelicensure students view themselves as evolving leaders and the ways in which graduates of such programs contribute to the creation of practice environments that embrace excellence?
- What are the most effective experiences in a transition-to-practice program for new graduates that contribute to those nurses' sense of empowerment and willingness to advocate for changes in practice?
- What is the impact on the development of nurse leaders when their mentors are within or outside their work environment?
- What is the relationship between measures of creativity and measures of leadership in advanced practice nurses?
- What characteristics of the work environment are most effective in encouraging nurses to function as leaders and effective followers?

Although there are many more questions that could be, and perhaps need to be, pursued through research, it is hoped that those noted here stimulate thinking about the many dimensions that influence how we prepare and nurture our leaders and followers. In conclusion, a contemporary piece of advice seems to capture the essence of leadership, excellence, and professional involvement:

> *Excellence can be attained if you ...*
> **CARE** *more than others think is wise,*
> **RISK** *more than others think is safe,*
> **DREAM** *more than others think is practical, and*
> **EXPECT** *more than others think is possible.*

We hope each student and nurse who reads this book will take on the challenges of excellence and leadership. You are the future of our marvelous profession. We have every confidence that you will take up this challenge with all seriousness and that you will succeed in creating a preferred future for nursing.

CRITICAL THINKING EXERCISES

Ask several children how they define excellence or what goes into something being called "excellent." Pose this same question to nurses in practice and to individuals engaged in other professional roles (e.g., teacher, physician, social worker). What common themes emerge in the responses you receive? Are there any differences in the way various groups (e.g., children versus adults, women versus men, nurses versus other professionals) talk about the concept? What conclusions can you draw about why the commonalities and differences exist?

_____

_____

Read a short story or poem or watch a film that has recently received a significant award for excellence, and do the same for a "nonwinner" in the genre. What sets the "winner" apart from the "nonwinner"? What were or seem to be the criteria used to determine excellence in the area? How do those criteria compare to your personal description/ definition of excellence?

_____

_____

Identify a nurse who recently received an award that acknowledges excellence—in clinical practice, in education, in research, in contributions to the profession, in the care of a particular population (e.g., the homeless), and so on. The award can be local, regional, national, or international. Interview the award recipient about his or her recognition. Talk about the individual's background, philosophy, accomplishments, contributions, and ideas about excellence and leadership. What have you learned from this interview that you can use to promote excellence and exert leadership in your arena of practice? Outline specific strategies that could lead you to receive such an award in the future.

_____

_____

References
_____

Astin, A. W., & Astin, H. S. (2000). *Leadership reconsidered: Engaging higher education in social change.* Battle Creek, MI: W. K. Kellogg Foundation.

Bossidy, L., & Charan, R. (2002). *Execution: The discipline of getting things done.* New York, NY: Crown Publishing Group (Random House).

Burns, J. M. (1978). *Leadership.* New York, NY: Harper Torchbooks.

Curtin, L. (1990). The excellence within (Editorial Opinion). *Nursing Management, 21,* 7.

Deming, W. E. (1986). *Out of the crisis.* Cambridge, MA: MIT Press.

Diers, D., & Evans, D. L. (1980). Excellence in nursing (Editorial). *Image, 12*(2), 27–30.

Gardner, J. (1961). *Excellence.* New York, NY: Harper & Row.

Herlinger, I. (1990). President's corner. *Phi Kappa Phi Newsletter, 16,* 4.

Hesselbein, F. (2002). *Hesselbein on leadership.* San Fransisco, CA: Jossey-Bass.

Mescon, M. H., & Mescon, T. S. (1984). Perfection: The possible dream. *Sky* (Delta Airlines magazine), *13*(9), 94, 96.

Richardson, W. C. (2000). Foreword. In A. W. Astin & H. S. Astin. *Leadership reconsidered: Engaging higher education in social change* (pp. iv–vi). Battle Creek, MI: W. K. Kellogg Foundation.

Robert Wood Johnson Foundation (2005). *Evaluation of pursuing perfection: Raising the bar for health care performance.* Retrieved from http://www.rwjf.org/pr/product.jsp?id=14954

Wergin, J. F. (2003). *Departments that work: Building and sustaining cultures of excellence in academic programs.* Boston, MA: Anker.

Annotated Bibliography

Adams, R. (1972). *Watership down*. New York, NY: Avon Books.

Watership Down is a book about the adventures of a group of rabbits who leave their comfortable warren in search of a better, safer place to live. Originally thought of as a children's story, this book is an excellent portrayal of leadership styles, leader–follower interactions, and the qualities of effective leaders and followers.

The group of rabbits that serves as the focal point of the story travels extensively to create a new life for themselves, and they encounter several different warrens along the way. They experience warrens that are leaderless, those that are headed by a totalitarian despot, and those where the "leader" provides direction and the basic needs of rabbits in the warren are met, but there is an aloofness between the leader and followers, and high-order needs are not met.

The Watership Down warren rabbits come to form a democratic, participating group where the talents of each rabbit are known and called upon as needed, where followers assume the role of leader when circumstances require a particular type of leadership, and where there is a constant exchange of ideas and support. In essence, this group of rabbits exhibits all that is good about leaders and followers.

This book exposes the reader to various types of leadership and leader–follower relationships. One sees risk-taking, acting in uncertainty, clarity of vision, clear communication, and many other behaviors of leaders . . . all within the context of a beautiful story that captures the imagination and holds one's attention.

Babcock, L., & Laschever, S. (2003). *Women don't ask: Negotiation and the gender divide.* Princeton, NJ: Princeton University Press.

When Linda Babcock asked why so many male graduate students were teaching their own courses and most female students were assigned as assistants, her dean said: "More men ask. The women just don't ask." It turns out that whether they want higher salaries or more help at home, women often find it hard to ask. Sometimes they don't know that change is possible—they don't know that they can ask. Sometimes they fear that asking may damage a relationship, and sometimes they don't ask because they've learned that society can react badly to women asserting their own needs and desires.

By looking at the barriers holding women back and the social forces constraining them, *Women Don't Ask* shows women how to reframe their interactions and more accurately evaluate their opportunities. It teaches them how to ask for what they want in ways that feel comfortable and possible, taking into account the impact of asking on their relationships. And it teaches all of us how to recognize the ways in which our institutions, child-rearing practices, and unspoken assumptions perpetuate inequalities . . . inequalities that are not only fundamentally unfair but also inefficient and economically unsound.

With women's progress toward full economic and social equality stalled, women's lives becoming increasingly complex, and the structures of businesses changing, the ability to negotiate is no longer a luxury but a necessity. Drawing on research in psychology, sociology, economics, and organizational behavior as well as dozens of interviews with men and women from all walks of life, *Women Don't Ask* is the first book to identify the dramatic difference between men and women in their propensity to negotiate for what they want. It tells women how to ask and why they should.

Bass, B. M. (2008). *The Bass handbook of leadership: Theory, research, and managerial applications* (4th ed.). New York, NY: The Free Press.

This is a classic volume that provides a historical perspective on leadership, an analysis of the meaning of leadership, descriptions of various categories or typologies of leadership, and an examination of leadership theories and models (including Great Man, trait, situational, psychoanalytic, and other theories). Beyond this introductory material, the major emphasis of this 1000+-page book is research that has been completed about leaders and leadership.

The research reported focuses on leadership traits, tasks of leaders, leadership styles, women and leadership, leader–follower interactions, and the significance of values to leaders. Concepts such as charisma, inspirational leadership, power, and conflict also are addressed.

This *Handbook* is an excellent resource for any serious student of leadership. Sadly, however, although the author notes that leadership and management are different phenomena, most of the studies reported use managers as subjects, thereby suggesting that one needs to be in a position of authority to be considered a leader. Despite these limitations, *The Bass Handbook of Leadership* is a classic that should be read and used as a reference source.

Bass, B. (1985*). Leadership and performance beyond expectations.* New York, NY: The
Free Press, MacMillan.

Written in 1985, this outstanding book describes leadership in terms of transformational
and transactional components and still has relevance. The author says transformational
leadership is found in varying amounts in everyone and needs to be tapped. He offers
traditional leaders—such as Moses, Buddha, Jesus Christ, and Mohammed—as well
as contemporary leaders—such as Theodore Roosevelt, John F. Kennedy, and Gandhi—
as examples for study. He also cites how each of these individuals depicted charisma,
individualized consideration, and intellectual stimulation. Bass gives behavioral examples of transactional leadership and defines the principles of management-by-exception
and contingent rewards.

Perhaps the most interesting aspect of this book is the description of the data collected from the author's classic study of 104 military officers who completed the author-
developed *Leadership Questionnaire*. This instrument asked the officers about their
perceptions of their immediate supervisor's leadership skills, and the findings regarding
what these individuals believe make someone an effective leader are extremely interesting. The results of this study also point out how an effective leader can influence the
followers in a group. (A copy of the *Leadership Questionnaire* and parameters for scoring
are included in the book.)

Beatty, J. (1998). *The world according to Peter Drucker.* New York, NY: The Free Press.

This book chronicles the life of Peter Drucker and delineates how he constantly pushed
himself to become a stronger and more successful person by thinking about what people **can** do, not only what they **cannot** do. Drucker is a firm believer in frequent self-
evaluation, which he calls "keeping score on self" (p. 14), and this theme is inherent
in all of his work.

Drucker is perhaps best known for his philosophy of "management by objectives,"
which emphasizes the significance of planning, goals, and evaluating results against
preestablished expectations. All of this clearly is management, but it is a crucial part of
being an effective leader . . . namely, having a vision and evaluating, on a regular basis,
the progress being made toward realizing the vision.

This book is easy to read and gives the reader a feeling that anyone can be whatever
one wants to be. It also stresses the importance of making a difference in people's lives
and not being remembered merely for writing a book or developing a theory. This book
is good for helping individuals develop their leadership abilities.

Bennis, W. (1993). *An invented life: Reflections on leadership and change.* Reading,
MA: Addison-Wesley.

This is a retrospective look by Bennis about his own life and work. He candidly
explains leadership through his lens as a social scientist and business administrator,
and offers thoughts on comparing leaders to managers: "I decided that the kind of
university president I wanted to be was one who led, not managed. That's an important

difference. Many an institution is well managed yet very poorly led. It excels in the ability to handle all daily routine inputs yet never asks whether the routine should be done in the first place" (p. 31).

Bennis speaks of a democratic leadership style as what is most promoted in U.S. industry and defines it as including: "1) full and free communication, regardless of rank and power; 2) a reliance on consensus rather than on coercion or compromise to manage conflict; 3) the idea that influence is based on technical competence and knowledge rather than on the vagaries of personal whims or prerogatives of power; 4) an atmosphere that permits and even encourages emotional expression as well as task-oriented behavior; and 5) a basically human notion, one that accepts the inevitability of conflict between the organization and the individual but is willing to cope with and mediate this conflict on rational grounds." He ends with the importance of leaders of all organizations, small and large, to partner with others and collaborate in order to best set the stage for change.

Bennis, W. (2009). *On becoming a leader: Leadership classic—Updated and expanded* (4th ed.). New York, NY: Perseus Books

Written by one of the foremost authorities on leadership, this book is a classic in the field. Beginning with the conviction that everyone can potentially be a leader, this book is a reflective exploration of the nature of this elusive phenomenon and the qualities and characteristics of those who serve as leaders. Bennis asserts there are few people answering our nation's call for leaders, and he worries about the impact of this lack of leadership because our "quality of life depends on leaders." He gives many examples of where leadership is lacking in our world, including American business and the Roman Catholic Church. Bennis says leaders tend not to seek a leadership position, but rather wish to express themselves.

Although leadership can be provided by almost anyone, leaders are not ordinary people, according to Bennis. They work everywhere; they serve as guides; they take risks, and they fail. Leaders always learn from those failures; they engage in continuous learning and self-development, and they know themselves.

By using many examples—from Norman Lear to Gloria Steinem and from the executive director of the American Association of University Women to the chairman and CEO of Johnson & Johnson—Bennis helps the reader understand how leaders need to master the contexts in which they find themselves, create new contexts, use their instincts and intuition, and be innovators who help others move through chaos, among other things. These examples also are used to illustrate the differences between leadership and management.

Serious students of leadership will want this classic reference in their collection. It is insightful and offers many practical suggestions for developing as a leader.

Bennis, W., & Biederman, P. (1998). *Organizing genius: The secrets of creative collaboration*. Reading, MA: Addison-Wesley.

This book starts out reminding us that "none of us are as smart as all of us." Charles Handy says in the forward that "Warren Bennis's great gift is the ability to find meaning and messages where the rest of us see only happenings" (p. xi). This is accurate because as one reads through this book, it is the everyday observations seen on a daily basis that Bennis and Biederman have used to convey their ideas of great leadership being made up of great followers and leaders who have the freedom to do their very best every step of the way and then to enjoy the "personal transformation" that such accomplishments bring. This book provides strategies for success by collecting a group of great people, led by a leader who facilitates each and every individual to perform his or her absolute best, in order to accomplish excellent results.

Bennis, W., & Nanus, B. (2003). *Leaders: Strategies for taking charge* (2nd ed.). New York, NY: Harper & Row.

This is the second edition of the seminal work in which Bennis first claimed that managers are those who do things right and leaders are those who do the right things. The authors speak to the dramatic changes taking place in our world and acknowledge the dire need for competent leadership and for more flexibility and awareness on the part of leaders and followers alike.

Based on the results of a 2-year study of individuals who were thought to be leaders, Bennis and Nanus identified four major themes/areas of competency/"human handling skills" that emerged. Those strategies are as follows: attention through vision (i.e., creating a focus or having an agenda, particularly one that draws others in), meaning through communication (i.e., expressing ideas powerfully so that others understand and want to support them), trust through positioning (e.g., making one's position known, being reliable, and being persistent with relentless dedication), and the deployment of self (i.e., having a positive self-regard, knowing one's strengths and weaknesses, and setting high goals). Each of these strategies is discussed thoroughly, and many ideas are offered as to how one can implement each.

The authors conclude by recommending that we must increase the search for new leadership to a national priority. They urge the purposeful and continuous development of leaders because without effective leaders, the best our society can do is maintain the status quo; at worst, our society could disintegrate.

Bennis, W., & Thomas, W. (2002). *Geeks and geezers: How eras, values, and defining moments shape leaders.* Boston, MA: Harvard Business School Press.

This book is a compilation of ideas on leadership development and the generational differences between the Geeks (people under 30 years old) and the Geezers (people over 70 years old). It focuses on the young and the old more so than on the people between 30 and 70 years of age. The leadership development model described in this book can help readers develop the four areas that these authors define as leadership: voice, integrity, adaptive capacity, and ability to engage others by creating a vision. A great emphasis is on what the authors call "crucible moments," which are life-changing experiences that people have throughout their lives and that call for leadership. This book is easy to read, worthwhile, and helpful to improve self-confidence and general self-concept regarding one's ability to achieve dreams and personal visions.

Bolman, L. G., & Deal, T. E. (2011). *Leading with soul: An uncommon journey of spirit* (3rd ed.). San Francisco, CA: Jossey-Bass.

Using the story of Steve, a dispirited leader in search of something more meaningful in his life than "the bottom line," these authors help the reader see and appreciate the spiritual dimensions of leadership and how work and spirit can and, in their opinion, need to be connected. They discuss the interrelationship of leaders and followers, the "gifts" of leadership (love, power, and significance), and the legacy of leadership. This book challenges the reader to look deep inside oneself and reflect on one's true self and values. Finally, the dialogue between the authors and an "interviewer" that concludes the book provides insights into why they examined the concept of the soul of leadership and how this work has affected individuals in various positions in diverse organizations.

Book, E. W. (2001). *Why the best man for the job is a woman: The unique female qualities of leadership*. New York, NY: HarperBusiness.

This book reports on intensive studies the author conducted with 14 women who have exhibited leadership, primarily in the corporate world. Among the strengths that were common to all women were "a gravity-defying level of self-confidence . . . a preternatural sense of exactly what their [followers] want . . . [and a tendency to] foster a more collegial environment" (p. xiii). The author claims that "evidence is mounting that the style of leadership women offer is beneficial not only to employees but also to the bottom line, [perhaps because] women are better at communicating, empowering people and being positive" (p. xv).

The author provides extensive descriptions of the key characteristics of what she calls "new paradigm leadership": selling one's vision, reinventing the rules, having a laser focus to achieve, maximizing high touch in an era of high tech, turning challenge into opportunity, and having courage under fire. She contrasts these with features of the old paradigm—masculine, hierarchical, command-and-control oriented, opposed to change, focused on individual efforts, and limited to communication—and describes the advantages of new paradigm leadership.

In conclusion, Book offers a number of tips on becoming a new paradigm leader and encourages women to assume such roles with enthusiasm. As such, this book provides a thoughtful analysis of women's leadership styles and serves as a helpful guide to those wishing to integrate such styles into their own repertoire.

Burns, J. M. (1978). *Leadership*. New York, NY: Harper Torchbooks.

This book is truly a classic! It was Burns who first acknowledged that "leadership is one of the most observed and least understood phenomenon on earth" (p. 2) and then proceeded to help us understand this complex concept.

He noted how little we knew at the time about leadership and how to develop it—despite the hundreds of definitions of the term!—and how little attention was given to the significance of followers and the "interwoven texture of leadership and followership" (pp. 4–5). He also analyzed the nature of power and the role of power in leadership and explored the ways in which leaders help release the potentials of others.

In his attempt to clarify the meaning of leadership, Burns offered distinctions between *transactional* and *transformational* leadership and introduced the notion of *moral* leadership. In recent years, many authors have "carried the banner" of transformation leadership, but Burns was the first to name it and describe it exquisitely.

As a result of Burns' seminal work on leadership, our understanding of this complicated concept has progressed enormously. This is a book that must be read as a foundation to subsequent works about leadership.

Burns, J. M. (2003). *Transforming leadership: A new pursuit of happiness.* New York, NY: Atlantic Monthly Press.

In this book, Burns expands on his notion of transformational leadership. He asserts that "to transform something . . . is to cause a metamorphosis in form or structure, a change in the very condition or nature of a thing" (p. 24) . . . a change of breadth and depth.

The primary focus of this book is an examination of how a number of leaders in the past, including the American Founding Fathers, embraced and lived the three standards or norms that Burns claims constitute a good leader: virtue, ethics, and transforming values. He then conducts an extensive analysis of how these standards shaped the Declaration of Independence's emphasis on life, liberty, and the pursuit of happiness, with particular emphasis on the latter (hence, the book's subtitle).

Although Burns offers many insightful comments about leaders, leadership, followers, empowerment, and other topics relevant to a study of leadership, they often are difficult to cull from the discussions of the pursuit of happiness. Leadership scholars will want to study this book carefully, but novices to leadership studies are likely to benefit more from other resources.

Chaleff, I. (2009). *The courageous follower: Standing up to and for our leaders* (3rd ed.). San Francisco, CA: Berrett-Koehler.

This book gets to the heart of what leadership truly is and how it grows from followership. The author describes followership in a very positive way and avoids the negative connotations often associated with being a follower.

Chaleff speaks to being an *effective* follower and how such individuals are critical to generating effective leaders. He offers many fundamental, commonsense, helpful ideas that could be most useful to the person interested in empowering her/himself and others, creating a vision, making a change, and preparing for a leadership role.

The author makes a point of explaining the significance of being a follower, supporting the leader's vision, and participating actively in change processes. A major point made by Chaleff is that followers do not do things simply at the bidding of leaders, nor do they hide behind leaders. Instead, followers do things because they think those things are best for themselves and for the organization. Followers, according to Chaleff, are not weak or passive. They are dynamic and passionate about many issues.

This book is a "must read" for understanding the relationship between leaders and followers and for appreciating the significance of followers in making change and realizing visions.

Clampitt, P., & DeKoch, R. (2001). *Embracing uncertainty: The essence of leadership.* Armonk, NY: M. E. Sharpe.

The authors make the case that embracing uncertainty is more effective and rewarding than trying to eliminate it. They advocate that leaders recognize that they will never have all of the right answers and that "not knowing" is quite legitimate. Leaders should never feel bad about not knowing but should attempt to foster this belief in their followers so that increased creativity and increased morale are the outcome. The *Working Climate Survey* developed by these authors to measure one's tendency to embrace uncertainty provides fascinating insight into one's comfort with uncertainty and ambiguity. This tool is included in this book, along with directions for interpreting results.

Cohen, W. (2004). *The art of the strategist: 10 essential principles for leading your company to victory.* New York, NY: American Management Associates.

This book is essential for those wanting to learn new strategies for fulfilling a group's or individual's vision. It emphasizes the importance of being aware of environmental influences and recognizes that it sometimes is necessary to change strategy or components of strategy to fulfill goals. The fact that the success of a strategy depends on the "judgment and leadership qualities of the individual responsible for the undertaking" (p. vii) is the underlying premise.

Cohen offers 10 essential principles that are worth reading and pondering: commit fully to a definite objective; seize the initiative and keep it; economize to mass your resources; use strategic positioning; do the unexpected; keep thing simple; prepare multiple, simultaneous alternatives; take the indirect route to your objective; practice timing and sequencing; and exploit your success. The author then gives excellent realistic examples of both successful and unsuccessful strategies and offers reasonable ideas about how to examine one's plan and make changes midstream so that success is the outcome. Ideas for strategizing in an escalating crisis and in emergencies also are discussed.

Coles, R. (2001). *Lives of moral leadership: Men and women who have made a difference.* New York, NY: Random House.

This book powerfully conveys the meaning of moral leadership using well-known and influential, as well as "ordinary," people as examples. The lives and work of individuals like Robert Kennedy, Gandhi, and Albert Jones, a Boston bus driver, are used to illustrate the bond that develops between true leaders and their followers, and how "moral energy" helps our society respond to crises and challenges. Coles asserts that "we need heroes, people who can inspire us, help shape us morally, spur us on to purposeful action" (p. xi), and he acknowledges that "from time to time we are called on to *be* those heroes, leaders for others, either in a small, day-to-day way, or on the world's larger stage"

(p. xi). Reading this book helps one appreciate what moral leadership is and how it is achieved. As such, it is a most significant resource in today's environment.

Conger, J. (1992). *Learning to lead: The art of transforming managers into leaders.* San Francisco, CA: Jossey-Bass.

Conger firmly believes that leadership can be "broken down" into specific behaviors, those behaviors can be taught, and they can be learned. In fact, this book is an account of the author's own experiences in learning to be a leader, specifically through his participation in the following innovative leadership development programs: Kouzes and Posner's Leadership Challenge, the Center for Creative Leadership's Leadership Development Program, the Experiential Pecos River Learning Center Program, and the Vision Quest Program.

The author explains the significance of leaders having a vision so that they can provide some type of direction and meaning, being inspirational, demonstrating charisma, being empowered, and acting as a transformational change agent. He asserts that one can learn these skills.

Work experiences, taking advantage of opportunities that present themselves, educational advancement, mentors, and experiencing hardship all are variables identified by Conger as fostering leadership. He explains the historical development of leadership training and points out the importance of having such programs focus on providing feedback to participants regarding their conceptual development, skill building, and personal growth.

Conger also explores some of the more "common" theories about leadership. He explains how situational leadership and the "task-versus-relationship" contingency model of the 1980s lack the strategic envisioning, inspirational speaking, and management of change that he feels is absolutely essential for an effective leader in today's environments. He believes that all aspiring leaders need to participate in the kind of personal growth programs that he discusses in this book.

Covey, S. (1992). *Principle-centered leadership.* New York, NY: Summit Books.

This book is grounded in the idea that having principles to guide one's life, like a compass guides one's journey, makes for a more productive, fulfilling life. Covey presents his ideas regarding the principles of vision, leadership, and human relationships as the way to make decisions in one's personal, interpersonal, managerial, and organizational lives. He offers suggestions on how to cultivate eight characteristics that facilitate the making of what he calls a "principle-centered leader."

This excellent book on self-leadership can be used as a rich resource to assist others in their development as leaders, particularly "principle-centered" leaders. Covey's ideas center around the importance of a leader being a pathfinder—someone who can align an organization's or an individual's structure with an individual's behavior, **not** the organization's behavior—and a facilitator or empowerer of others. By pathfinder, Covey means being able to move an individual or group down a path or to realize a vision. The pathfinder is an individual who, by using leadership, moves individuals or organizations in new directions, an approach that is vastly different from making changes merely in response to revised organization policies and expectations.

Covey, S. (2004). *The 8th habit: From effectiveness to greatness.* New York, NY: Running Book Press.

This book is an excellent sequel to *The 7 Habits of Highly Effective People.* The author has added the idea of "finding your voice and encouraging others to find theirs" as the eighth habit. He describes how all individuals can discover the voices that evolve from three gifts at birth: freedom to choose, natural laws, and the four intelligences (mental, physical, spiritual, and emotional). He gives multiple examples of how people can use these ideas to improve themselves and become more holistic people and leaders.

Covey discusses how leadership roles have changed and gives examples of how individuals can maximize their leadership skills with new roles. He also describes what he sees as new roles for leaders: modeling, path-finding, aligning, and empowering. He discusses the value of vision, discipline, passion, and conscience in leaders and gives many real-life examples for using the new roles of leadership. The book also offers advice on how a person can change from being a "want to" person to a "can do" person, and the section on Frequently Asked Questions about his ideas of leadership is helpful.

Csikszenthihalyi, M. (1996). *Creativity: Flow and the psychology of discovery and invention.* New York, NY: Harper Perennial.

The major purpose of this book is to remind the reader that creativity is a process that unfolds over a lifetime. It is "based on histories of contemporary people who know about [creativity] firsthand" (p. 1) because they have experienced the challenges, disappointments, and joy in promoting creative ideas or approaches. As an outcome of scholarly, in-depth interviews with selected individuals known for their creative endeavors, the author offers several conclusions: creative ideas arise from the synergy of many sources and not from the mind of a single individual; it is easier to enhance creativity by changing conditions in the environment than by trying to make people think more creatively; and a genuinely creative accomplishment is almost never the result of a sudden insight but comes after years of hard work.

Reading about creativity in the young, middle-aged, and elderly is inspiring and informative, and anyone wishing to better understand this phenomenon that is "a central source of meaning in our lives" (p. 1) is encouraged to explore this book.

Denhardt, R., & Denhardt, J. (2006). *The dance of leadership: The art of leading in business, government, and society.* New York, NY: M. E. Sharpe.

This book emphasizes the need for each individual to lead, no matter what his/her role. The authors assert that each person should use his/her leadership ability to improve the work setting, home situation, or other circumstance. They offer a view of leadership that originates from the arts, noting that "artists see the world in a way quite different from others . . . they see the world in terms of an especially intense and textured interplay of space, time, and energy" (p. 6). Denhardt and Denhardt weave an interesting story about how one cannot really have a single operational definition of leadership, and they assert that "the only thing that really counts in leadership is that which you can't explain" (p.10).

This book is interesting and entertaining and challenges the reader to seriously think about the emotional aspects of leadership and the importance of the leader's audience (i.e., followers). The authors explore various concepts such as rhythms of human interaction, communication, spontaneity, and creativity; and they share their rendition of the difference between leadership and management. These authors make a strong argument that leadership originates from art, not science.

DePree, M. (2004). *Leadership is an art* (2nd ed.). New York, NY: Doubleday Currency.

This book is about how the art of leadership frees people to do what is required of them in the most effective way possible. As an art, leadership is something one learns over time. This second edition includes a new foreword by the author, who stresses the importance of having a mentor in one's life to assist in developing one's leadership ability.

One of the most significant aspects of leadership, according to DePree, is a genuine concern for and about others. Leaders understand the diversity of the talents, gifts, and skills others possess and find ways to allow each individual to contribute to a cause or purpose in her/his own way.

The author asserts that leaders serve others. They are responsible for identifying, developing, and nurturing future leaders, and they bind people together to accomplish great things. They provide and help to maintain the momentum of a group, and they keep the group focused on the values and visions that guide them. DePree describes the three most important themes of the book: integrity, ability to build and nurture relationships, and community building. He relates all of these components of leadership to knowing who we intend to be in the future, which, he says, will help us to generate exactly what we will end up doing with our lives.

This easy-to-read book includes many insightful points about leaders and leadership that stimulate one's thinking in new ways. The conceptualization of leadership as an art, but an art that can be learned, is a useful one for the would-be leader.

DePree, M. (2008). *Leadership jazz: The essential elements of a great leader* (2nd ed.). New York, NY: Doubleday.

This is the second edition of a classic book on leadership that was described by Sam Walton as "one of the best books I have ever read in my life on the subject of leadership and business management philosophy." The basis for this book is an assertion that without followers, leaders can do nothing but play solo. The book tells how leaders can facilitate leadership in others because DePree believes in developing leaders and not directing them. He expands on four questions that he believes assist him in gaining insight on leaders and leadership: 1) How can I know what's in the hearts of my followers?, 2) What gifts of leadership have I come to treasure most?, 3) What questions do I know wish I had been asked? and 4) What questions would I ask you? He believes these four questions underlie one's future in becoming a global citizen prepared to take advantage of multiple opportunities.

Dreher, D. (1996). *The Tao of personal leadership*. New York, NY: Harper Business.

This book is a rich blend of the principle of centering and balancing one's life and the Taoist philosophy of engaging in compassion while remaining detached. It emphasizes the importance of realizing the power of living systems that generate energy all around us, and it reinforces the appreciation of all people potentially becoming leaders, regardless of their "station" in life.

Communication, team building, having an appetite for constant change, credibility, risk taking, and the ability to facilitate others in accomplishing goals/vision are necessary assets of a strong leader, according to Dreher. The author describes the Tao leader as being a pioneer, a pathfinder, a person who guides with intuition, someone who constantly faces the unknown with excitement, and someone who turns conflict into opportunities for stronger relationships, greater knowledge, and better solutions. The author has written an exhilarating account of how one can develop one's leadership capacity in exponential fashion.

Gardner, J. W. (1990). *On leadership*. New York, NY: The Free Press.

John Gardner is one of the experts on the topic of leadership, and he reports, in this book, insights gained from a 5-year study of the phenomenon. He distinguishes leadership from management and expresses the great need we have for true leaders, individuals "who are exemplary, who inspire, who stand for something, [and] who help us set and achieve goals" (p. xi).

One of the most significant contributions Gardner makes through this book is helping the reader understand what he calls "the tasks of leadership." Included in those "tasks" are the following:

Envisioning Goals . . . pointing us in the right direction or asserting a vision

Affirming Values . . . reminding the group of the norms and expectations they share

Motivating . . . stimulating and encouraging others to act

Managing . . . planning, setting priorities, and making decisions

Achieving a Workable Unity . . . managing conflict and promoting unity within the group

Explaining . . . teaching followers and helping them understand why they are being asked to do certain things

Serving as a Symbol . . . acting in ways that convey the values of the group and its goals

Representing the Group . . . speaking on behalf of the group

Renewing . . . bringing members of the group to new levels

In fulfilling these tasks, leaders must work collaboratively with followers, whom Gardner refers to as constituents. He acknowledges that "followers often perform leaderlike acts" (p. 23) and recognizes the significant role that followers play in accomplishing change and realizing a vision.

Finally, Gardner draws on the work of many researchers to identify several attributes of leaders, including the following: physical vitality and stamina (i.e., a high energy level), intelligence and judgment-in-action (i.e., ability to identify and solve problems, set priorities, etc.), willingness to accept responsibilities (i.e., exercise initiative, bear the burden of making a decision, and step forward when no one else will), task competence (i.e., knowing the task at hand and the system), understanding followers/constituents and their needs, skill in dealing with people, a need to achieve, the capacity to motivate others, and courage. He also discusses how leaders need to use power and how they need to be morally responsible.

Gladwell, M. (2005). *Blink: The power of thinking without thinking*. New York, NY: Little, Brown.

Although this book is not about leadership *per se*, it nevertheless offers valuable insights for anyone who strives to fulfill the role of leader. It is a book about how we think without thinking and how this process can be very valuable or have disastrous consequences.

Gladwell notes that "our world requires that decisions be sourced and footnoted" (p. 52). He then challenges that approach and labels it a mistake, asserting that "if we are to learn to improve the quality of the decisions we make, we need to accept the mysterious nature of our snap judgments. We need to respect the fact that it is possible to know without knowing why we know" (p. 52).

While somewhat unorthodox, Gladwell's perspective is congruent with much of the leadership literature, which notes that leaders often rely on their intuition and do what they believe . . . in their hearts . . . is right. As such, the reader interested in developing herself or himself as a leader could benefit from these ideas that help one see the world in a different way.

Goleman, D. (1998). *Working with emotional intelligence*. New York, NY: Bantam Books.

This is an interesting book describing how emotions affect one's life even more than one's intelligence quotient. The author asks the question, "Have you known leaders who are smart and experienced, but failed because they could not form collaborative relationships?" Goleman says a leader must be a master of emotional intelligence, and leaders must build their relationships with commitment and empathy. He suggests that emotional intelligence influences one's success at home, work, and school, and it affects how people interact with others and work in teams. Goleman discusses how one can improve one's emotional intelligence and how it increases with age. Essentially this book explains how people can be more successful if they can deal with their own emotions, learn to work with other people's emotions, and respond appropriately to others.

A leader must be visionary and capable of getting people motivated to participate in new ideas, making change, and working in totally different ways than ever before. Goleman explains how having emotional intelligence will help leaders be successful in these and other areas.

Goleman, D., Boyatzis, R., & McKee, A. (2002). *Primal leadership: Realizing the power of emotional intelligence.* Boston, MA: Harvard Business School Press.

This book speaks to the concept of resonance, which is defined as "a reservoir of positivity that frees the best in people" (p. ix). The authors expand on this concept as they explain that at its root, the primal job of leadership is emotional. Being intelligent about emotions is extremely significant to leaders being successful, and the authors discuss how maximizing the power one derives from being emotionally intelligent improves performance. The relationship between neurotransmitters and mood is exciting to read about because it illustrates how leaders' moods affect their behavior and the behavior of those they lead.

Examples of how emotionally intelligent leaders are successful in guiding organizations during chaotic times are excellent and well worth reading. The leadership competencies of emotional intelligence—self-awareness, self-management, social awareness, and relationship management—are clearly explained, and the idea that "there are many leaders and not just one" (p. xiii) pervades the book.

Greene, R. (1998). *The 48 laws of power.* New York, NY: Viking.

This author claims that "all of us hunger for power, and almost all of our actions are aimed at gaining it" (p. xix), and he asserts that "if the game of power is inescapable, better to be an artist than a denier or a bungler" (p. xix). Given these perspectives, Greene then goes on to describe thoroughly 48 laws that, he claims, will help one attain and retain power. Among those laws are the following: conceal your intentions, learn to keep people dependent on you, keep others in suspended terror, play all the way to the end, and preach the need for change, but never reform too much at once.

It is obvious that these laws reflect a Machiavellian perspective on power, and the author fails to discuss more positive sources or uses of power. For those who find themselves in "cut-throat" environments where one must do anything to survive, these laws may be helpful. For those who aspire to providing leadership in the way it has been discussed in the *New Leadership Challenge: Creating the Future of Nursing* and proposed by most authorities on the subject, such actions will not empower followers, create a sense of unity, or renew leaders or followers. Perhaps reading this book serves as a good lesson in what *not* to do as a leader.

Grossman, S. (2006). *Mentoring in nursing: A dynamic and collaborative process.* New York, NY: Springer.

This book is helpful for nurses who are interested in empowering others, whether in academic or health-care settings. The author offers a new definition of mentoring in nursing that encompasses the multiple components of the mentoring process. Examples of various mentoring models are described, and perspectives of both mentors and mentees are shared.

Various tools to assist in developing mentoring are cited, along with precepting models and programs. The idea is reinforced that young and old need to mentor each other in the nursing profession if the profession's covenant with the public is to be kept.

Hames, R. D. (2007). *The five literacies of global leadership: What authentic leaders know and you need to find out.* San Francisco, CA: Jossey-Bass.

As noted in the Foreword of this book, "The future is shaped by the quality of leadership" (p. xvii). With this caveat in mind, Hames proceeds to examine the current state of leadership throughout the world and create "a manifesto of a group of remarkable people who are intent on creating better futures" (p. xxi). The remarkable people highlighted in this book are well-known politicians, scientists, and "the man next door," but whether they reside in rich, powerful nations or very poor ones, the author claims they have five things in common: they are passionately optimistic, their curiosity and craving for wisdom drives them to continually explore new possibilities, they acknowledge the power of collective action, they embrace uncertainty and system-wide change, and they are compassionate.

Through the narratives and stories provided, this book helps the reader appreciate what individuals can do to mobilize and collaborate with others to create a preferred future. It is inspiring and reinforces the commonalities among us.

Harvard Business Review on Leadership. (1998). Cambridge, MA: Harvard Business School Press.

This collection of eight articles reflects some of the foremost thinkers in the area of leadership, including Mintzberg, Kotter, and Zaleznik. Many of the articles are accompanied by an executive summary, and most are followed by a retrospective commentary by the author. Mintzberg, for example, even offers some self-study questions after his chapter.

Clearly, these writings are significant in that they raise key questions such as the following: Are managers and leaders different? What do leaders really do? How do chief executives really lead? Why is providing leadership difficult?

At the end of the text is a short paragraph describing all of the contributing authors and their accomplishments since their seminal pieces were originally published. This book is definitely a "must read" for those wishing to develop a comprehensive understanding of the complex phenomenon of leadership.

There are additional books of compilations of *Harvard Business Review* articles that relate to leadership that may be of use to readers. Examples of "subtitles" are Leadership in a Changed World, Breakthrough Leadership, and Leadership at the Top.

Heifetz, R. A., Grashow, A., & Linsky, M. (2009). *The practice of adaptive leadership: Tools and tactics for changing your organization and the world.* Boston, MA: Harvard Business Review Press.

This book by authorities on organizational leadership discussed the concept of adaptive challenges and how leaders can help groups be effective when faced with those transformative types of situations. The authors distinguish between leadership and authority and provide numerous examples of how leaders and followers need to collaborate to thrive in a constantly changing world that calls for both adaptation and the need to up-end the status quo, regardless of its tenacity. The book is filled with stories and examples from business and public life, offers many practical tools and realistic tactics, and is designed to help readers better understand the systems in which they operate, put ideas into action, understand themselves, connect with their leadership purpose and those who are critical in realizing it, and continually grow and be renewed.

Hein, E. C. (Ed.). (1998). *Contemporary leadership behavior: Selected readings* (5th ed.). Philadelphia, PA: Lippincott.

This book is a collection of articles that were originally published in a variety of journals, and although it is somewhat "dated," it still provides a good resource for the student of leadership. The articles are organized into categories that focus on the culture of nursing (e.g., caring and gender socialization), theories of leadership and attributes of leaders, leadership behaviors (e.g., assertiveness, advocacy, and mentoring), the organizational setting, and shaping nursing's future.

This is a good resource of varied articles and differing perspectives on topics relevant to leadership. Chapters can be read out of sequence, and no chapter depends on the preceding, thereby giving readers a great deal of flexibility in how to use the book.

NOTE: Previous editions of this book contain some of the same readings and some different ones. They also are helpful references. The publication dates of those editions are as follows: first, 1982; second, 1986; third, 1990; and fourth, 1994. E. C. Hein and M. J. Nicholson edited the first three editions.

Helgesen, S. (1990). *The female advantage: Women's ways of leadership*. New York, NY: Doubleday Currency.

In this book, one of the few that deals specifically with women as leaders, Helgesen describes ways in which women lead differently than men. Based on a study of women leaders in the workplace, she found patterns of behaving and approaches to making decisions and setting priorities that were quite different from what had been reported in studies of male leaders.

Women in Helgesen's study were very concerned about being involved in the work of the organization, keeping relationships healthy and productive, making time for activities that were not directly related to their work (e.g., parenting responsibilities), and maintaining a "big picture" orientation. They also viewed their jobs as only one element of who they were, not as *the* factor that defined who they were, and they preferred to see themselves at the center of things, rather than at the top.

As a result of these values, perspectives, and preferences, women tended to create operational structures that were more web-like rather than hierarchical. Such structures provide for more interaction among members of the group, allow for more participation of all players in goal setting and decision making, and result in greater inclusion.

Helgesen views these differences in the ways women lead as great strengths, strengths that are having and will continue to have dramatic effects on the nature of our organizations. The book provides a provocative analysis of women leaders and the way they can use their different perspectives and values to change organizations.

Hesselbein, F., Goldsmith, M., & Somerville, I. (1999). *Leading beyond the walls.* San Francisco, CA: Jossey-Bass.

This book, which is a collection of writings by leaders in the field of leadership, is a publication of the Drucker Foundation. It "explores what is needed to transcend the personal walls that inhibit effectiveness and the organizational, social, and political boundaries that inhibit reaching out, [and it calls upon leaders to] forge partnerships that are essential in the increasingly challenging period ahead" (p. xii). The authors acknowledge that each of us is surrounded by walls—walls of policy, procedures, assumptions, safety, familiarity, and security—but these walls that protect us also can "inhibit movement, limit understanding, restrict engagement, and diminish our relevance in the wider world" (p. 2). For these reasons, leaders are challenged to move beyond the walls that bind individuals, organizations, and institutions.

Among the strategies offered to help individuals lead beyond the walls are the following: be courageous, take risks, be passionate, trust in people, affirm our past but celebrate our present and future, "challenge the gospel" (p. 4), engage in long-term collaboration, create community, be aware of and be true to your core values, develop systems rooted in freedom of choice rather than in coercion and control, share information, and seek unity rather than competition. These and other themes are woven throughout this book and serve as guideposts for the would-be leader. As such, this book is a valuable resource for those wishing to fully understand this complex phenomenon.

Houser, B. P., & Player, K. N. (2007). *Pivotal moments in nursing: Leaders who changed the path of a profession* (Vol. II). Indianapolis, IN: Sigma Theta Tau International.

This book spotlights 11 nurses who moved the discipline ahead in significant ways. Included among those studied are Mary Elizabeth Carnegie, Imogene King, Ruth Watson Lubic, and Margaret McClure. Each nurse was interviewed and her "history" analyzed, and from these analyses, the authors drew conclusions about leaders. Their work helps the reader appreciate how leaders meet and overcome barriers and challenges to the ideas they propose that are "out of the mainstream," how they use their high energy level and passion to keep moving forward, how they are willing to always "go the extra mile" for their colleagues and for the profession itself, and how they become politically astute to deal with influential people in their environments.

It is clear from the study of these nurse leaders that they viewed themselves as rebels and were comfortable with that role. In addition, each of the individuals spotlighted had a vision and was able to see a bigger picture than others were able to see. The book, therefore, helps define what leadership is and offers insights into how one develops as a leader.

NOTE: The first volume of this book was published in 2004. It followed a similar format but presented 12 different nurse leaders, including Joyce Clifford, Luther Christman, Vernice Ferguson, Rheba de Tornyay, and Claire Fagin, among others.

Jaworski, J. (2011). *Synchronicity: The inner path of leadership* (2nd ed.). San Francisco, CA: Berrett-Koehler.

This author calls on Jung's classic definition of synchronicity—"a meaningful coincidence of two or more events, where something other than the probability of chance is involved"—to discuss what he refers to as "the most subtle territory of leadership, creating the conditions for 'predictable miracles'" (p. ix). Thus begins this fascinating book that focuses on how leaders shape the future instead of simply responding to the present.

Jaworski notes that most contemporary institutions are leaderless and bemoans this state of affairs in light of his expressed belief that there is leadership potential in everyone. Using his own personal journey, he describes how "we can shape our future in ways that we rarely realize" (p. 9) and "participate in the unfolding process of the universe" (p. 44), not merely accept what comes our way. By facing and overcoming personal challenges (i.e., being afraid to step outside one's own narrow circle, being afraid to take the risk of stepping into the unknown, fearing that one cannot make a difference anyway), Jaworski responded to the "call to redefine what is possible, to see a vision of a new world and . . . undertake, step-by-step, what [was] necessary . . . to achieve that vision" (p. 58).

The personal journey described in this book helps the reader appreciate the risk taking inherent in a leadership role, as well as the rewards of serving in such a role.

Kellerman, B. (2008). *Followership: How followers are creating change and changing leaders*. Boston, MA: Harvard Business Press.

Recognizing that the preparation of leaders has become an industry while attention to followers has been virtually nonexistent, Kellerman sets out to help the reader appreciate how "people without obvious sources of power, authority, and influence are far more consequential than we generally assume" (p. xxi). She is clear in asserting that good followership matters and acknowledges that we are more willing now than ever before to recognize that followers are integral to the leadership process.

Through a careful analysis of Germany during the Nazi regime and other real-life situations, the author guides us to think about five different kinds of followers: isolates (who are completely detached and alienated); bystanders (who observe but make a conscious decision not to participate), participants (who invest some of what they have [e.g., time] to try to have an impact), activists (who are fully engaged and energetic, either in support of or against the leader), and diehards (who are prepared to "put everything on the line" for the cause). She points out the value and concerns about each type of follower, acknowledges clearly that all of us are followers at some point, and suggests that self-reflection regarding the type of follower one is in various situations is in order.

Kelley, R. E. (1992). *The power of followership: How to create leaders people want to follow and followers who lead themselves*. New York, NY: Doubleday Currency.

Robert Kelley presented one of the first and best discussions of followership that is available in the literature. His goal in writing this book was to "shift the spotlight toward followership as *the* important phenomenon to study if we are to understand why organizations succeed or fail" (p. 5), and he achieves that goal extremely well.

This author talks about the increasing emphasis on teams and collaboration and the kind of power that followers can and do have in groups and organizations. He notes that "followers determine not only if someone will be accepted as a leader but also if that leader will be effective" (p. 13), and he asserts that effective followers are critical for success.

The term "effective follower" is not used lightly in this book. Indeed, Kelley describes five different followership styles: passive, conformist, pragmatist, alienated, and exemplary/effective. He offers ways to help the reader identify her/his followership style, argues for the importance of developing one's followership skills, and offers very convincing arguments why individuals should become followers.

This book, therefore, is unique in its attention to a critical but frequently ignored role in the leadership process. It is one that must be read to gain a better appreciation of the concept of followership.

Keohane, N. O. (2010). *Thinking about leadership*. Princeton, NJ: Princeton University Press.

Written by a former president of Wellesley College and Duke University, where she was the first woman to hold that position, Keohane offers a perspective on leadership "from the inside." This book is a masterful combination of theory and practical points that incorporates political theories, literature, biographies, and other sources to examine the leader–follower dialectic, the need for balance in leaders, the importance of vision, and whether gender makes a difference in leadership. This is a thoughtful, scholarly, informative book about leadership that challenges leaders to consider the ethics of their behaviors, how power can be easily abused, and the uniqueness of providing leadership in a democratic society that values equality, involvement of its citizens, and expertise.

Koestenbaum, P. (2002). *Leadership: The inner side of greatness* (2nd ed.). San Francisco, CA: Jossey-Bass.

This book is a philosophical analysis of individuals and what it takes for successful leaders to achieve specific goals. It is not a synthesis of stories about people who have been successful but rather a compilation of how to create environments and societies that will facilitate the achievement of goals. Koestenbaum describes his Leadership Diamond Model, which revolves around the concepts of time, democracy, motivation, teamwork, and salesmanship.

This is a good book to read if one wishes to analyze one's leadership ability and/or develop one's leadership skills. There are some excellent cases, such as the Enron scandal, that examine marketing morale and history, and the exercises and checklists to assist the reader in leadership development are helpful.

Komives, S. R., Wagner, W., & Associates. (2009). *Leadership for a better world: Understanding the social change model of leadership development*. San Francisco, CA: Jossey-Bass.

This book is unique in that it shares the voices of students who are engaged in activities designed to help them develop as leaders who can influence social change. It provides a set of principles about how knowing oneself, engaging in meaningful ways with others, and adopting a systems perspective can promote the socially responsible leadership many argue is so desperately needed in today's world.

Through case studies, thought-provoking questions and scenarios, pointed content, and a clear commitment to social change being at the heart of the leadership experience, this book is an excellent resource for educators who are in search of learning activities related to leadership development, service learning directors looking for meaningful ways to engage students in the life of their communities, or individuals desiring to make a difference in the world.

Kotter, J. (2008). *A sense of urgency.* Boston, MA: Harvard Business Press.

This book—a sequel to Kotter's previous books on change such as *Leading Change, The Heart of Change,* and *Our Iceberg is Melting*—points out the absolute necessity for leaders to help others appreciate the urgency for change. In fact, Kotter believes the biggest error that people make in implementing a change is not being able to create a sense of urgency for a specific change. He points out how most successful people become complacent and do not want to "rock the boat" by instituting a change, but soon find themselves not being successful because they actually did miss out by not implementing change. He further points out that some embark on change, not because they feel the urgency, but because they are motivated by anxiety, anger, or frustration; as a result, they create a frantic culture that does not allow a clear focus on the needed change. Kotter offers several strategies to assist in acquiring the skills to lead change. This skill is especially important today when change seems to be continuous and not episodic in occurrence.

Kouzes, J., & Posner, B. (2003). *Encouraging the heart: A leader's guide to rewarding and recognizing others.* San Francisco, CA: Jossey-Bass.

The main theme in this book is that people who are recognized for their good work and encouraged are more likely to achieve higher levels of success. The authors recommend how leaders can support the human need to be appreciated for what we do and who we are. They describe the process of "encouraging the heart" with four ideas: leaders must follow general principles that reward people for work well done; leaders will not be perceived as being "soft" for encouraging the heart; leaders have multiple methods they use to encourage the heart; and all leaders must be aware of the soul and spirit involved in any organization. This book gives the reader ideas on how to keep hope alive and explains how ordinary people can actually be effective leaders by being encouraging to others. This is a good book for all to read, especially when the organizations in which we function appear to be losing their edge and failing to be responsive to all those involved in the work of the organization, and there is still a need to get extraordinary things done.

Kouzes, J. M., & Posner, B. Z. (2005). *Credibility: How leaders gain and lose it . . . Why people demand it* (2nd ed.). San Francisco, CA: Jossey-Bass.

The purpose of this book is to explore, in depth, the quality of a leader whom constituents (i.e., followers) would want to follow: credibility. Based on extensive research, the authors conclude that people have very high expectations of their leaders, wanting them to "hold to an ethic of service, [be] genuinely respectful of the intelligence and contributions of their constituents, [and] put principles ahead of politics and other people before self-interests" (p. xvii).

Kouzes and Posner view leadership as a relationship and a service, with credibility clearly at its foundation. This book examines leadership as a relationship, talks about the benefits of credibility, and discusses the behaviors that convey and establish credibility. Among those behaviors are the following: knowing yourself and your values, appreciating the strengths and talents of followers, reinforcing shared values, developing others to reach their fullest potential, making meaning out of the work or tasks to be done, and sustaining hope in the followers. Strategies for how leaders develop/gain and can even lose credibility also are discussed.

This analysis stimulates the reader to thoughtfully reflect on her/his own actions and how they establish or undermine credibility. Although other writers imply the significance of credibility in the leader–follower relationship, Kouzes and Posner make a most valuable contribution to our understanding of how leaders can be most effective by their careful study of the concept. Any discussion of leadership would be incomplete without a discussion of credibility; this book, therefore, is an excellent resource for enhancing such understanding.

Kouzes, J., & Posner, B. (2007). *The leadership challenge* (4th ed.). San Francisco, CA: Jossey-Bass.

This fourth edition of an excellent book reflects the authors' observations of what leaders do to encourage extraordinary accomplishments when they are leading, not managing. This edition includes interviews with some of the most significant leaders around the globe and shares a new and more global perspective of leadership. Kouzes and Posner's classic "five sets of behavioral practices" and "ten behavioral commitments" are described fully, and the importance of leaders having perseverance, having direction, empowering others, being role models, and recognizing others' contributions are all discussed thoroughly. Each of the five behavioral practices are correlated with two of the behavioral commitments and discussed with reality-based examples.

The book describes leadership as a skill that can be developed by coaching and through experiential learning. In fact, this fourth edition has been described as "a personal coach in a book" and gives excellent examples of how to apply coaching skills in assisting others to gain leadership ability. The necessity of purposefully developing one's leadership is advanced, as is the notion that leadership is more important today than ever before if we are to achieve success in the future. The authors remind us that leadership is everyone's business and, therefore, that everyone should accept the leadership "challenge" on a daily basis.

Kritek, P. (2002). *Negotiating at an uneven table: Developing moral courage in resolving our conflicts*. San Francisco, CA: Jossey-Bass.

This book relates important lessons to people who want to be involved in decisions being made in an organization or personally. It gives sound advice on, as well as good examples of, how to negotiate conflicts, especially when the players are not "equal," and hints to assist the reader in being able to recognize when there is an uneven table are discussed. Conflict resolution or management is the theme of this book, and the author (a nurse) applies it to nursing situations as well as to her mother's long death. The author addresses the inequalities and diversity with her "ten ways of being," which are helpful in opening one's mind to creative ways of managing conflict.

Krzyzewski, M. (2000). *Leading with the heart: Coach K's successful strategies for basketball, business, and life.* New York, NY: Warner Business Books.

"Coach K," as the author is known, is the winningest basketball coach in NCAA history. He has been head coach at Duke University since 1980 and coached the gold-medal-winning 2008 U.S. Olympic men's basketball team. In this book, Coach K shares tips for being a successful leader, one whose players say they learned lessons like the following from him: "setting the bar high so that you can strive to be the best you can be; the value and rewards of a hard-work ethic; building close relationships based on trust; setting shared goals; sacrificing; giving of yourself; winning with humility; losing with dignity; turning a negative into a positive; being a part of something bigger than yourself; [and] enjoying the journey" (pp. x-xi).

Among the guiding principles offered by Coach K are the following that have implications for those aspiring to provide leadership: know your team, help the entire team think in terms of "we" rather than "I," build on the strengths of team members and expect everyone to help one another achieve full potential, be clear about shared goals and expectations, be honest, be passionate about what you do, strive to do your best 100% of the time, and have fun. By following such principles, leaders will constantly be energized, team members will grow, and great things can be accomplished.

Leadership in Nursing. (1994). *Holistic Nursing Practice, 9*(1), entire issue.

This journal issue offers a thoughtful collection of articles about the nature of leadership, particularly as it relates to nursing. It is a useful resource since each article can be read independently of the others. The articles focus on many significant areas, all of which facilitate an understanding of the complex nature of leadership. Included among those areas are the following: the nature of leadership and ways to conceptualize it that make sense for 21st-century practice; the holistic nature of leadership; transformational leadership, particularly as it relates to women leaders; the significance of followers; ethical aspects of leadership; the preparation of leaders; an exploration of the leadership that is needed to shape a preferred future for nursing; and an analysis of 10 years of nursing leadership research.

All the articles in this issue are intended to "provide new insights and to explore important issues related to leadership" (p. vi). They accomplish that goal in a stimulating way that has relevance for our profession.

Loue, S. (2011). *Mentoring health science professionals.* New York, NY: Springer.

This is an interesting book that provides examples of mentoring of faculty, students, and junior professionals in health fields. It provides an overview of the concept of mentoring, highlights and critiques various formal mentoring programs, and shares the journey of a mentor and protégé as they collaborate to help the protégé develop a successful career trajectory as a faculty member in an academic medical setting. Although the foundations of mentoring presented in this book are similar to those offered in other works, the fact that the examples provided reflect the uniqueness of health fields and health settings may be particularly useful to those in nursing.

Lowney, C. (2003). *Heroic leadership: Best practices from a 450-year-old company that changed the world.* Chicago, IL: Loyola Press.

This book was written by an individual who lived for 7 years as a Jesuit seminarian then moved into the corporate world, namely JP Morgan. The author uses what he learned about the Jesuits (the 450-year-old company referred to in the book's subtitle) as a model for understanding leadership. It is exceptionally well written and presents many insightful ideas that focus on true leadership.

From his experience at JP Morgan, the author concluded, "It was clear that only a handful of banks would emerge as winners in our changing, consolidating industry. And the winners likely would be those whose employees could take risks and innovate, who could work smoothly on teams and motivate colleagues, and who could not only cope with change but also spur change. In short, *leadership* would separate winners from losers" (p. 3).

Throughout this fascinating, informative, and historically grounded book, the author highlights numerous examples of true leadership and illustrates the concepts most effectively. This book is highly recommended for those who wish to learn about leadership from a nontraditional source, as well as for those who wish to learn more about "those radical Jesuits." He recommends leaders look for a "competitive advantage" and to use it at all times so that the leader does something different but also adds value.

Malloch, K., & Porter-O'Grady, T. (2010). *The quantum leader: Applications for the new world of work* (2nd ed.). Sudbury, MA: Jones & Bartlett.

This book describes how leadership can be understood using quantum mechanics. Ideas that leaders can use to develop themselves and their followers are explained using various technological innovations while integrating the personal touch. The purpose of the book is to depict how leaders can be courageous and assist others by coaching for achievement, eliminating toxic behaviors, and having a future-perspective. A great emphasis of the authors is to delineate the significance of organizations having quantum-age characteristics, such as being multilateral, multidirectional, relational, interacting, intersecting, and integrating. The book focuses on the "fully engaged leader" who is defined as someone with competence and intelligence, someone who is engaged in her/his work and other aspects of life, and someone who is conscious of his/her own and others' feelings. The case studies and scenarios offered in this book relate specifically to health care and are particularly helpful to the nurse or nursing student reader.

Marshall, S. P. (2006). *The power to transform: Leadership that brings learning and schooling to life.* San Francisco, CA: Jossey-Bass.

This book focuses on the need for change in education and the kind of leadership that is needed to create a "new landscape for deep and integral learning" (pp. xi–xii). Such leadership is critical, Marshall notes, because "how we engage the minds of our children in learning profoundly shapes the patterns of their thinking and their thinking shapes the world" (p. xvii). Thus, one could conclude that the development of future leaders who think broadly and in innovative ways and who can help society create preferred futures is at stake if our education systems do not change.

This is an incredibly powerful book that should be read by all those involved in the educational process. It challenges long-held assumptions, presents challenges that must be taken up by leaders, and provides insight about the kind of leaders needed to transform education.

McBride, A. B. (2010). *The growth and development of nurse leaders.* New York, NY: Springer.

This is an interesting book focused on leadership, not management. McBride divides the book into three parts: personal leadership, leadership as it pertains to organizational goals, and transformational leadership. There are multiple examples that illustrate various aspects of leadership development both personally and professionally. Each chapter ends with a list of "Take-Away Points," which further serve to assist the reader in gaining insight into one's own leadership style. The book is written with the idea that one will want to reflect on one's own lived experiences regarding leadership and how best to augment one's success with leading and inspiring others to also lead. After reading this book, readers will have many ideas that will hopefully transform their own leadership and ultimately help them to lead in a more productive fashion.

McCall, M. W. (1998). *High flyers: Developing the next generation of leaders.* Boston, MA: Harvard Business School Press.

The major emphasis in this book is on corporate executives who have a "bent" toward management more so than leadership. Despite this emphasis, however, McCall presents many interesting ideas about leaders and what needs to be done to prepare individuals to be effective in leadership roles.

The author asserts that "organizations not only overlook people with the potential to develop but also frequently and unintentionally derail the talented people they have identified as high flyers by rewarding them for their flaws, teaching them to behave in ineffective ways, reinforcing narrow perspectives and skills, and inflating their egos" (p. xi). He notes that we often keep people from developing their full potential as leaders, and as a result, neither they nor their organizations progress as much as they otherwise could.

McCall firmly believes that leadership can be learned and points out that "the development of leaders is itself a leadership responsibility" (p. xii). Learning leadership, he says, is a "lifelong journey, with its lessons taught by the journey itself" (p. 17). He challenges each of us—as aspiring leaders who must take responsibility for our own growth, and as practicing leaders who must take responsibility for the leadership development of others—to attend to the conscious development of ourselves and others as leaders.

Meyerson, D. E. (2001). *Tempered radicals: How people use difference to inspire change at work.* Boston, MA: Harvard Business School Press.

""Tempered radicals' are people who want to succeed in their organizations yet want to live by their values or identities, even if they are somehow at odds with the dominant culture of their organizations. Tempered radicals want to fit in *and* they want to retain what makes them different. They want to rock the boat, and they want to stay in it" (p. xi). So begins this fascinating book about those who walk the fine line between (a) resisting the majority culture and becoming an outcast for not being part of the team, and (b) wanting to fit in but not wanting to "sell out" on their values and principles.

Meyerson conducted interviews with more than 250 individuals in several different organizations, people who were seen as change agents. These individuals continued to operate in environments where their values were sometimes in conflict with those of the organization while they effected slow, incremental change in their organizations to achieve a closer alignment between personal and organizational values.

The author asserts that tempered radicals' acts "represent a crucial form of leadership, what [she] call[s] 'everyday leadership'" (p. xix). She describes why people act as tempered radicals, the many ways people may be different from their colleagues or coworkers, and how quiet resistance can lead to significant change. These discussions are most helpful to those who would aspire to be leaders in their organizations because they help one realize that change can come from within and that organizations can be altered to align with the values of the individuals who comprise them.

Nanus, B. (1992). *Visionary leadership: Creating a compelling sense of direction for your organization.* San Francisco, CA: Jossey-Bass.

This is an excellent book about the concept of vision and its importance in the leadership process. Nanus asserts that vision is the key to leadership and that without it, an individual cannot be considered a leader, nor can significant progress be made in our organizations, professions, or societies.

A leader, Nanus explains, must be attuned to the external environment (perhaps more so than the internal one) and be focused on the future, not merely on the present. This kind of direction setting is what vision is all about, and it is what "attracts commitment and energizes people" (p. 16). Vision also serves to create meaning in the lives of the followers and establish a standard of excellence.

In addition to discussing what vision is, Nanus also helps the reader understand what vision is not. It is not, he says, prophesy, a mission, factual, true or false, static, or a constraint on actions. Instead, it is a view of the future that arises from one's values, passions, dreams, hopes, and desire to create a better world (or piece of the world).

Nanus offers many realistic and helpful strategies for how leaders can develop a compelling vision for the future of their organizations or groups. He also helps the reader think about ways to implement the vision.

Pandya, M., & Shell, R. (2005). *Lasting leadership: What you can learn from the top 25 business people of our times.* Philadelphia, PA: Wharton School Publishing.

The Nightly Business Report (NBR), the most watched daily business program on television in the United States, collaborated with these authors to identify the most influential business leaders in the past 25 years. Some of the leaders are Mary Kay, John Bogle, Warren Buffett, Peter Drucker, Steven Jobs, Sam Walton, and Oprah Winfrey.

This book is a compilation of each of these leaders' business ventures, their leadership skills and styles, and the results or impact of their efforts. Reading how various leaders reacted, planned proactively, and learned from their success and mistakes is inspiring, and the attributes they identified as portraying lasting leadership are most helpful. Those attributes are as follows: "building a strong corporate culture, truth telling, finding and catering to under-served markets, 'seeing the invisible' (i.e., spotting potential winners or faint trends before their rivals or customers do), using price to build competitive advantage, managing and building their organization's brand (which, in some cases, may be their own name), being fast learners, and managing risk" (p. xx).

The authors noted that no one leader possessed all of these attributes, but each of the 25 leaders studied had more than one of these characteristics. This is a good book to learn how to develop and use one's talents at leading.

Porter-O'Grady, T., & Malloch, K. (2011). *Quantum leadership: Advancing innovation, transforming health care* (3rd ed.). Sudbury, MA: Jones & Bartlett.

The third edition of this book is directed toward individuals wanting to develop their own and others' leadership skills, particularly those in health care who wish to maximize the leadership abilities of others in this era of transformation. The authors present their idea of how quantum mechanics is applied to human dynamic behavior and give useful examples of how important this idea is to assist leaders in delivering health care successfully. This edition is completely revised and offers two new chapters, *Creating Context: Innovation as a Way of Life* and *Evidentiary Leadership: An Expanded Lens to Determine Healthcare Value.* Examples of how to deal with "toxic" people in organizations are helpful, as are the ideas presented about how to apply successful conflict management strategies. The authors reinforce several times how important it is that readers review multiple books on the phenomenon of leadership because the concept of leadership is always changing; hence, it is best for people interested in learning about leadership to read all that they can and not just this book.

Rath, T., & Conchie, B. (2008). *Strengths based leadership: Great leaders, teams, and why people follow.* New York, NY: Gallup Press.

This book challenges the reader to think about and assess her or his own leadership. Based on the assumption that each of us will have many opportunities to lead during our lifetime, the authors want us to be able to seize those opportunities and be effective as leaders. They analyzed decades of Gallup data (in-depth interviews with more than 20,000 senior leaders, Gallup Polls about most admired leaders, and studies of more than 1 million work teams) and combined that information with the findings of their own study of more than 10,000 followers to summarize three key findings about the most effective leaders: 1) they always invest in strengths, 2) they surround themselves with the best people and then maximize their team, and 3) they understand the needs of the followers.

Given that "the path to great leadership starts with a deep understanding of the strengths [one] bring[s] to the table," (p. 3), the authors provide the StrengthsFinder (2.0) Assessment for readers to identify their strengths as a leader. Once that personalized "report" is received, the book provides an explanation of each of the three key findings and how one's own strengths can be used to meet followers' needs, to lead others who themselves are strong in various areas, and to continually grow as a leader. The assessment is easy to complete, the customized "report" is informative, and the self-reflection prompted by this analysis is revealing. Anyone who works collaboratively with others could benefit from learning about their own strengths and how to use them most effectively.

Robinson-Walker, C. (1999). *Women and leadership in health care: The journey to authenticity and power.* San Francisco, CA: Jossey-Bass.

This book reports on intensive dialogue with nearly 100 women and men responsible for managing a significant portion of America's health care. It is clear that "women are simply not present in the numbers we would expect, nor do they ascend at the rate we would expect to the most senior leadership roles in health care" (p. ix). Given this reality, the author—who co-created the national Center for Nursing Leadership in the late 1990s—examines the significance of gender in the 21st century; stumbling blocks faced by women in reaching "the top"; and relationships among gender, values, and leadership.

The author asserts that the characteristics most commonly exhibited by women, particularly women interviewed for this book, are precisely the qualities needed by those providing leadership in health care: an ability to tolerate ambiguity, a collaborative style, dispersed power, consensus building, integrity, "doing the right thing—even when the price is high" (p. 185), and others. She then offers a number of "antidotes" to help women be more effective leaders: defusing gender's role in conflict, negotiations, and power; using communication as a bridge; renewing our careers; nurturing ourselves; and mentoring others.

Although this book acknowledges the difficulties women often have with taking on the leader role, it also is positive and offers specific strategies to overcome those difficulties. As such, it is an excellent resource on gender issues related to leadership.

Rosenbach, W. E., Taylor, R. L., & Youndt, M.A. (Eds.). (2012). *Contemporary issues in leadership* (7th ed.). Boulder, CO: Westview Press.

This book (and all previous editions) is one of the best collections of readings about leadership. None of the articles—many of which have been published originally elsewhere, and several of which are classics in the field—has focused specifically on nursing (to date), but each offers many rich ideas that could easily be applied to a nursing context. The seventh edition reemphasizes followership as an integral component of leadership, discusses the importance of leaders as mentors, helps navigate the hazards of leadership, and presents a renewed framework for understanding leaders and leadership from a contemporary perspective The book, therefore, continues to be a most valuable one for students and teachers of nursing.

This book draws on experts in various areas and includes original articles as well as ones previously published in the *Harvard Business Review, Leader to Leader, World Futures,* the *Wall Street Journal,* and *Compass: A Journal of Leadership.* It is, therefore, exciting and inclusive of diverse perspectives. Although several of the articles are from management journals, they clearly are focused on leadership, and this is one of the things that makes this collection of reading so valuable—it does not confuse management and leadership.

NOTE: All previous editions of this book also are quite valuable and include collections of different readings. The first edition was published in 1984, the second in 1989, the third in 1993, the fourth in 1998, the fifth in 2001, and the sixth in 2006.

Schiff, K. G. (2005). *Lighting the way: Nine women who changed modern America.* New York, NY: Hyperion.

Written by the daughter of former Vice President Al Gore, this book chronicles how nine extraordinary women worked behind the scenes and against the odds in the major political movements of the last century. It tells powerful stories of women who influenced women's suffrage, the decision to enter World War II, the struggle for civil rights, environmental health, the AIDS crisis, and other significant issues of the past 100 years.

In telling these stories, Schiff points out that women have always been consequential, if often unrecognized, political leaders and have been responsible for many of the most creative ideas that helped shape history. This book is uplifting and powerful and is an excellent resource for the study of women as leaders.

Senge, P. (2006). *The fifth discipline: The art and practice of the learning organization* (2nd ed.). New York, NY: Doubleday Currency.

This newer edition of Senge's seminal work, *The Fifth Discipline,* describes how many of his ideas regarding leadership and management have been operationalized in organizations since the original 1990 publication. He shares the outcomes of his interviews with people from companies such as Intel, Ford, BP, and HP, as well as organizations such as The World Bank, Roca, and Oxfam. Some new and particularly interesting chapters in this edition are *Impetus,* which describes how to build learning-oriented cultures instead of staying in one's comfort zone, *Leaders' New Work,* and *Frontiers for the Future.*

Through this book, Senge teaches the reader how to see things differently (e.g., seeing the forest **and** the trees), how to deal with the constant struggle of being tugged by personal **and** work issues, and how to maximize one's creativity. This is perhaps a more management-focused book, but because being a good manager serves to strengthen one's leadership ability, it is a valuable resource.

Sinetar, M. (1998). *The mentor's spirit: Life lessons on leadership and the art of encouragement.* New York, NY: St. Martin's Press.

This book is another excellent publication by the best-selling author of the following books: *Do What You Love . . . The Money Will Follow* and *To Build the Life You Want, Create the Work You Love: The Spiritual Dimension of Entrepreneuring.* It discusses the art of encouragement, which is the word Sinetar uses to mean mentoring. She describes 12 lessons of mentoring, explains how one can be mentored and how one can mentor others, and offers realistic strategies and easy-to-follow plans for both mentors and mentees.

This valuable book is easy to read, and it encourages the reader to want to be involved in a mentor–mentee relationship. Sinetar's main point, which constantly echoes throughout the book, is that no matter what one might think, a single person is not the center of the world . . . it really is much more worthwhile to reach out to, network with, encourage, and mentor others.

Soder, R. (2001). *The language of leadership.* San Francisco, CA: Jossey-Bass.

The author suggests that management is a larger, more encompassing concept than leadership; however, he goes on to say, "This book deals with elements of leadership as applied to those in elected and other public offices . . . and those in the private sector" (p. xv), meaning, largely, that the focus is on individuals in management positions.

The author asserts that persuasion is "a critical aspect of leadership" (p. 3) and focuses most of the book on an analysis of the concept of persuasion and how leaders can use it to get others to do what they want. In addition, the author makes leadership seem like little more than political maneuvering (p. 28), almost as if one needs to be quite Machiavellian (e.g., use devious means to get information) to be successful as a leader. These perspectives are contradictory to most other literature on leadership.

In addition, the author seems to want to "impress" the reader with his knowledge of a wide range of literature by inserting quotes and "snippets" from various philosophers, historical figures, etc. A few such quotes and examples are helpful to illustrate a point, but after a while, it seemed that the author was inserting such items simply to impress the reader. Instead of accomplishing this goal, however, this style may obfuscate the real point of the book.

Spears. L. C. (Ed.). (1995). *Reflections on leadership: How Robert K. Greenleaf's theory of servant-leadership influenced today's top management thinkers.* New York, NY: John Wiley & Sons.

This collection of 27 essays—written by some of the leading thinkers and practitioners of servant-leadership—brings together into one volume some of the most significant ideas about the concept and the growing influence of Robert K. Greenleaf's legacy. It begins with several chapters by Greenleaf himself, describing the evolution of his thinking and the development of his "theory."

This book is an excellent source of information about servant-leadership and how a variety of people have interpreted and lived the concept. It is inspiring and uplifting, and helps one think about leadership in a different way.

Spears, L. (Ed.). (1998). *The power of servant leadership: Essays by Robert Greenleaf.* San Francisco, CA: Berrett-Koehler.

This book captures the vision and writings of the late Robert K. Greenleaf, who was the first to use the term "servant-leadership." According to Greenleaf, "servant-leadership" is a way of leading that puts serving others (e.g., customers, patients, employees) first. This collection includes the following eight essays written by Greenleaf throughout his career: *Servant-Leadership: Retrospect and Prospect, Education and Maturity, The Leadership Crisis, Have You a Dream Deferred?, The Servant as Religious Leader, Seminary as Servant, My Debt to E. B. White,* and *Old Age: The Ultimate Test of Spirit.*

All of the essays in this collection reflect Greenleaf's ideas about spirit, commitment to vision, and wholeness. Given this focus, this is a most reflective book that leaves the reader with a feeling of "wanting to do things right."

Spreitzer, G.M., Bennis, W. (Ed.), & Cummings, T.G. (Ed.). (2011). *The future of leadership: Today's top leadership thinkers speak to tomorrow's leaders.* San Francisco, CA: Jossey-Bass.

This book is a collection of essays written in tribute to Warren Bennis for his distinguished life and career by present leaders (short bibliographies of whom are included in the book). It is divided into six parts: setting the stage for the future, organizations of the future, leaders of the future, how leaders stay on top of their game, insights from young leaders, and some thoughts on the leadership challenges of the next generation. Bennis also added to this book his thoughts on challenging issues that leaders must be able to understand and manage if they are to be successful in the future: how organizations collaborate, whether future leaders will be comparable to present leaders, whether employees will be calling all of the shots, how the inequalities of different people and organizations will affect leadership, demographics, what loyalty will exist between employees and organizations, what organizational change will ensue, personal and career balance, and where the new leaders will come from.

Staub, R. E. (2002). *The heart of leadership: Twelve practices of courageous leaders* (2nd ed.). Greensboro, NC: Staub Leadership Consultants.

This comprehensive book provides step-by-step advice on how to develop effective leadership skills, as well as skills for becoming a productive follower. The author advocates the following practices of leadership: provide guidance through shared vision, focus on purpose, create followership, set standards while eliciting goals, read and understand others, provide resources, liberate motivation, support others, provide feedback, practice principled flexibility, solicit personal feedback, and cultivate the heart of courage.

Staub is a strong believer in everyone working together to lead an organization or group, not just one or two leaders "at the top." Reading this book reaffirms the notion, expressed by so many other experts on leadership, that true leadership is possible for everyone who can master her or his attitudes, express her or his ideas, and act on her or his dreams.

Vance, C., & Olson, R. K. (1998). *The mentor connection in nursing.* New York, NY: Springer.

This book is not presented as a "leadership" book, but the nature of its focus—mentoring—makes it quite relevant in any study of leadership and followership. In addition, the book is one strategy used by these authors to realize their own vision of nurses mentoring each other. Its roots were in the 1977 and 1984 doctoral dissertations of the two authors, and it crystallized more than a decade of collaboration between the two.

Mentoring, these authors say, is a unique type of developmental relationship. It involves colleagues helping each other grow and learn. It empowers each person in the relationship. It is a means to "strengthen the profession by ensuring an adequate supply of competent practitioners and leaders" (p. 3). As such, mentoring must become a natural part of the practice of all nurses.

Through the use of personal "stories," many of nursing's accomplished leaders help the reader understand the nature of mentoring, the value of such relationships, and the relevance of mentoring to nursing. A variety of contributing authors talk about negotiating the mentor relationship, peer mentoring, the privilege and responsibility of mentoring, mentoring in the practice and the academic setting, and global and cross-cultural mentoring. Many of these discussions incorporate personal experiences and are, therefore, particularly moving, meaningful, and memorable.

This is an excellent resource for understanding the phenomenon of mentoring. It also is a valuable collection of personal stories that present a positive view of our profession and that serve as "anchors" for neophytes who are looking for or hoping for a mentoring relationship. It is, in essence, an informative and an inspiring book.

Ward, M. (2001). *Beyond chaos: The underlying theory behind life, the universe, and everything.* New York, NY: Thomas Dunce Books.

This book presents an interesting discussion of the phenomenon of universality, or how physics explains "how inert lumps of matter conspire and self-organize to produce life" (p. ix). The book title is a bit lofty perhaps because, of course, one book cannot answer the underlying theory behind life, the universe, and everything! It does, however, present an excellent discussion of how patterns emerge in various systems, it is helpful in understanding chaos theory, and it is applicable to how organizations and individuals lead their organizations or professions through tumultuous times.

Wheatley, M. (2006). *Leadership and the new science: Discovering order in a chaotic world* (3rd ed.). San Francisco, CA: Berrett-Koehler.

This third edition of Wheatley's seminal work on the New Science reinforces ideas presented initially in 1992 and offers many new ideas to challenge our thinking. Contrary to the scientific or Newtonian model of step-by-step planning, the New Science emphasizes the importance of exploring and accepting things the way they occur, as viewed from the perspectives of quantum physics, chaos theory, and biology.

Wheatley speaks to how leaders and those responsible for running organizations can benefit from application of the New Science. She asserts that by moving toward holism and appreciating the intricate relationships that exist between and among all things, one can develop and effectively use methods to change how people act, how they work, and how they view life. As a result of this interconnectedness between every single thing in the world [actually everything *plus* the world, according to Wheatley], every moment of one's day is dynamic and unpredictable. She emphasizes the importance of relationships, even at the subatomic level. Also, the idea that change and chaos are the most significant way to transform positively is integrated throughout the book.

This edition offers examples of how self-organizing networks can flourish in our new world, and it presents information on how best to respond to disasters and stop terrorism. The author concludes that the fundamental work of our time centers around all of us discovering new ways of working and being together.

Wheatley explains how order and chaos can be seen as identical images and how these two seemingly opposite forces actually drive each other. Using natural phenomena (such as the evolution of the Grand Canyon, a babbling brook, and stormy weather), Wheatley creates complexity from simplicity and excites the reader with ideas of how the future will evolve from the whole, rather than from the parts. This is an essential book for anyone interested in learning more about chaos theory and the New Science.

Wheatley suggests people organize their own "Leadership & the New Science" discussion groups by going to *www.bkconnection.com* or joining the listserv group.

Wheatley, M., & Kellner-Rogers, M. (1996). *A simpler way*. San Francisco, CA: Berrett-Koehler.

This book offers a way of thinking about life in a dynamic and totally different way, and it is critical reading for those who wish to better understanding the New Science of Leadership. The authors share a magnificent collection of photographs of life, poems that convey the importance of being oneself, and narratives about simpler ways of viewing what most people define as a stress-filled, nonenjoyable life.

This is a remarkable book about how to view life within the vastness of the universe. The authors speak to how life "self-organizes" without our planning every minute of every day, and how this organization creates our identities. The advantages of seeing the world self-organize without human manipulation is challenged, and ways to foster more creativity, freedom, and "real" meaning in life are generated. In addition, the notions of play, organization, self, emergence, and coherence are explored.

Yudkowsky, M. (2005). *The pebble and the avalanche: How taking things apart creates revolutions*. San Francisco, CA: Berrett-Kohler.

The basic premise in this book is that revolutions—in how we think, how we do business, how we use technology, and so on—can be relatively easy to create by taking things apart, a process the author calls *disaggregation*. Disaggregation and innovation, the author asserts, have positive results such as heightened creativity in organizations, healthy competition, cost reduction, greater simplicity, and synergy, all of which "sweep aside old infrastructures" (p. 22).

The notions of taking things apart and questioning basic premises or assumptions are valuable ways to stimulate change, and they can be helpful to leaders. In addition, the idea that a small change can trigger a huge avalanche of change has merit to the leader who attempts to influence complex, tradition-laden systems. This book, however, suggests that revolutionary change is relatively easy to achieve, which is a conclusion that must be questioned.

Yukl, G. (2010). *Leadership in organizations* (7th ed.). Upper Saddle River, NJ: Prentice Hall.

Much like the classic reference by Bass (2008) noted earlier, this book is an excellent resource about leadership. It summarizes research related to key leadership concepts—followership, power, transformation, change, gender considerations, developing leadership skills, and others—providing the reader with a rich and comprehensive overview of the field. Although much of the book focuses on management, rather than leadership, it still serves as a worthwhile, scholarly book on the latter and would be a useful addition to any library on leadership.

Zaleznik, A. (1977). Managers and leaders: Are they different? *Harvard Business Review, 55*(3), 67–78.

This article is indispensable reading. It is one of the earliest works in which leadership is clearly distinguished from management, and as such, it is a classic in the field.

Zaleznik talks about the differences between managers and leaders in terms of how they relate to other people, to the organization, and to goals. He explores the different conceptions of work, different perspectives on solitary activity, and different views about conflict and status quo held by leaders and managers. For purposes of illustration, the author talks abut leaders and managers in the extreme, but he does acknowledge that managers can also be leaders . . . and leaders also can be managers.

This article is clearly written and is extremely helpful in clarifying the distinctions between these two related phenomena. It is an essential reading in one's quest to understand leadership.

INDEX

Note: Page numbers followed by b indicate box; page numbers followed by f indicate figure; and page numbers followed by t indicate table.